PENGUIN BOOKS

BREAKING ALL THE RULES

Nancy Roberts was born in New York City in 1945. She attended the High School of Music and Art, the City College of New York, and New York University, where she studied fine arts and political science. From 1969 through 1985, she lived in England, where she worked in the fashion business and in public relations before becoming a founding member of the Spare Tyre Theatre Company in 1979. She hosted her own program for Thames Television and continued her vigilant campaign against fat discrimination. She and her husband, Uwe Blanken, now live in New York, where she hosts a weekly radio program about health issues on WYNY, "Large as Life."

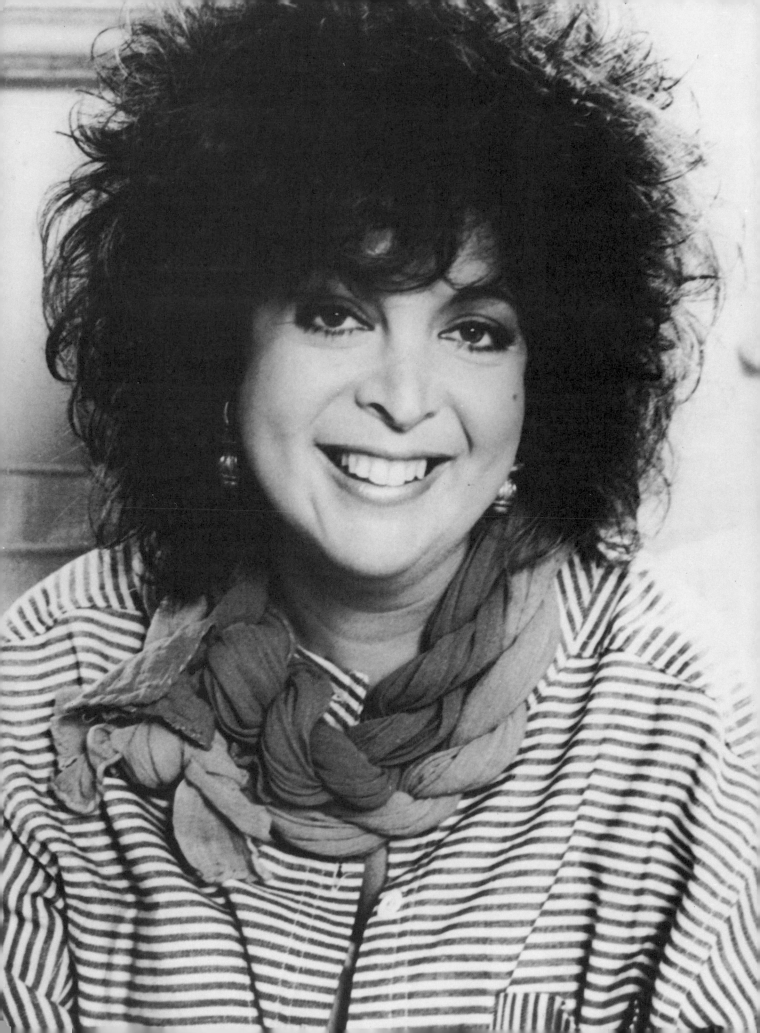

BREAKING ALL THE RULES

NANCY ROBERTS

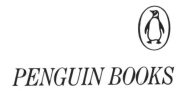

PENGUIN BOOKS

For Mom and Dad—with love

PENGUIN BOOKS
Viking Penguin Inc., 40 West 23rd Street,
New York, New York 10010, U.S.A.
Penguin Books Ltd, Harmondsworth,
Middlesex, England
Penguin Books Australia Ltd, Ringwood,
Victoria, Australia
Penguin Books Canada Limited, 2801 John Street,
Markham, Ontario, Canada L3R 1B4
Penguin Books (N.Z.) Ltd, 182–190 Wairau Road,
Auckland 10, New Zealand

First published in Great Britain by Penguin Books Ltd 1985
First published in the United States of America by
Viking Penguin Inc. 1985

Published in Penguin Books 1987

Copyright © Nancy Roberts, 1985
All rights reserved

Illustration acknowledgments appear on page 220.

LIBRARY OF CONGRESS CATALOGING IN PUBLICATION DATA
Roberts, Nancy, 1945–
    Breaking all the rules.
    1. Beauty, Personal.   2. Obesity.   3. Reducing.
I. Title.
RA778.R528   1987   646.7′042   86-15144
ISBN 0 14 00.7463 5

Printed in the United States of America by
The Murray Printing Company, Westford, Massachusetts
Set in Cheltenham

CONTENTS

With thanks to my good friend Jan Dally, who first had the idea for this book, and then convinced me that I could do it! Her guidance, her expertise and her unflagging enthusiasm were invaluable to this project.

*   *   *

With special thanks also to my friends at the Spare Tyre Theatre Company, then and now, and to Caroline Eves; Sheri Safran; Michael Manning; Carole Jones, Wendy Dagworthy; Margaret Dawson; Bonnie Spencer; Julia Fletcher; Lynne Franks and her team; Sally Gaminara, Tony Lacey, Pat Mulcahy, Esther Sidwell, Yvonne Dedman, Caroline Bugler and everyone at Viking US and UK; and to all the women whose experiences and feelings make up such an important part of this book.

And, of course, to my darling Uwe, who, for the past six months, put up with a state of chaos even worse than usual!

INTRODUCTION

Have you ever woken up in the morning, jumped out of bed, looked in your mirror and thought, 'Yuk, I'm too fat'? If your answer is 'yes', I've written this book for you.

Whether you are a size 12 compulsive dieter who hates her body, or a size 26 woman who has never been on a diet in her life, but who is sick of being treated like an outcast by a society that despises 'fat', you will find help and support within these pages.

This book is the answer to every diet book, every 'health and beauty' guide, and every fashion magazine that tells women that the only way we can look good and feel healthy is to be pencil-thin.

This is also a book about power. The power to make yourself look and feel great, the power to change the way you think about yourself and the way other people think about you, and the power to change your own life.

Most of us do not look like the models in *Vogue* or *Cosmo*, and those of us bigger than a size 10 never get the chance to see other women who look like us looking great. It is disheartening, at the very least, and downright undermining and destructive never to see a bigger woman dressed well and looking gorgeous. The only big women who do occasionally creep into the women's magazines are there as 'before pictures' for a diet or exercise feature, and they are inevitably portrayed as dumpy and miserable. This book shows these women as they could and should be and as they are – attractive, successful, happy. This is a book that says you can feel good about yourself the way you are right now.

When I see a big woman who has really put herself together with style and imagination my immediate reaction is that she must be very strong. I know the obstacles that she has had to overcome…the ridicule of our society, the practical difficulties of finding decent clothes in bigger sizes, and above all the overriding feeling that somehow she is not entitled to look good or to feel good. All the rules of our contemporary culture say she should be hidden away, dreaming of the day when she will be thin enough to care about her looks and about her life.

This kind of thinking has gone on too long. Enough is enough! We big women are fed up with being treated as second-class citizens. We want to lead our lives to the full, no matter what our size. We want to stop postponing our lives until we lose weight and start living now!

This is a book to help you do just that. It is a book not just about fashion and style, but about pampering yourself, about taking care of yourself, about doing the things for yourself that other women take for granted, but that big women, and women who may only *think* they are big, do not do, simply because they feel they don't deserve it!

This is not a book about rules, about what to wear and what not to wear, about 'putting on your face' before you leave the house every day. It is a book about suggestions, about experimenting, about having fun with your clothes, your make-up, your hair, about being brave enough to try anything. It says you can look and feel terrific without losing weight. Every picture in this book will prove it.

This is a book to help women of all shapes and sizes to face the world feeling stronger and prouder. It is about confidence and self-respect. It's also about compulsive eating – the tortuous diet/binge addiction that affects so many women of all weights and that ruled my own life until the age of thirty-three, when I 'broke the habit', overcame a lifetime of dieting and self-loathing, and changed my life.

Many women have spoken to me through the years about their own lives. Some of them were compulsive eaters, both fat and thin. Some were big women who were normal eaters – whatever problems they had came as the result of living in a world that ostracized them and treated them as outcasts. To all these women I give my heartfelt thanks for sharing their experiences with me. Without them I could not have written this book.

Within these pages you will meet many big women who are leading a full, healthy, satisfying life. Some feature as models in the series of specially commissioned fashion photographs that you will find in the style section. All of them gave a great deal of their time and energy to talk to me and tell me their stories. At intervals throughout the book you will find examples of their good sense and of their humour. Their practical advice and their encouraging words will, I hope, help you to deal successfully with the day-to-day problems we all face.

The women whose stories and pictures feature throughout this book are:

Elizabeth Osborne *(thirty)*	Teacher
Mandy Crane *(late twenties)*	Fashion designer for her own company
Liz Birru *(twenty)*	Dancer
Angela Troak *(mid-thirties)*	Owns a women's clothing shop
Vicki Pepys *(mid-twenties)*	Public relations executive
Carole Burton *(late twenties)*	Toy librarian
Denise Smith *(late twenties)*	Television production assistant
Jan Murphy *(mid-thirties)*	Personal assistant
Sue Formston *(mid-forties)*	Costume designer
Helen Terry *(late twenties)*	Singer
Kate Franklin *(early sixties)*	Owns her own public relations company; mother of two and grandmother
Kathy Beard *(late twenties)*	Model and actress; one daughter
Meredith Etherington-Smith *(late thirties)*	Author, journalist, and British representative of French *Vogue*
Annette Badland *(early thirties)*	Actress
Claire Rayner *(early fifties)*	Author, advice columnist, and broadcaster; mother of three
Janis Townes *(late thirties)*	Nursery-school teacher; one son
Professor Joanne Brogden *('over forty-five')*	Head of the School of Fashion Design – Royal College of Art

But before we hear from them, I want to tell you something of the long, sometimes painful, and always bumpy journey that inspired me to write this book.

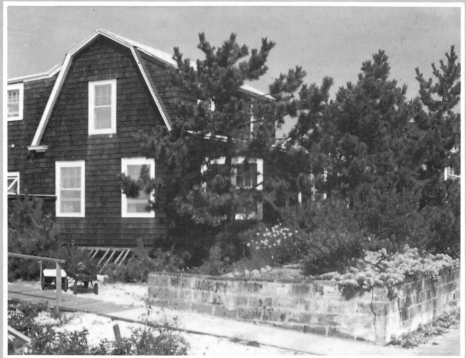

The house at Ocean Beach, Fire Island

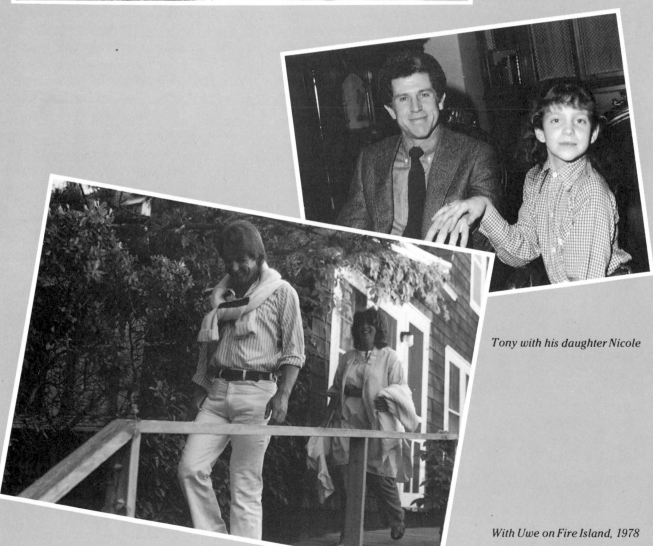

Tony with his daughter Nicole

With Uwe on Fire Island, 1978

1

THE OBSESSION BEGINS

The house still had that musty out-of-season smell and the floor under my bare feet was sticky with dampness as I changed into my sneakers. This was my brother Tony's room. I had watched him emerge from it every summer morning since 1953 when my parents first bought the house on Fire Island, that wind-swept strip of sand off the southern coast of New York. Eyes clogged with sleep and wrapped only in a towel, Tony would stumble through the living-room towards the rear bathroom and fling himself under the heavy shower for what seemed an eternity before returning fresh and dripping water to his room. There he'd change into shorts and a T-shirt, and the day would officially start in our house. In this flimsy wooden beach house built at the turn of the century and floated over to Fire Island on a barge, only a rickety set of louvre doors separated my brother's bedroom from the main living-room, and, until he was up and about, we all kept very quiet lest we wake him.

I slept in his room now, sharing it with my husband, Uwe, on our rare trips home to America from England where we lived. We were there on this rainy May weekend in 1984, our suitcases with the London Heathrow labels piled on the beds. My parents were here too. So was Tony and his teenage daughter Nicole. This weekend was the first time in five years that we had all returned together to the place that I still think of as home.

Together we'd pulled the two wagons piled high with summer clothes and food through the main street of Ocean Beach and up the slight slope of Bungalow Walk to the brown shingled house of my childhood summers.

I was in the kitchen helping my mother unload the food bags when my father called from the back deck. My brother sighed, put down his *New York Times* and followed me out.

My father stood in the middle of the deck, hands on hips, jeans sagging, contemplating the surrounding foliage. This spot was his pride and joy, his little bit of paradise carved out of the sandy wilderness of Fire Island, and most of his summer weekends were spent tending it, watering it, and carting huge bags of peat moss to enrich the arid soil.

He stood now looking up at the pine trees which surrounded this haven. They stretched high above the telegraph poles and got lost in the wires. Unchecked,

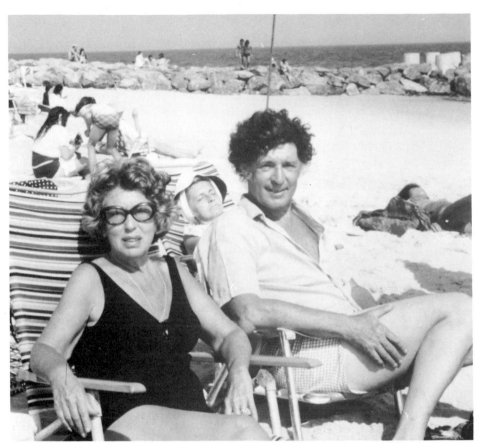

Mom and Dad on the beach at Fire Island

With my mother and brother pulling the wagon down Bungalow Walk, Fire Island – early teens

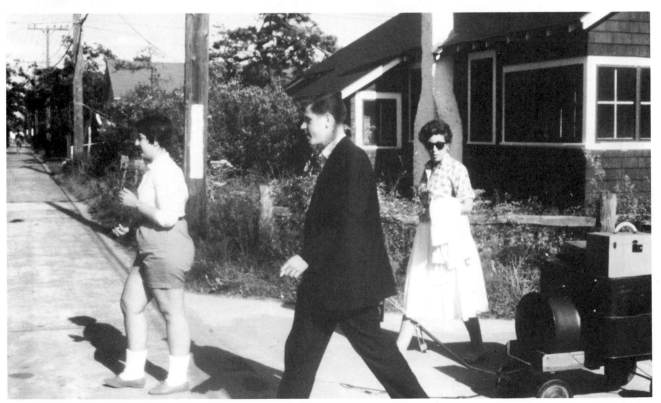

their winter growth had spread over the perimeters of the deck and the new branches hung over the wrought-iron garden furniture, blocking out much of the light. 'We've got to cut some of this back, kids, give me a hand.' He was holding the special long-handled pruners that he used every spring. He grabbed the long wire that operated the shears and pulled. Each sharp clip was followed by the dull thud of branch dropping. Soon we were surrounded by a light blanket of pine which my mother would later gather into large containers of water, and place around the house, where they would give to this first weekend of the new summer the incongruous scent of Christmas.

I was eight years old when my parents bought the house on Bungalow Walk. The island was more primitive then, no electricity in many places, a bathtub was still a luxury, and the only telephones were party lines. It was more barren too, and our new house was surrounded by flat, empty sand dunes which spread over the narrow walkway that ran behind the house and led to the outside shower.

It was on a blustery, clear, early spring day in 1953 that my father and I knelt together in the sand and carefully planted the fragile pine seedlings that I came to think of as 'my trees'. For thirty years I've watched them grow and alter the landscape around our house. On each trip home I'd rush outside to check their progress and as I looked up at them I'd think 'These are mine, I planted them, and they're still here…they'll always be here…in this, my place.'

The year I planted my trees, the year I was eight, was also the year I went to my first diet doctor. I can't pinpoint the moment in time when I started to gain weight. My mother tells me I was a very skinny toddler. I can't remember

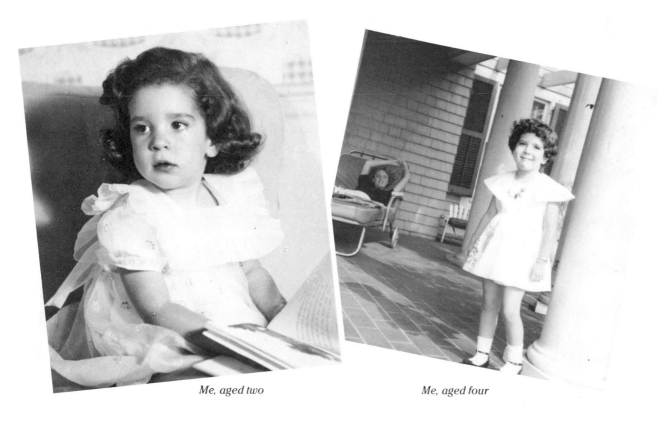

Me, aged two   *Me, aged four*

when it changed. It's almost as if overnight I blew up like a balloon. I can't remember ever being thin as a child but I know, because I've been told, that I *was* thin, and that it was at around the age of six that I got fat.

Until that time I'd had a nanny named Ethel. My older brother Tony was only an infant when Ethel came to work for our family and my mother often told me the story of how nervous she was about entrusting the care of her little boy to an inexperienced seventeen-year-old girl. But Ethel turned out to be one of the most capable, competent and loving of women, and she adored my brother. He was a gorgeous little boy with white blond curly hair and blue eyes and a very pale white china skin.

When I was born, six years later, my mother was frightened that I might be neglected by Ethel. What happened couldn't have been more different because from the moment that I was born I became Ethel's girl, and she became mine. She slept in my room, she cooked my food, she even made my clothes, and then, when I was six years old and just starting to go to school full-time, she left. My parents decided that I was old enough to do without her and she moved out of our apartment in New York to a small place of her own on 16th Street. I was allowed to spend weekends with her occasionally, and to me those weekends stand out so crystal clear that I might have been there, with her, just last week.

My father would drive me downtown on Friday evening after school. He'd carry my overnight bag upstairs in the old self-service lift with the heavy gate. Ethel would greet me with bear hugs at her front door, chat with my father for a few seconds, and then we'd close the door on our own private world.

Our weekend was spent strolling through the streets of Greenwich Village, the people and the shops so exotic and so different from the straight-laced elegance of the Upper East Side. There was always a stop at Sutters, the bakery, where we pulled a cardboard number from a machine on the counter and waited in the long narrow shop for our turn to choose from the glassed-in selection of cakes and pastries and cookies. Ethel must have been watching my weight by this time because there was always a feeling that we really shouldn't be there in Sutters. We always went there, and I was always allowed to pick something, but there was an undercurrent of wickedness, a sense that this was a forbidden fruit to be carefully rationed.

The highlight of these weekends was going out late on Saturday night to buy the Sunday papers. At 10.30, after 'The Hit Parade' and before the 11 o'clock news, we bundled ourselves up and headed for the all-night newstand on Sixth Avenue, whose lights shone out like a beacon across the pitchblack streets. We'd buy the *Sunday News* and maybe the new *TV Guide* and then stop off at Max's delicatessen for a loaf of fresh bread or some orange juice for the morning, before heading back to the cosy refuge of the apartment.

Upstairs, I'd put on my nightgown and sit propped up in the big bed, the newspapers spread all around me, and devour the Sunday comics. I'd stay awake as long as I could on Saturday night, fighting sleep. But Sunday always came. Sometimes my father would come and pick me up with the car, but usually Ethel would take me home, and we would ride uptown together on the Fifth Avenue bus. There was very little traffic as the bus sped past the empty department stores and the Sunday strollers, past Central Park, towards 88th Street and our apartment, where Ethel would soon be leaving me. We'd go straight into my room, which, until recently, we had shared, we'd unpack my few things and then

Ethel on Fire Island

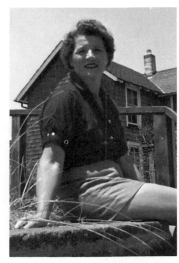

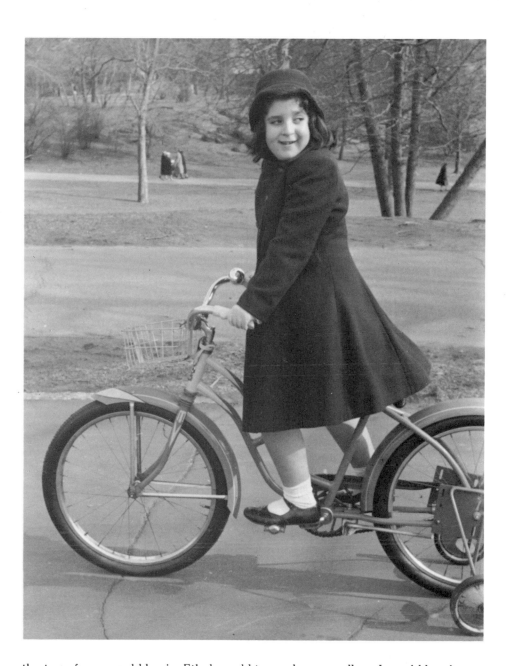

In Central Park, aged eight

the tug-of-war would begin. Ethel would try and say goodbye, I would beg her to stay, just five minutes please, just ten, just fifteen, just an hour. She would always say no at first, then allow herself to be convinced, and finally would stay until I was in bed. Even then I couldn't let her go easily and as she sat on the edge of my bed and kissed me goodnight, I would beg her not to go. But of course she had to leave, and as my mother took her to the front door, I could hear them saying goodnight, and thank you, and that they would speak during the week. Then I heard the heavy clunk of the New York City apartment door closing, and Ethel was gone. That's when I would start to cry. My poor mother would rush in and try to comfort me. She'd sit on the same edge of the bed where Ethel had sat, and stroke my face and make soothing sounds, but I was not to be consoled and, eventually, she had to give up and leave me alone to cry myself to sleep.

It was about this time that I got fat. Eventually my parents thought the problem serious enough to take me to a diet doctor, a man who spent his whole professional life weighing people and giving them pills and handing out diet sheets.

Of course it was usually adults who went to him. I don't remember ever seeing another child in his waiting-room.

My mother and I took a taxi across town to my first appointment with Dr Stein. I sat in the back seat huddled and quiet next to her. It was winter and I clung fearfully to her arm through her fur coat sleeve as the taxi drew up in front of the doctor's entrance to 187 Central Park West. I can't drive by that building, even now, at the age of thirty-eight, without looking, without wondering, 'Is he still there? Is he the richest doctor in New York?'

Is his office the same as it was that terrible day, thirty years ago when I first set foot inside it? Is his nurse still sitting stiffly just inside the door, all starched white and unyielding, and is there some other little girl staring fixedly across at the gorgeous array of tropical fish in their illuminated blue aquarium, and is she, as I was, too terrified actually to get up and go over to look at them?

After what seemed an interminable wait my mother and I were led into a white and chrome laboratory, all slides and test tubes and equipment and scales. My blood pressure was taken and my pulse, my full name, Nancy Jane Roberts, was printed at the top of my file card, my age, eight years old, and my weight. We were then ushered into the doctor's private enclave, wood-panelled and dark and plush, everything was leather and brass and wood and diplomas, and there was another scale next to his desk. I was weighed on this scale too, the result being checked against the figure on my card. Did they think that perhaps I had gained an ounce or two *en route* from the examination room? Or were they merely checking their equipment?

I sat dwarfed by the enormous leather chair next to Dr Stein's polished desk while my mother sat in another chair obviously meant for the mothers of people who were the prime suspects in this particular operation. He took out little boxes of pills that the nurse had brought out to him, already counted out in the weekly prescribed dose. Each little matchbox contained a different colour pill and had instructions handwritten across the top stating·how many pills to take before each meal. He showed me these pills, spilling some of them out on to his desk blotter and then he put them back into their boxes.

He handed them to my mother and he handed me a printed sheet of paper with my own special eight-year-old's diet typed out on it. My mother nodded seriously, taking it all in, and I nodded seriously, taking it all in and I can't honestly say which was the stronger feeling. On the one hand there was the sense of relief that the worst was over, I'd been weighed, they'd written it all down, it could only get better now, couldn't it? I was on the road to recovery, to being a better person, to making everyone happier with me, wasn't I? It was like going to the dentist, you dread it, and you lie awake the night before and tell yourself that your fears are groundless, and then you go. When it's finished you walk out sagging with relief and the joy that you don't have to go back – you've gotten through it. In Dr Stein's womb-like leather sanctuary that day there was an element of this familiar relief. But on the other hand there was also somewhere the dawning awareness that there was a terrible struggle ahead of me, that it wasn't all going to end with this visit.

I went back to Dr Stein's office every week. I was weighed and slight alterations were made to my diet, and the combinations of my pills were changed, a few

At the Hoffman School aged eleven – with my mother

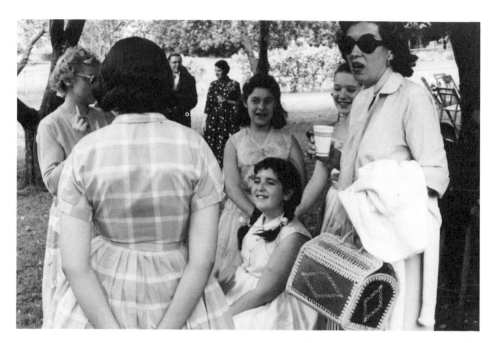

yellows added here, a blue switched from breakfast to dinner there. I always lost weight. I was a good dieter even then, and I always took my pills in the proper order, even at school. I went to a small school in Riverdale at that time, the Hoffman School, the kind of place where you called your teachers by their first names and there were less than a hundred children in the whole place. Lunch was cooked by two enormous, cheerful women named Emma and Estelle, and served in the small-home-like atmosphere of the dining-room. We sat at long, low tables of yellow formica while the teachers circulated to make sure that everyone was all right and behaving. I sat in my small child's chair in that dining-room, day after day, and counted my pills. I counted them out and washed them down with a swallow of skimmed milk and, as large steamy platters of spaghetti and meatballs and macaroni and cheese were passed down the table and around me, I would slowly, self-consciously, unwrap my own lunch. I opened the waxy plastic container holding the day's ration of cottage cheese or white meat of chicken or dry tuna fish, the tinfoil packets of carrot sticks, celery, and soggy cucumbers. And I would eat and pretend that I didn't care.

I can remember more of what I didn't eat from those days than of what I did. I wanted that food so badly, almost as much as I wanted to be just like everyone else. For my pills and my wrapped, nutritionally balanced little lunches made me different, made me stand out even more than my fat did.

I was always a good student at the Hoffman School, bright and hard-working and reliable. I was also popular with the other children and had lots of friends, and yet my happy memories of those times are marred by the feelings of separateness and isolation that I experienced at every meal in that relaxed, inviting dining-room, which for me had become a hell on earth.

It was in that same dining-room that one awful day a visiting medical team came to set up a mobile clinic, complete with an enormous doctor's scale. I stood in line with my friends, all happy to be excused from a few minutes of class, as we waited our turns on the scale. There were to be many times when I

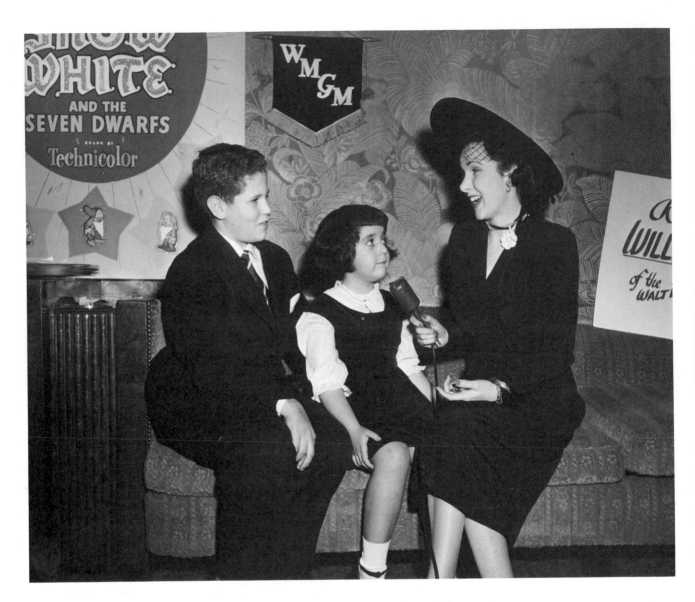

With Tony at the premiere of Snow White

had to be weighed in front of other people, when I had to stand trembling and blushing in line, joking and trying to cover up my intense embarrassment, but that was the worst, that first time in the dining-room of the Hoffman School, where not only did I have to endure the torture of eating a different lunch from everybody else but now I actually had to be weighed in front of all my classmates, who would, at last, know the horrible truth.

The Hoffman School was in Riverdale on the outskirts of the city, but I lived, for all of my life before coming to England, in a large rambling old apartment right in the centre of Manhattan. Lots of people say that New York City is no place to bring up a child, it's much better to live in the suburbs and have a garden, or better yet, some place in the country, but for me, as a little girl, New York was a magical place. I guess you could say that I was the child of a show-business family. My father, Kenneth, was a radio broadcaster who did everything from presenting one of the first big radio game shows 'Quick as a Flash', to hosting his own pop music show on radio WMGM, one of the first of the DJs. My mother, Norma, had been, before her marriage, the first-ever female story-writer in the cartoon business. In the days before Walt Disney, she worked for the Max Fleischer studios and wrote the story-lines for such immortal hits as Popeye and Betty Boop. My father's cousin, Everett Sloane, was one of the most respected actors in Hollywood. And my older brother, Tony, seemed always to have known what he wanted to do, and that was to be an actor. All my parents' friends and, later on, my brother's were 'in the business', actors, and writers, and directors, people who worked on Broadway or on television; often at my parents' parties, amidst the chat and the laughter, there would come a hush as one composer or another would sit down at the piano in the living-room and play a selection of songs from his latest score.

One of my greatest treats as a child was to go with my father to a Saturday matinée. My father loved the theatre and together we went to plays, we went to the ballet, we even went to the opera; I remember the thrill of seeing *Aida* for the first time at the Metropolitan Opera House and my amazement when they led a live elephant on to that great stage. But my favourite thing of all was to go to a Broadway musical. The first show that I ever went to see as a little girl of five was the original production of *South Pacific*. We sat up front in the fourth row, and I was mesmerized by the sight of Mary Martin actually washing her hair with real water right there on the stage. For years afterwards I ran around the apartment singing 'I'm gonna wash that man right out of my hair', and 'I'm as corny as Kansas in August'. I was hooked. From the moment that I sat in that darkened theatre and watched the curtain go up on that, my first show, a hidden part of me dreamt of being up there, on that stage.

As the years went by and I got older, I sat in one theatre after another with my father, watching *West Side Story*, *My Fair Lady*, *Carousel*, and *Oklahoma!*, and wanting so badly to be up there myself singing and dancing. My father and I usually stopped off at a record store on the way home and bought the album of the show that we'd just watched, I would rush into the living-room, put the record on and, sitting in the large beige wingchair, listen to it over and over again, until I knew every word by heart. I sang all the parts, acted all the roles, and I never admitted to anyone that I wanted to be an actress. I somehow couldn't speak those words out loud. I was afraid that people would laugh at me, because, already, by this time, I was struggling with my weight, and I was fat. I knew enough about 'the business' – I'd heard all my life about how hard it was for even those actresses with beautiful faces and faultless figures to get work, so who was I, fat and dumpy, to even dare to imagine that I could be a part of that special world.

My brother Tony used to tease me whenever he caught me singing. He said I was tone deaf, and, as he was incredibly musical, singing perfectly, playing the guitar, the piano, and even writing songs, I believed him. Sometimes I would sit alone at the piano in the empty apartment and, staring intently at the open pages of the Rodgers and Hart songbook, I would pick out with one hand the melody line of 'Ten Cents a Dance' or 'My Funny Valentine' and sing along, in a voice that I was sure was hopelessly flat, off-key and out of tune.

So I decided early on to risk no further ridicule and I pushed my dreams so far to the back of my mind that, with time, I almost forgot them myself.

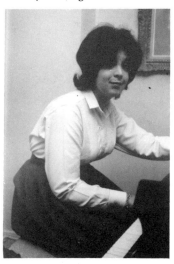

At the piano, aged sixteen

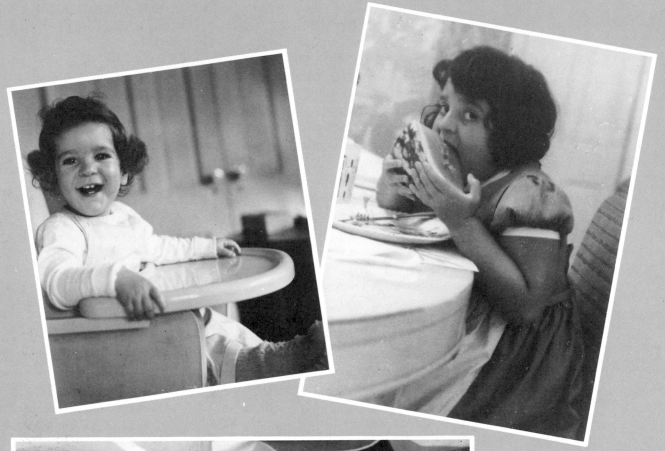

Above left: Before food became a problem

Above right: At my place at the table, aged six

Lunch at the Zoo in Central Park with Tony and Mom

2

EATING

The ritual surrounding dinner time at home started the second I came in the front door from school. I was inevitably hungry, and, after dropping my coat and my books on the chair by the door, I would head for the kitchen. Now, if my mother was not already there, she would get there pretty fast from whatever she was doing at the other end of the apartment. As I pulled open the door to the fridge her voice would greet me down the long corridor 'What are you eating? You mustn't eat anything. We're going to have dinner soon. You'll spoil your appetite.' Of course, the fact that it was 4.30 and we didn't eat dinner for two hours made no impact whatsoever on her. Mealtimes were sacrosanct in our house and eating between them was frowned upon. I don't know how I did it but I somehow always managed to sneak something past her and into my room, where I would close my door, eat whatever it was that I had managed to procure, and watch TV or do my homework until 6.30.

At 6.30 on the dot, every night of the week, there would come the resounding cry throughout the apartment of 'DINNER, DINNER'. I was always first out of my room, first through the large foyer, and first at the table, in my chair, waiting for the rest of the family to assemble.

The dining-room at 40 East 88th Street, where I grew up, was very light, very beautiful, very elegant and strictly for dining. This was no combination living-dining room, no kitchen-dining room, it was a dining-room pure and simple, all you did in it was eat, and fight. It was all pale colours with silky wallpaper and a marble patterned floor that may have been real but was more likely vinyl. We had a large antique inlaid table that my mother had 'picked up for next to nothing' at an auction, with cream stained chairs for my brother and me, and elaborately carved orange armchairs at either end for my parents. One whole wall was windows, hung with floor-length cream drapes that my grandmother Fanny had made years ago.

On either side of the wall of windows and Fanny's drapes were two rectangular art deco cabinets, with enormous lamps on top. In the left-hand cabinet, filled with old games and pieces of silver that needed polishing, was one of my mother's secret hiding places for candy and nuts. I would often creep through the darkened apartment in the dead of night to rummage through this cabinet. And there, behind

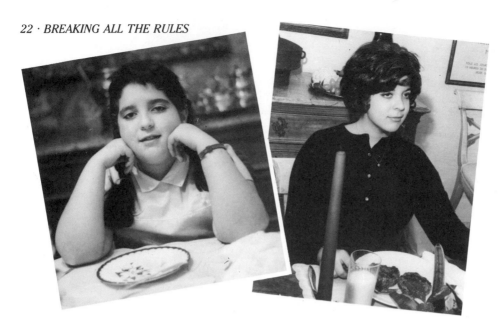

At my place at the table opposite the mirror, (left) aged ten, and (right) aged sixteen

the tarnished sugar bowl, amidst ancient boxes of stationery that no one used any more, and a Scrabble set with a lot of the pieces missing, my night-time prowlings would be rewarded as I found a bag of peanuts or some chocolate-covered almonds from Barton's Bonbonnière. I would always take only the smallest sample, for of course I was terrified of being caught.

My place at the dinner table was opposite Tony, and behind Tony's chair there hung a large gilt mirror. By waiting till Tony's head was bent over his plate or by slightly straining my own head a bit to the right I could see my own reflection there. I could see my face and my shoulders and the top of my glass of milk, and in that mirror I watched the changing face of my youth. I saw myself grow up in that mirror. My hair grew long, was braided, was cut again, was curled, straightened and curled again, according to the prevailing fashion. My face went through its million metamorphoses from fat to thin and back again. I started to wear make-up and tweeze my eyebrows, and everything was reflected back at me, night after night, over my brother's shoulders, as we sat there at dinner. I can't recall seeing myself actually eating in that mirror. Even though I must have only looked up between mouthfuls, I know I spent a lot of time 'me-gazing'. My parents were always saying, semi-jokingly, 'Stop looking at yourself, Nancy', and I always vehemently denied that I was. I think that's when I learned how to catch myself at just the right angle, with just the right expression on my face to look my best. In that moment of preparation before I looked at my own reflection, the mind and the imagination took over from the eyes and I altered my perception to something I could accept. I still do it, and still get a shock when I catch a glimpse of myself suddenly and unprepared in some shop window. But in those days I was careful and never looked up and into the glass unless I was ready.

The first image I remember seeing in that mirror was myself at the age of eight or nine. I had long thick, heavy braids, and hair that was parted in the middle with a very fat little face bulging out between these two long braids hanging down the front of my blouse. Around that time I looked in another mirror at Michael's barbershop where I had gone with my mother to have my long hair finally cut. I stared miserably as the barber chopped my hair off to just above shoulder length, all the time encouraging and exclaiming on the vast improvement that this was making, as it 'made my face look so much thinner'.

My mother always came next into dinner, followed by my brother a bit late and slightly distracted, and then would start the waiting for my father. Now, as I've already said, dinner was at 6.30, not 6.15, not 6.45, but 6.30, every night without fail for as long as I can remember. We all knew it. My brother knew it, I knew it, my mother certainly knew it. Even now, thirty years later, at 6.30 every night, a certain something goes off inside of me, a slight twitching, a conditioned response; I prick up my ears and wait for that call; no matter where I am, or what I'm doing, some internal alarm clock rings now, as it rang then, for all of us. All of us that is, except my father. For my father that 6.30 call was a call of another sort. Yes, it was a call to action, but not to the same kind of action as the rest of us. For my father it was the signal to leap up from whatever he was doing, and immediately engross himself in any one of five million other incredibly important things that he absolutely had to finish off before he could join us at the table. There was always just one more bill to pay, one more envelope to address, one more stamp to affix in his collector's album, one fast phone call he had to make.

And regardless of whatever small chores he found to do each night there was the inevitability of his two favourite pre-dinner occupations, which every single night filled that gap between the cry of 'Dinner, dinner' and my father's arrival in the dining-room. The first of these was the 'putting on of the music'. My father loved to have background music to eat by, usually operatic, and as my mother, my brother and I sat waiting, he would race off to his elaborate hi-fi system at the other end of the apartment, and fiddle around with his complicated reel-to-reel tape recorders, flicking from one to the other, looking for the perfect aria, and as he switched from one machine to the other the house was filled with the scratchings and screechings of feedback and the shrill snippets of sopranos cut off in mid-note, until my mother, her knuckles turning white from the tension of her fists gripping the edge of the table, would call out to him, 'Kenneth, I don't like music on while we're having dinner!' Because she didn't. About 50 per cent of the time she won, half the time we had music, half the time we didn't, but at least she usually won about the type of music, and when my father finally came within sight through the large double dining-room doors, it was to the strains of Frank Sinatra or Ella Fitzgerald that he appeared. The next and last stage in my father's preparation for dinner was the 'selecting of the wine'. My father gets pleasure from anything concerning a bottle of wine, from the label, which he reads aloud in his rather halting French, to the sniffing of the bouquet and the rolling around on the tongue of the first sip. Once again, this was a delight that was his alone.

Although my father had done his best to encourage my brother and me to share his pleasure by always bringing us a wine glass and urging us to taste, the most we would do was begrudgingly take a sip and turn up our noses in disgust. And my mother was not a wine drinker. If you put a glass in front of her she would drink it, but without any real gusto. She really couldn't care less about whether or not there was wine with dinner. What was important to her was that everyone should be sitting down at the same moment, sitting down and ready for this meal, which had in most cases already arrived at the table.

When my father finally sat down to join us, his hands full of glasses, the rest of us had already finished our grapefruit. He'd gobble his up at tremendous speed so that he'd be ready for the main course. This was in the days before cholesterol awareness struck and it was still thought to be healthy to eat lots of red meat,

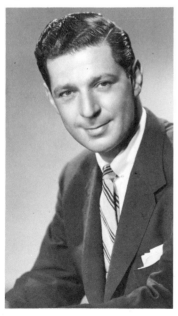

My Dad – known as 'The Voice'

and so our dinner consisted of steak or chops and always lots of salad. The occasional chicken sometimes found its way on to our table, but apart from that it seemed to be an endless round of rare steak, lamb chops and hamburgers.

So here we are at the table. The steak is carved, my own slices put on my white plate with a spoonful of the thin blood which I loved, my string beans with no butter lie next to it, a rather sad-looking salad is heaped on a side plate and next to this is a glass of skimmed milk.

That was our dinner. We never had bread, or potatoes, or rice or pasta. No sir, the only starch that found its way on to the table at 40 East 88th Street was the starch that went into the white linen napkins.

So my skimmed milk is sitting there staring me in the face, and I'm sitting there staring at myself in the mirror, and dinner has begun. The first remark of the meal is usually directed at me by my father.

'And how was school today, Nancy, darling?'

Me, sullenly, 'OK.'

'What did you do?'

'Nothing.'

'Well, you must have done something?'

'We did what we always do.'

'Did you have art class?' he struggles bravely on.

'No.'

'Well, you must have done something special.' Poor man, he is determined to get an answer, to get a dialogue going between us, a happy family-type conversation around this dinner table, just like the kind you see in a Hollywood movie, but I'm not playing. No way. And my last answer is delivered with such an undercutting snideness, with such a twinge of withering disdain, that my mother can contain herself no longer and interjects sharply, 'Don't be rude to your father!' And the unfairness of this, the total and complete unjustness in my eyes of me being made the victim in this little scenario, was too much for me to bear and I stand up, throw my chair back, sometimes literally crashing it over backwards against the sideboard, and go tearing through the big double doors and through the long length of the apartment to my room, where I slam the door and throw myself down on my bed in a rage of tension and anger and tears.

Some time later one or the other of my parents would come to my room. I never knew whether they would be angry or apologetic; my door would either fly open with a crash, or inch gently open a bit at a time, but whatever way it was I would usually soon find myself back at the table, the fight sucked out of me like air from a balloon, picking at the remains of my now cold dinner.

My mother, sitting to my left, is clearly not enjoying this meal. She will be as happy as I am when it is over. She watches carefully what everyone else is eating but she never eats very much herself. She thinks she's fat. She isn't, of course, but she truly believes she is, and she's always trying to lose just a few pounds. To me this seems like an excuse to cover up her anxieties about my own weight, which by this time has become a recurring theme in the family dialogue. I can't believe her concern with her weight is genuine, because with the exception of a very few times in my life, my mother has always been thinner than me. Her weight hovers 5lb/2kg north or south of 9½ st/133 lb/60 kg, which is about 'normal' for her height. My father's weight constantly threatens to creep up to about 10 lb or even 15 lb/4.5–6.8 kg above his own 'ideal', and although they both express regular dismay at their fluctuating waistlines, to me they have always appeared thin.

Now that I am back at the table, we can begin our dessert. We don't have real dessert in our house. We have what passes for dessert. We have a constantly changing array of diet jello, the flavour changes every night, and on those evenings when we haven't had grapefruit to start off with, we have it to finish. But we never have what I called dessert, bread and butter puddings, or chocolate custards whisked up with milk from a supermarket packet, or fudge cake, or any of the other delights that seemed to form a staple part of the diets of my friends at school. Oh, there was always a cake hidden somewhere at the back of the fridge, or high up on the top shelf of the kitchen cupboard, but that wasn't for us, that was for company, and my mother would get extremely upset if one of us happened upon it and took a slice. Sometimes my father or I would bravely venture, 'Well, why do you buy it if you don't want us to eat it?' And her answer, which she thought was eminently sensible, was, 'I buy it so that in case anyone comes over I have something to give them!' So there was this sense of good food, delicious food, fattening food, being something for other people, for people who for some reason didn't have to worry about their weight as we did. I had to worry every day, for somewhere I had strayed from the road of righteous eating, and now I was in a culinary prison from which I could escape only by denying myself day after day the things that I most craved.

But, of course, I couldn't go on denying myself for ever, and I was still quite young when I discovered the miraculous spending power of my allowance. There was a candy store on the corner of Madison Avenue and 88th Street called Saul's that became my salvation. We had a charge account there, and Saul sold a variety of childhood items from comic books to school stationery. So, many afternoons after school, I would casually announce that I needed some drawing paper or maybe a new pencil or two and off I would go to Saul's where I would charge the art supplies and pay cold cash for the Hershey Bars. Yes, it was deep, dark, chocolate Hershey Bars with almonds that were my downfall. I kept them stashed in the middle drawer of my night table and devoured them, sticky and melting, under the covers at night. Lying in bed, with only my flashlight to guide me, I would carefully break each bar into small pieces, always sure to include just one almond in each mouthful, and as the chocolate slowly dissolved on my tongue, I hated myself. I was filled with guilt and self-loathing. How could I be so weak, so naughty, so bad, and still only nine years old? I was sure no one would ever love me, would ever marry me, this terrible creature, who, totally lacking in willpower and self-control, lay alone in the night and greedily stuffed her little mouth with an unending stream of Hershey's chocolate.

I don't know if my parents ever found out about these secret binges. It's conceivable that Saul told them about my purchasing patterns, or even that they did find my hiding place. I always assumed that they must know, as I assumed at that point that they must know everything. And I was sure that it was my own behaviour that had brought into being the state of constant dieting that existed in our house. My brother, six years older than me, was also fat at this time, and there are pictures of us standing together, looking miserable and fat, but I still thought that everything to do with the eating restrictions was my fault. I don't know if Tony ate secretly. I suppose he must have done and there were times when we were older, he late teenage, me about twelve, when we would meet in the kitchen late at night, and concoct marvellous sandwiches, tomatoes on Pepperidge Farm bread, sloopy with mayonnaise, or his own particular favourite, egg noodles melting with cottage cheese. But Tony went to the diet doctor too, at the age of sixteen and lost a lot of weight very fast, weight that he never really put back on.

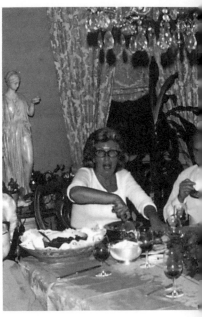

A dinner party at 40 East 88th Street

M y mother also had her own private eating. Her time was late at night, and she would sit alone in the study, watching the Johnny Carson show, and eat steaming hot bowls of chilli, with thick slices of white bread. Chilli and soup, those were my mother's favourites. She loved to make soup, which she always started cooking at night. After dinner, as soon as the dishes were washed and put away, out would come her huge soup pot and into it would go the slabs of meat, the vegetables, and the bones. Sometimes I would awake in the middle of the night to the delicious steamy smells of cooking, and find her sitting in the study, in front of the TV set, hunched over an enormous bowl of cabbage soup with sour cream and marrow bones.

My mother's soups that she made for herself were her own great private pleasure. I would sometimes join her, but more often than not I would come out in the morning to get ready for school and find the kitchen counter covered with enormous jars of soup still cooling, waiting to be put in the refrigerator, and the sink full of big, dirty pots. My mother ate her soup in private, but there was no way that her eating could be kept hidden from the rest of us; it's hard to hide ten gallons of cabbage soup.

T here were wonderful dinner parties in that cream dining-room, when candles would glow and reflect off the good china and my father's favourite wine glasses. My mother would cook for days ahead of time and, at the back of our large fridge, bowls of sauce and platters of hors d'oeuvres, all covered tightly with aluminium foil, gathered waiting for the big night. I was always dressed up and brought out to meet the guests before dinner while they had their drinks in the living-room and, then, when they went in to dinner, my mother would prepare a plate for me of all the different things that she had cooked, and I would take it off into my room. I always came back for my dessert, and was usually invited to sit and listen to the grown-up conversation while I ate my strawberry shortcake or chocolate mousse. I would sit at my mother's side, listening to the joking and the laughter, and wish that every night could be like this.

When my mother cooked, she inevitably made too much of everything. She loved to quip, 'You can never accuse me of not having enough', and for days afterwards we would eat the leftovers from those dinner parties. It was heaven. The night after, we'd have a complete re-run of the party menu and then for the next few nights as things got finished up, our regular dinner would be supplemented with the leftovers from some potato dish, or a crusty bit of lasagna, or the very last dabs of chocolate mousse.

I learned early on that eating with gusto, with delight, was something that you did only on a social occasion, when the presence of other, 'normal' people gave you licence to do so. Eating with crowds, with groups, at parties, was the only

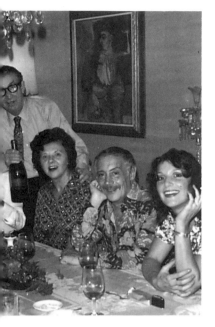

eating that was not accompanied with guilt at that early age and so I looked forward to these dos with tremendous anticipation, and was correspondingly depressed when the very last vestiges of these dinners had disappeared from the fridge and we returned to our normal regime.

Luchows v. the House of Chan

Of course we didn't always eat at home. We had a ritual in our family of going out to dinner on Sunday night. It was one of those family habits that became institutionalized through the years and there was one aspect of it that remained the same whether I was eight or eighteen, and that was that I never wanted to go to the place that my parents had chosen. The arguing would start early in the day and continue as a low grumble as we got dressed and ready for departure. I would wear my patent leather shoes and my white ankle socks, and my black velvet dress with the white lace collar and cuffs, and I never wanted to go. We would leave the house at about 7 o'clock and the dispute would rage in the car. I always wanted to go to a large popular Chinese restaurant called the House of Chan, and my parents always wanted to go to Luchows. I don't know where my brother wanted to go. I think he just wanted us to stop arguing.

My parents usually won, and we would continue on downtown along the quiet Sunday night length of Park Avenue, and head for 14th Street and Luchows. Luchows was a German-style family-run restaurant serving enormous portions of very rich eastern European food, roast duck and Hungarian goulash and potato pancakes and red cabbage, and wonderful strudel with whipped cream. Luchows was also, in those days, *the* place to go on Sunday nights.

We were shown to our large round table covered with the starched white linen cloth, and as we passed through the various dining-rooms my parents would greet their friends who were also there with their children. There was always a gipsy orchestra playing music and wandering around among the tables or sitting on the bandstand, and at Christmas time there was an enormous tree with wonderful hand-carved ornaments hanging from it, and shiny wrapped presents underneath, and at all times of the year the atmosphere on a Sunday night was incredibly bright and festive.

The real trouble started when the smiling maître d'hôtel passed around the large, yellowed cardboard menus, and scurried away to get my parents' before-dinner drinks. I was immediately thrown into the most terrible state of conflict about what to order. Oh, I knew what I wanted to order. What I wanted to order was roast duck and mashed potatoes, and all the other things that were the specialities of Luchows. And I also knew that I wasn't supposed to order those things. I knew that I was supposed to scan the endless menu and find there, among the mass of tempting, tantalizing, heavy, fattening foods, the one or two choices that had been placed there especially for people like me, the chopped steak pattie, the broiled chicken, the poached fish. And I went through unbelievable agonies in the few seconds before my father turned to me and asked brightly, 'What are you having, Nancy?' If I did, on the rare occasion, pluck up the courage to answer 'I'll have the duck, please', there was an almost imperceptible moment of stony silence while my parents caught each other's eye across the table and one of them would say, 'Oh, do you really want to have the duck, it's so much. It's such a big portion. You don't really want to have the duck.' And my mother, trying to be helpful, would add, 'Why don't you have the broiled chicken, that looks good, yes I'm going to have the broiled chicken.' And she would put her menu down, the matter settled. And I was caught in that terrible space between the roast duck and the broiled chicken, and I didn't know which way to turn. Because I didn't want to make them angry at me, and, more than anything, I didn't want to look like a pig. There was pig on the menu and pig at our table, and I didn't want anybody to know.

I wasn't the only one in the family who suffered these problems. We all worried about what we ate and felt guilty if we actually gave in to our baser instincts and ordered from the gluttons' column at Luchows. It was warm and cosy and homy, and the whole atmosphere was one of pleasure and enjoyment and eating. Except at our table, where the atmosphere was one of restraint. We were there, but we weren't actually there to eat. We were there to have dinner out, but not to go through the menu and choose what looked good – we were there to eat as little as was humanly possible under the circumstances.

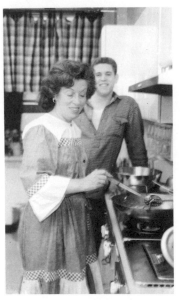

My mother cooking Chinese food with Tony, 1960 – the one cuisine we could all enjoy together without guilt!

Our other Sunday night restaurant option couldn't have been more different. My own favourite choice, and the reason for all of that pre-dinner Sunday quarrelling, was the House of Chan. The reason was simple. There is no way that you can be careful in a Chinese restaurant. You can't be good – there is no grapefruit, no broiled fish with no butter, there are only dishes of such complexity and such unknown calorific content that it's impossible not to gorge yourself, and we did, because being good New York City Jews, we loved Chinese food. This was the one time that my parents gave in and gave way. At the House of Chan we had *carte blanche* to eat and enjoy. No problem choosing from the menu here. Everything was equally tempting, equally threatening, equally fattening and we went haywire. We had everything from spare-ribs and egg rolls to start, right through lobster Cantonese, and chicken with cashew nuts, and sweet and sour pork, and there was absolutely no way that we could restrict ourselves. There was also the wonderful feeling of communal eating, with everyone sharing all the dishes, and offering little morsels to each other and exclaiming over some new first-time delight. We sometimes had Chinese takeaway at home and would all gather around the dining-room table and eat directly out of the soggy cardboard containers and drink small cups of Chinese tea, which my father would bring to the table with the same pride as he showed in his wine. And so, by crossing a cultural barrier, we did manage to find a cuisine that we could all enjoy together without guilt. Even now, thirty years later, when I arrive home in New York, the first family meal is usually Chinese takeaway, delivered straight to the door and eaten around the same inlaid table of my youth.

So those were the patterns of eating as a child. There was always the sense of food as falling into two distinct categories. If I ate the foods that were good for me then I was good, worthy, acceptable. If I didn't, if I strayed into the no-man's-land of pasta, and potatoes, and sweets, then I became, after the merest mouthful, an outcast, a failure, a freak. Because the inevitable consequence of cheating, of bingeing, of indulging in those foods that I loved, was that I would put on weight, I would get fat, fatter, fattest. And that was, of course, the ultimate failure. All of that denial, all of that haggling over menus and restaurants, all of those grapefruit and broiled chicken dinners were ostensibly about one thing. They were about ridding me of my excess tonnage. And to be thin became my one ambition. Then everything would fall into place. I would be happy, I would be successful, I would be loved. And I did lose weight, pounds and pounds of it, and my clothes would gradually get looser and looser, until I would be able to go shopping for a smaller size, and my mother would stare in wonder as I tried on my new jeans, or my new dress, and exclaim, 'It's fantastic, the weight is just falling off of you. I can always see it in your face, first. You're so lucky because you're still young and your face gets so beautiful when you lose a few pounds; when you get old like me, you just look haggard.'

But if my face looked beautiful when I lost weight, what did it look like when I didn't? Because for most of the time when I wasn't losing, I was of course gaining, never really staying the same for more than a few days at a time, always on a diet or breaking one. I look back at photos of myself taken during my growing-up years and I am amazed. In some of them I see the Nancy that I remember so well. She is fat and ungainly and shy before the camera. She is squeezed tightly into her clothes which make her seem too old for her years. But then, in other pictures, there is a thin, delicate, dare I say beautiful girl staring out at me, and I'm shocked and saddened, because I don't remember ever feeling that I looked like that. No matter how thin, how pretty I was, I always felt too fat. I never felt that I had arrived at my goal of thin, or that my body was slim enough to be proud of. Even when, in my early twenties, I had managed by months of careful dieting to get down to a size 8 in dresses, I still had to buy a size 12 or 14 in trousers, and that seemed like a disaster, a personal failure, and I kept dieting, kept trying, in the hopes that all the rules of nature might be reversed and I would wake up one morning to find my thighs had miraculously disappeared in the night. They never did. But that never stopped me hoping.

In fact, every morning, for most of the years of my life, I woke up, and as my hand crept down to feel the swell of my stomach, my first thought of the new day was, 'What did I have for dinner last night?' And if I could proudly answer, 'Six ounces of dry fish, four ounces of green vegetables and one fruit' then bliss, paradise, perfection. I'd spring out of bed, joyous and strong and ready for anything. The clothes that fitted snugly only yesterday would be hanging off my bony limbs and I was sure I had lost at least ten pounds overnight. Life and opportunities seemed limitless, I was complete. BUT let that first question of the day be answered differently, let the answer this day be 'two enormous plates of spaghetti followed by a hot fudge sundae, followed later by the scrapings of the sauce pot and the last few strands of drying spaghetti picked from between the gaps of the colander,' and here we have my own personal recipe for disaster. My wandering hand would recoil in horror from my ballooning stomach, that had seemed so flat only yesterday, but today could have contained the Dionne quintuplets and a few extra siblings as well. I needed all the energy I could muster to drag my laden body from the bed, and I painstakingly avoided the mirror as I slumped through to the bathroom. And what could I wear? Nothing, absolutely nothing would fit, and everything that I tried, and I tried everything, looked terrible. I was disgusting. I was revolting. Surely everyone I passed on the street would be snickering inside at this horrifying slob, who had done it once again, who had let everyone down once again, who had committed the unpardonable sin, the final indignity against myself and the entire human race, who had for the one thousand, two hundred and seventy-third time, BROKEN HER DIET!

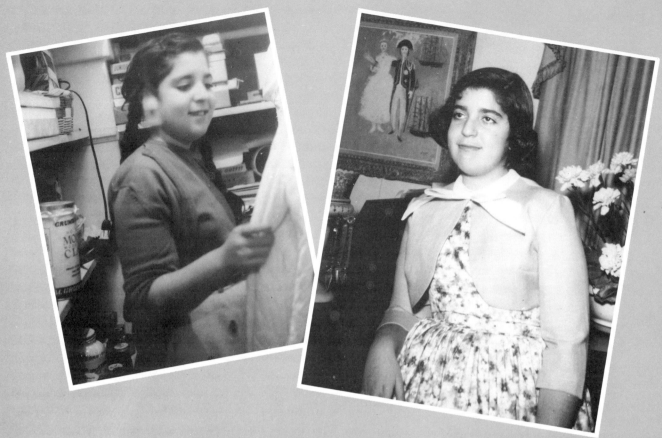

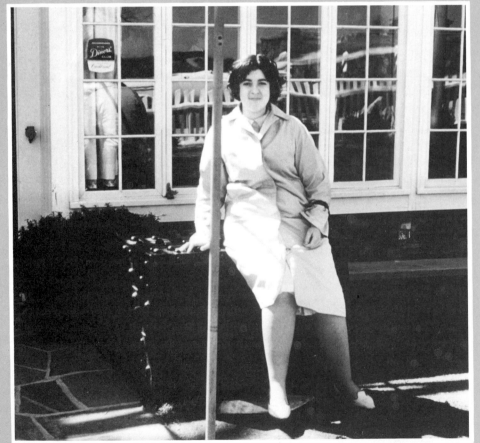

Above left: Before my braids were cut off

Above right: My new 'slimming' haircut!

Covering up, aged thirteen

3

DIETING–A WAY OF LIFE

I became an expert in the ways of dieting. It was my vocation. The well-balanced, nutritionally sound childhood diets of Dr Stein were not drastic enough when I entered my teens, and I soon replaced them with calorie-counting. I carried a little notebook with me everywhere and entered everything I ate in one column with the amount and the calories per ounce across the page. I would start out planning to eat 900 calories a day and my greatest feelings of satisfaction came on those days when I kept well under that limit. To end a day at 500 calories was my ultimate triumph. I discovered the foods that were the lowest in calories and would eat those constantly, often more than once a day. Boiled chicken became a favourite at that time and I would have it for lunch *and* dinner. Although it drove my mother crazy to have to keep a bowl of pallid unseasoned chicken breasts constantly at hand, she was at the same time delighted with the rapid weight loss that was the result of this colourless regimen.

With the exception of my boiled-chicken phase, every time I was on a diet, everyone else in the family would be on an approximation of that diet, and I was happily never faced with the situation of having to watch my brother and my parents eat one thing while I ate something else. My father always supplemented his meal with a bit of cheese, but, apart from that, it was the diet of the day that governed the menu of the night.

My favourite of that period, if not of all time, was the Stillman diet, known to its devotees, who included half the population of New York, as 'the water diet'. It was so popular not because of its culinary variety (you could only eat meat, fish, chicken, cottage cheese, and certain condiments, such as ketchup) but because you could lose fifteen pounds in under ten days, no problem! You could actually lose more weight on this regime that you could by fasting.

There was only one drawback. In order to get rid of that terrible dry taste that developed in your mouth after a day or two, and to keep yourself from dropping dead from dehydration, you had to drink about thirty gallons of water a day. This meant that Stillman was rather limiting. It was hard to get on a bus or go shopping or maybe take in a movie, because you simply couldn't be more than ten steps from the nearest bathroom at all times. But the Stillman diet worked like a treat for me. I lost tons.

Another diet that came around at that time, and that is still with us, in one form or another, is Atkins. Now Atkins had the same high-protein base as Stillman, but on Atkins, you were also allowed slatherings of fat: mayonnaise, butter and oil. You also got two tiny green salads a day, on which you could lavish as much oily salad dressing as you liked. The Atkins diet was unique because it actually required you to enter into the world of science. On the Atkins diet you were pulled into the complex scientific analysis of what you were eating and your own body's particular chemical reaction to it. The theory was that when you had been eating the prescribed foods, and only the prescribed foods, for a couple of days, your body would enter the state known as *ketosis*, a state in which you were, surprise, surprise, burning up your own fat stores. In addition, once again, to that awful taste in the mouth, and a dragon's breath, there was another way of checking for this heavenly state. You went off to the drugstore and you bought yourself a little brown jar of Ketostix, and on to one of these tiny litmus-paper-tipped plastic strips you would let fall, at least once a day, your pee. And when you had achieved the blessed state of ketosis, this wonderful little gauge hanging there between your thighs would turn a bright shade of purple. It was the greatest feeling, I can tell you, and I used to use a Ketostick, not just once a day, but every time I went to the loo, just to see that colour change from beige to pink to lavender to purple and to have this indisputable proof that I was losing weight even as I sat there. It really gave me the incentive to go on.

There were two things that Atkins and Stillman had in common. The first was their very rapid initial weight loss. I would be on either of these diets for three hours and feel that I'd lost ten pounds and that my life had changed completely. I'd wake up that first morning after I'd begun the diet and practically break my neck running to the scale, to see the inevitable weight loss of at least three pounds, and I would feel just great. Oh, wondrous new life, I'm on my way now and nothing's going to stop me, I'm going to stay on this diet until I lose all of this weight (even though it's recommended for only two weeks at a time), I'm going to stay on it for ever!

The other added additional bonus of both of these diets was that, of the things you could eat (with the exception of the salad), you could eat as much as you wanted. You could eat all the steak, all the fish, all the chicken, unlimited quantities. Now the idea of unlimited quantities to a dieter is irresistible. If you're used to a diet on which you're restricted to four ounces of this and two ounces of that, and someone comes along and says, 'Right, you can have unlimited quantities', well, you think you've landed in culinary heaven. It doesn't matter in the slightest what the unlimited food is. I mean, if someone says you can have unlimited quantities of horseradish sauce, it seems like the greatest thing in the world, and believe me, you get through a lot of horseradish sauce.

You could say that these diets encourage a somewhat unnatural attitude towards food, and some rather bizarre eating habits. All New York went crazy for each new diet, and the apex of this was reached with the now infamous Scarsdale diet. The Scarsdale Clinic's Dr Tarnower, he of the murdering mistress, dictated, before his untimely death, a diet in which not only the types of food were restricted but you actually had to eat certain meals on certain days only. So, because New Yorkers are used to getting good service, and, because New Yorkers are what might be called food junkies and we expect this good service in restaurants above all other places, you could walk into some local bistros on a Tuesday, or a Thursday or for that matter on a Sunday, announce to your waiter, 'I'm on Scarsdale', and he would bring you that day's perfect Scarsdale meal, complete down to the paper frills on your lamb chops.

The other diet that featured big in my past is Weight Watchers. Weight Watchers was started by a suburban housewife in the early sixties who rightly judged that it was easier to diet *en masse*. I was nineteen years old when I attended my first meeting. I took the Lexington Avenue bus to 79th Street and climbed a steep, dark flight of stairs to a cavernous room above a delicatessen to be greeted at the door by a large hand-lettered sign reading 'WELCOME TO WEIGHT WATCHERS'. Inside the meeting hall there were rows of folding chairs set up facing a large blackboard at one end. At the back of the hall was a table at which two women sat filling out filing cards and collecting money. And just in front of them was a large professional doctor's scale and a big crowd of women lining up waiting to be weighed. I obviously knew that this was going to happen, and although, as ever, I dreaded stepping on the scale, I also had that good feeling of relief that I had finally decided to 'do something about it'. I was awash with that familiar feeling that always came at the beginning of a diet, that at last I was giving myself up to a greater control, to someone or something that would tell me just what to eat, and when to eat it, to an authority to whom I could abdicate all responsibility for my own disgraceful eating habits. I always had that feeling at the beginning of any diet, but that night walking into Weight Watchers it was especially strong. For it took a lot of courage to go to a meeting full of strangers; it was a big step to take, and now that I was there I was prepared to give myself up to it completely.

I weighed in at 13st 1lb/183 lb/83 kg and was told that my goal weight was 10st/140 lb/64 kg. I filled out my registration card, paid my fee and sat down. I watched the hall fill up with many women, some bigger than me but many already smaller, already aglow with the achievement of their losses. Soon that would be me, I knew it, I felt that I belonged here, that here at last I would be taken care of. There followed a talk by our 'lecturer', a small blonde named Sylvia, who I thought was enormously funny. She told us that first evening about how to stick to the 'programme' (because you never ever referred to Weight Watchers as a diet) if you found yourself at a wedding or a bar mitzvah, faced with the inevitable laden buffet table. It was easy. You simply took along your own specially prepared Weight Watchers skinless roast chicken in a little plastic bag, which you ate while everyone else was eating their disgusting party fare. It all seemed eminently sensible to me at the time.

Later on everyone's name was called with their weight loss for that week, they were applauded, or in the few cases where someone had gained a pound or two, gently reprimanded. Several women had reached a 'plateau' after losing great amounts of weight, and they were given encouragement and a round of applause for their past achievements. I stayed on after the meeting with the other new recruits to learn the 'programme'.

Sylvia patiently explained the intricacies of 'legal' and 'illegal' foods, and answered our questions on such burning issues as why when everyone loathed it so, did we have to have liver once a week. Nothing was left to chance at Weight

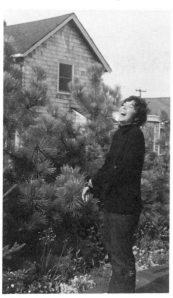

Above: With 'my trees', aged twenty-two – thin after a strenuous bout of 'weight watching'

Watchers, and the illegal foods you just didn't touch at any time. So, like most people, the second I was out of there and on my way home, I went straight to the list of forbidden foods at the back of my Weight Watchers pamphlet, and immediately developed an insatiable craving for all the things on that list. You can understand *some* of those cravings, for listed there were such popular favourites as peanuts, chocolate, and mayonnaise. But ketchup? Can you believe that I can remember wanting ketchup more than anything else in the whole world, and just because it was there on that list as something that I couldn't have?

I did very well on Weight Watchers. I lost a lot of weight and I felt good and healthy. I adored going to the meetings and looked forward to the moment every week when I would take off my shoes and my belt and my jewellery and my cardigan and anything else that moved and step on to the scales, and watch that little metal weight as it slid down and down, closer to my goal.

I also loved the preparation of the food. The total commitment that one had to make to getting it all right, because every portion had to be weighed. You could even buy a little Weight Watchers scale at the meeting. Six ounces of fish and four of tomatoes, and one of hard cheese, and two or four of cottage cheese, depending on whether it was breakfast or lunch. And of course, you had always to be sure to include just one number four vegetable with your dinner, and as many as you wanted of number three, and fresh fish at least three times a week and canned as many as you wanted, but without the oil.

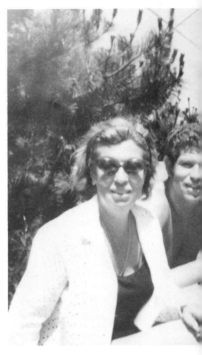

Above: With my parents and Tony on the deck at Fire Island – one of the few pictures of me in a bathing suit

Weight Watchers gave you licence to think food twenty-four hours a day; when you weren't eating it, you were preparing it, and when you weren't preparing it you were weighing it, and when you weren't weighing it you were shopping for it. But the strange contradiction about all of this concentration on what was going into your stomach was that *hunger* never entered into it! Hunger was the last thing on your mind when you were on Weight Watchers, because in those days the golden rule of this organization was 'Never Skip a Meal'; never, even if you weren't hungry, even if you woke up at noon on a Sunday and thought that it was a good time for brunch, that wonderful combination of breakfast and lunch, no way, not on Weight Watchers. What those of us on the programme in those days were expected to do, and what we did in fact do, was first have our Weight Watchers breakfast at twelve and then, say an hour or two later, our lunch!

What seems glaringly obvious to me now, although I would have considered it blasphemous then, is that the greatest thing about Weight Watchers, the thing that kept me coming back for more, year after year, is that it allows people already obsessed with food to develop, enhance and perfect that obsession. And what's more, it rewarded this obsession with institutionalized kudos, certificates, and diamond chip pins, and the truly overwhelming applause of one's colleagues. Yes, the lure of Weight Watchers was, without doubt, that winning combination of group dynamics and sanctioned obsession.

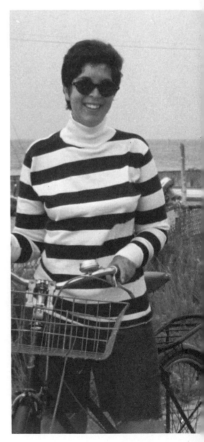

I was a member of Weight Watchers on four separate occasions, first in New York, and then later on after I had come to live in London, and the pattern of the meetings and of my weight loss was always the same. We were weighed, lectured to, applauded – the programme was gradually altered through the years to fit in with new dietary discoveries, one-time illegal foods like potatoes and rice becoming legal – and I was always the model Weight Watcher, I never cheated and I always had a nice surprise for my lecturer when I stepped on the scale.

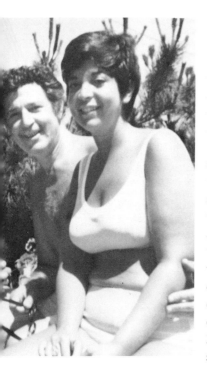

Below: With Tony – I'm twenty-four, he's thirty, we're both thin, but not for long!

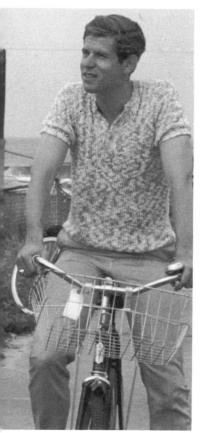

There were other diets that I tried through the years. With every new dietary discovery came the corresponding diet book. One moment it was high-protein, next high-fat, and most recently high-fibre. I tried them all, and I lost weight on all of them. Some were fast-acting and extreme, others well-balanced and slower, but steadier in their results. But there were two factors common to them all. The first was the constant, never-ending preoccupation with food that any and all of these diets presupposed. Because, as sure as night follows day, it is impossible to be on a diet without thinking most of the time about what you should and shouldn't eat, about what you just ate, and about what you are about to eat. Whether I was making an entry in my small calorie-counting notebook or selecting my day's assortment of pills from Dr Stein or running to the bathroom to check my Ketostick or carefully weighing out my fresh fish, I was thinking food and eating and weight. Now, weight is something that I have rarely mentioned up to now. And there's a good reason for this. It's because although the loss of weight, the getting thin, was supposedly the aim of all of these years of food obsessions and dieting, when I did on many occasions manage to get thin, the craziness didn't stop. It seemed to make no difference whatsoever to my need to diet and to my feelings of ugliness and lack of self-worth whether I weighed in at 200 lb/91 kg or 130 lb/59 kg. I always felt fat, and I always stuck with my dieting syndrome. And always to think about food, to 'watch yourself', to put the diet of the week first and plan around it, I took to be quite normal, even commendable behaviour. It showed that I was 'taking care of myself', that I was 'in control'.

The second thread that ran through all my dieting experiences, was the cruel, soul-destroying fact that no matter how hard I tried, no matter how quick the weight loss or how slow and steady, no matter that I had been on Stillman for six days, or Weight Watchers for six months, I always, but always, put the weight back on and always, eventually, even more than I had lost to begin with. And this fact, which formed the pattern of much of my life, from the earliest days of my childhood right up to my mid-thirties, I did not take to be normal in any way. I felt alone in my weakness. I felt that I lacked some vital component of self-control that had been given to others. I lacked that most important of all womanly graces, willpower. And this lack of willpower, this extreme helplessness when faced with the recurring mutiny of my own fat cells, became the one thing in life that I strove to overcome. If only I could get thin, once and for all, then every-thing would be all right! Then all the important things in my life like home and job and marriage would fall into place, and all the smaller day-to-day problems, like what to wear to the supermarket on a hot day, and how to get from the sand to the sea unnoticed, would disappear. And my life stretched ahead of me along two roads and I myself could choose every morning the direction I would take. To eat the wrong thing, to break my diet, meant going down the road to fatness, ugliness, failure in every sense. But to deny myself that smear of mayonnaise, that scoop of ice cream, that skin of chicken was to follow the road to happi-ness, to acceptance into a world that I coveted more than anything else, a world inhabited by the beautiful, the successful, the thin!

And so with each new day came the decision, my decision, would it be a good day or a bad day? It was up to me, and it all depended on what I chose to have for breakfast. If I stuck to whatever diet I happened to be following at the time, if I had my egg on dry toast (Weight Watchers) or my fried egg and bacon (Atkins), or my straight cottage cheese (Stillman), then I was strong, proud, worthy of respect, my own and everyone else's. If I strayed and indulged in some forbidden fantasy food, and it's important to realize here that this forbidden food didn't have to be fattening, merely forbidden, well if I indulged in that, then I was lost, a self-indulgent, worthless failure.

And sometimes this feeling of failure and despair would lead to a binge. Now bingeing is relative. It can mean having two slices of bread when you are trying to stick to a no-carbohydrate diet, or having ten chocolate bars when you're on no diet at all. And of course, I binged a lot, because it's impossible to diet without bingeing. Bingeing is only the other side of dieting, and when I was growing up anything that was forbidden was a binge; three peanuts were a binge. So was a tomato sandwich with Hellmann's mayonnaise. A binge doesn't have to mean sitting down in front of the TV with a package of chocolate-chip cookies and another one of Ritz crackers and going through the both of them without even coming up for air. It can mean overdosing on stoned dates and wholemeal bread and any other 'healthy' foods that you can lay your hands on, and that you devour until you are ready to burst. One of my own particular favourites from my teenage years was based on Graham crackers. My mother always kept Graham crackers in the house because they were, of all the cookies on the market at that time, the lowest in calories. By themselves, maybe one or two at a time, I'm sure they were, but I had devised a way of boosting the calorific content of Graham crackers beyond all the expectations of the manufacturers. At the back of the fridge, behind the skimmed milk and the lettuces, my mother also kept a small jar of Scrafft's hot fudge sauce, that rich chocolate syrup that is poured warm over ice-cream, preferably vanilla, where it slowly goes hard and sticky and chewy, and incredibly delicious. Not having vanilla ice-cream at my disposal, I would instead begin by breaking my Graham cracker in half along its ready-made perforations (could Nabisco have had this in mind, perhaps?) and then, gingerly dip it directly into the warmed jar of fudge sauce. But that's not all. I would finally coat the now chocolate-covered cookie with a layer of Ready Whip, the first whipped cream that you could shoot out of an aerosol can and an invaluable aid to the binger. I would always begin with a half of a cracker and then go on to a whole and then two or three or more before the guilt would become unbearable or I would run out of the ingredients, whichever came first.

The guilt and sense of failure that follows a binge is hard to describe. I felt that I'd thrown it all away, that I had undone all the good that I had done, that I had, yet again, lost this most important battle, and that I had better get myself back on to something the next day, and something more rigid, more restricting, to make up for my lapse.

There is another kind of binge, and that is the 'night before the diet binge'. And this binge is almost guiltless, because it is the overture to a new diet, to making a new start; even though you go through every cupboard and devour whatever you can find in peculiar combinations of salty and sweet, it is somehow all right to do it, because you have decided beforehand that it is positively the very last time in your life that this is ever going to happen.

There is always this sense of 'paying for your mistakes' when you are a dieter, of having to even up your own personal scoreboard, with you on the one side and food on the other. If I did let go, if I did have something that I enjoyed, there

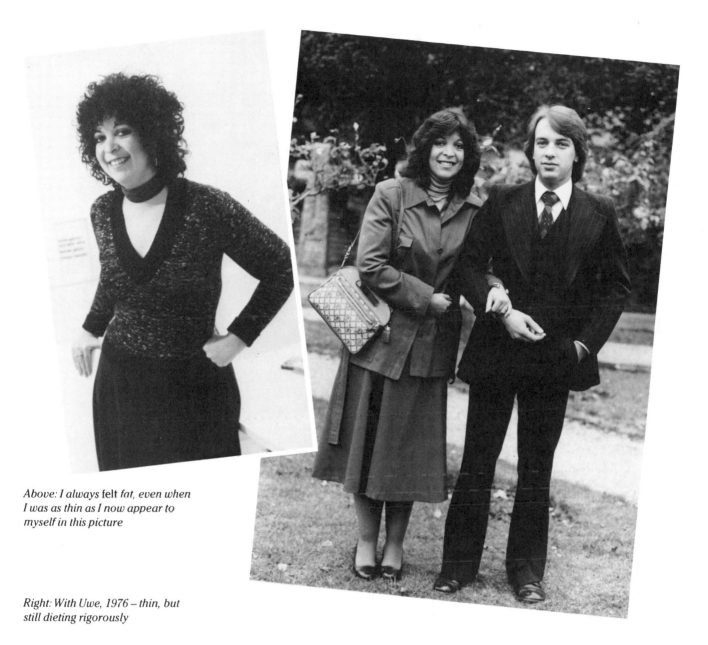

Above: I always felt fat, even when I was as thin as I now appear to myself in this picture

Right: With Uwe, 1976 – thin, but still dieting rigorously

was the immediate need to put a stop to it as soon as possible. And I did. I was, truly, what I ate and the only way I could face myself was by constantly winning in my war against food.

This pattern of appraising myself totally in terms of what I ate and what I weighed became the mainstay of my existence. I grew up, went to college, fell in love, got my first job, came to live in England, fell in love again, moved into my first flat, started my own business, but, everywhere and always, the predominant theme was my diet and my weight. When things didn't go so well with the current boyfriend, when the latest job fell through, I could always get myself together by starting a new diet. And it did make me feel better. For a while. Until the inevitable moment when I would slip off those familiar rails and have that one forbidden titbit, and then all was gloom and despair until I found my way back again on to the straight and narrow.

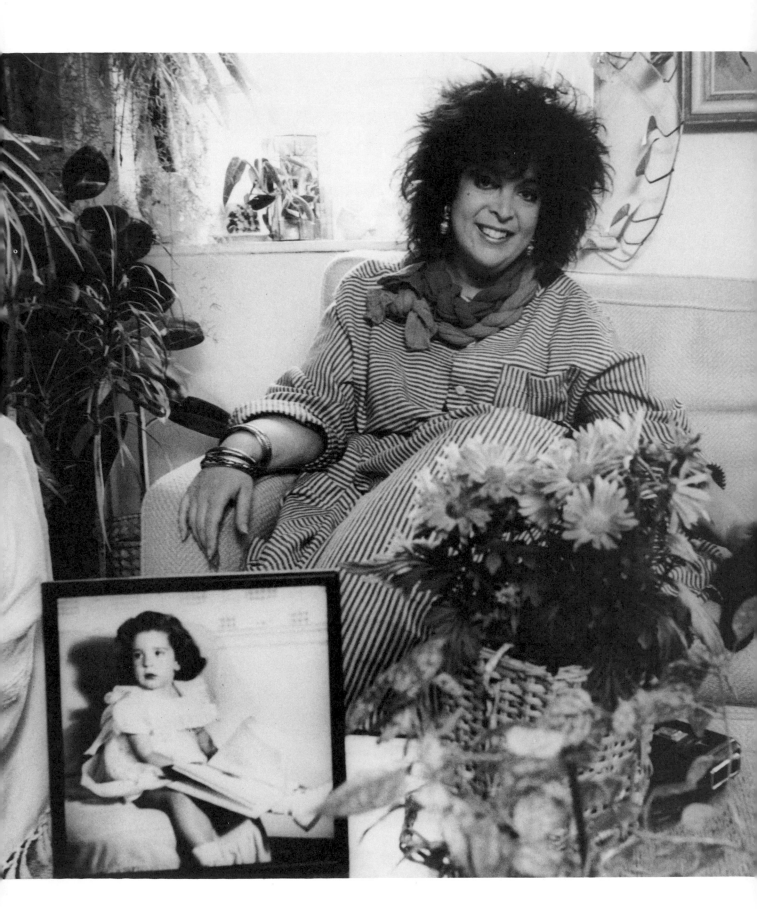

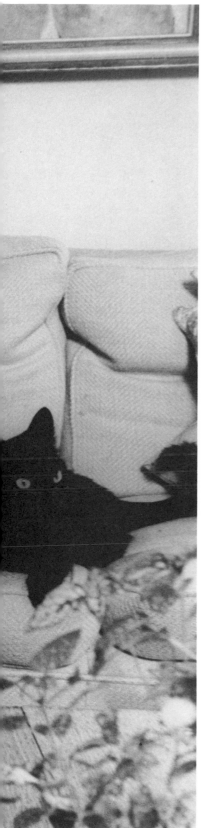

4

DIETS DON'T WORK

And then, one day in the spring of 1979, at the age of thirty-three, I turned a corner. I had been living in London for ten years and had gone from job to job. My most recent venture had been as a fashion buyer for some American retailers who sold English designer clothes, but unfortunately my employers had gone bust and I found myself filling in the time before I found something else doing part-time typing at the offices of a classical records company. I only worked there in the mornings and one afternoon as I headed home to my tiny flat near Marble Arch, I stopped off at my local newsagent to buy the evening paper. As I stood at the counter waiting for my change, my eyes strayed to the single paperback display case which stood just inside the door, and there, stuck in among copies of *The Shining* and *The Thorn Birds*, and looking like just another good read with its cover picture of a naked lady emerging from layers of gauze, I spotted the book *Fat is a Feminist Issue*. Hadn't I heard of it? The title was familiar but I couldn't remember anything else about it. Well, you can't really go wrong for 85p.

Later that afternoon I settled myself in my favourite chair and began to read. Four hours later I was still reading and had moved from the chair to the sofa and back again. I'd consumed endless cups of coffee and cut off all phone callers after their first hello. I literally couldn't put it down. I was dumbstruck. For here was a book all about women just like me. Women whose lives revolved around food, women who hated their bodies, women who were addicted to dieting and to weighing themselves, women who dieted one day and binged the next, women who were good if they ate right and bad if they ate wrong. So I wasn't the only one! There was even a name for us: 'compulsive eaters'. But the most staggering, the most revolutionary part of this whole book was that the writer, Susie Orbach, who actually taught at my old *alma mater*, New York University, was saying, in black and white, on page after page, that dieting was BAD for you! Not good for you, as I had always believed with a belief that had become the cornerstone of my life, but bad. It encouraged all kinds of negative feelings about yourself. She even suggested that there were other ways of evaluating oneself as a person that were more genuine and more long-lasting than your waist measurement. As I read page after page of this heresy, the foundations of my world slowly began to crumble. Because there, in the pages of this small paperback book, was the medical statistic that was to change my life for ever. Hidden in the footnotes at the back of the book was the following note: 'Diet organizations will not release figures on recidivism. However, various sources put it at 95 per cent.' (Recidivism – what's that? I rush to the dictionary: 'to fall back, to relapse'.) Ninety-five per cent! The weight came back! So it wasn't just me. It wasn't that I was greedy or out of control or lacking in willpower. I was simply fighting a losing battle, and there were millions of other women just like me, every one of us gaining weight again and hating ourselves for it. But if ninety-five out of every hundred women put the weight back on again, then surely *we* were the normal ones, and just as surely there must be something wrong with a method of losing weight – i.e. dieting – that fails in so many cases. And with that realization came the most incredible feeling: My God, if this is true, if dieting doesn't work, then I don't ever, ever have to go on another diet for as long as I live.

But wait a minute, if I stopped dieting, I knew what would happen. I'd blow up like a balloon. It had happened countless times before. I'd break my diet and whoosh, up would go my weight, always heading for new heights like some off-course rocket. But Susie Orbach said no. She said there was a distinct difference between breaking your diet and simply giving up dieting. When you give up dieting you gradually stop wanting to binge and when you stop bingeing your weight will stabilize and your eating become normal. Normal, what is normal? It seemed that normal eating was eating because you're physically hungry. Yes, folks, it's as simple as that. Eating when you are physically hungry, and not because you've just had a fight with your boyfriend or because it's lunchtime at Weight Watchers, or because you're going on a diet the next day, but simply because your body is hungry.

It sounded good. And I wanted so much to believe it, and I could, surely, because all the other things she was writing here about growing up, and relationships, and feelings about yourself were what I had read in many other books and had experienced for myself. So I was ready to believe this latest eating gospel, because after all the diet books, all the years of thinking food and weight and scales and measurements, here was someone saying stop! And I was ready. But how could I break the patterns of a lifetime? And the answer was there. Join a group of other women with the same problems and meet regularly to discuss and discover how we got like this in the first place. Find out the origins of your own compulsive eating problem, just what triggers you off, what makes you head for the fridge at all hours of the day or night, and you could beat it. And there was the address of a place called the Women's Therapy Centre in northwest London, where compulsive eating self-help groups were regularly held.

Well, I wanted to talk to this Women's Therapy Centre more than I have ever wanted to talk to anyone in my life. After several attempts, I finally got through. 'Hello, I'd like to join a compulsive eating group, tomorrow please.'

'I'm sorry, all our groups are full and there won't be any new ones starting till September. If you send us a stamped self-addressed envelope, we'll send you an application form, but there's no guarantee you'll get into a group. We are over-subscribed and it's first come, first served. Thank you for calling.' Click. I looked at the dead phone in disbelief. September, that's six months. I could be dead in

Previous page: Me, aged two, and aged thirty-six, in London, 1982. For most of the years in between I was dieting

six months! I could weigh 400 lb in six months. This is terrible. I call back. 'Look, you don't understand, this is really an emergency. Can't you make an exception? You see, I've had this problem for twenty-seven years, for Christ's sake, I'll go nuts waiting for September. Please?'

'I'm sorry, but you'll have to send a stamped self-addressed envelope...' she repeated apologetically. 'Thank you for calling.'

After waiting half a lifetime for this kind of help to arrive, I couldn't possibly wait another six months, I just couldn't. I didn't mail my self-addressed envelope. I took it by hand all the way to Holloway, and dropped it though the letterbox of the large grey stone house that was the Therapy Centre, hoping that the day or two saved would gain me a position a few places nearer the top of that waiting list.

I continued going every morning to my job at the record store and gradually, just slightly, food began to be less important. I was not on any particular diet, just trying to eat only when 'physically' hungry and waiting for the day when the letter from the Centre would arrive to tell me that help was at hand. And then, on a warm afternoon in early June, purely by chance, I saw the ad in *Time Out*.

I had skimmed through all the main features, passed through the pages of pine beds and community service jobs when the following small ad at the top of the theatreboard section caught my eye:

WOMEN INTERESTED IN WRITING A PLAY
ABOUT WOMEN AND WEIGHT,
AND BASED ON 'FAT IS A FEMINIST ISSUE',
CONTACT CLAIR, 176 LOFTHOUSE PLACE, NW5

Well! If you just imagine for a moment that I had never even READ the theatreboard section of *Time Out* before, you will realize what an impact this advertisement made on me. So much of an impact that I did absolutely nothing about it. But the next week, the ad was there again – as if specifically placed to break down my resistance. And so I put pen to paper and wrote to Clair. What did I have in mind? Certainly not anything to do with writing a play. But I thought that maybe they would let me address envelopes or lick stamps, and that somehow these women writers about weight, this Clair, would be my own particular route into a compulsive eating group.

A few days later I had a reply. 'Clair and Rina would be holding workshops at the Roundhouse [a real theatre!] on Saturday 29 June, RSVP.' OK, I'm coming, sisters. With much trepidation, I got myself up there on the day. I kept telling myself it was a mistake to go, what would they want with me, what good would I be to them, I'd never written a play, I'd never written anything, it would just be embarrassing. This kind of reasoning went on right up to the moment when Uwe pushed me out of the car door in front of the theatre.

I walk down a flight of damp stone steps into the basement of the Roundhouse and see that apart from two women who are moving chairs into a large circle I am the first to arrive. The two of them are thin. I am not. I feel very fat and very conspicuous. I'm wearing my favourite outfit of the moment – white slacks and a Victorian nightshirt of blue and white stripes that comes down to just below my knees and hides my most unappealing body area from view, or so I think.

After strolling nonchalantly up and down the side aisle three or four times staring intently at the floor, the ceiling and every detail of the paintwork, I decide that I am even more obvious than I would be just sitting down, so I casually slump into a seat at the back of the room.

'Why don't you come up and sit here?' This from one of the chair arrangers. And do I detect an American accent? Not like my Manhattan nasal perhaps, but...Now that my attention has been diverted from the strenuous task of making myself invisible, I can see that there is something American about her appearance that shines through even the distinctly un-American Dr Scholl's exercise sandals.

'I'm Nancy Roberts. I'm here for the workshop.' And I instinctively go for the largest of the straight-back chairs.

'I'm Clair. The others should be here soon. You're a bit early. And this is Rina.' She motions towards the dark-haired, exotic-looking beauty in the red boiler suit who is scanning a list on her clipboard. She smiles and checks off my name. I clear my throat and try to look busy. What am I doing here? Why did I listen to Uwe? Just the day before, I'd pleaded, cajoled, made every excuse I could think of, but he just stared at me with his wise Nordic eyes. 'Maybe you're not ready to give up your problem,' he'd said. 'Of course I'm ready,' I shrieked, 'but what kind of nut answers the ads in the back of *Time Out*, for God's sake? They'll be a bunch of loonies. It'll be a waste of time.' He just smiled. So I thought, OK I'll show him, I'll go.

And so here I am, and now, thank God, there is another arrival. Someone they call Katina rushes in, bubbling over with apologies for being late. She too is thin. She's dressed in bright pink trousers, a purple and pink striped sweater and lime-green basketball sneakers. She drops her enormous canvas bag on the floor where it immediately disgorges a multicoloured collection of notebooks and cardboard files and diaries. Removing an apple from this cornucopia of efficiency she plops down next to me, smiles broadly and says 'Hello'. I can tell instantly that I'm going to like her.

The room is beginning to fill up now and as one woman after another comes down the aisle towards our circle of chairs, Rina checks their names off the list. Then Clair calls the meeting to order. 'Hi, I'm Clair. I want to welcome you all and thank you for coming. I thought we could begin by telling each other a little something about ourselves.' A ripple of unease runs through the circle. 'I'll start, I'm Clair, I'm twenty-six, I'm American, and for most of my life I was a compulsive eater.' My God, I thought, it's like Alcoholics Anonymous, let me out. She continued, giving a rundown of her life to date, including the kind of details about her eating behaviour that had most of us in the room smiling bitterly in recognition. She finished off with a résumé of her theatrical credits.

We continued around the circle telling our stories, and although the women were of all sizes and shapes from very thin to very fat, the stories about food and dieting and guilt, about eating, and about dismay at the shapes of their bodies were the same. Most of the women had had theatrical or writing experience and by the time my turn came, I was wondering anew what in the world I was doing here. I was shaking with fear when Katina finished speaking and all eyes turned to me. I started hesitantly with Dr Stein at the age of eight, and soon I was telling it all, the years of dieting, the self-loathing, the covering up, both

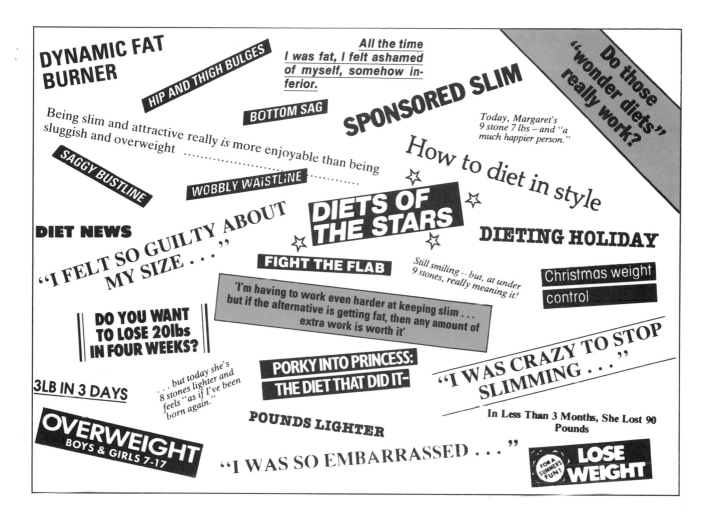

emotional and physical, and they smiled and urged me on, and, for the first time I felt that I was sharing all of that past pain with people who really understood. I finished my story: 'So I've never written or done anything like that, but I'd be happy to do typing or administration or anything else that may need doing.' I sighed with relief. The worst was over.

By the time all thirty women had spoken, we were relaxed and laughing and felt as if we'd known each other for ever. We broke for coffee, but not before Clair had spoken the words that sent a stab of ice down my spine. 'After coffee, we're going to do improvisations, so please find yourself a partner.' What? Improvisations? I couldn't. Surely, she didn't mean me, I was only going to be the typist, for God's sake.

I weighed up the possibilities. One, I could leave, cut out, make my exit. This would undoubtedly be the easiest solution. It would also be slightly embarrassing and what's more important, would surely cut off, now and for ever, my contact with this bunch of women whom I was counting on to get me into a compulsive eating group. Two, I could stay and do an improvisation, hopefully with Katina, who certainly seemed sympathetic, and wouldn't let me make a fool of myself, would she? I was saved by Katina's approach. 'Would you like to be my partner? We could work on this together.'

We did a scene about two old friends meeting each other on the street after not having seen each other for a couple of years. One had lost twenty pounds, the other had gained. I played the thin one; how's that for type-casting?

The interesting thing was that I had been both of those friends at some time or other, one year thin and preening, the next fat and ashamed, and I knew just what to say in both cases, for hadn't these things been said to me? Hadn't people praised my hairdo, and my shoes, and my jewellery, anything to divert attention from my body itself, which was unmentionable. And now, I said these same things to Katina, as she gushed over my new svelteness. When we finished, everyone laughed and applauded, and I returned to my seat, heart pounding and shirt sleeves drenched with sweat.

The meeting broke up shortly afterwards with Clair inviting everyone to her place the following night to talk further about the project. Well, the following night was Sunday, and if there's one thing I hate, it's having to go someplace slightly work-tinged on a Sunday, particularly a Sunday night. So later on, telling the whole story to Uwe, I finished off with, 'So, can you imagine, they actually want to have a meeting on Sunday night? No way. I'm not getting involved.' And that was that.

Until the next afternoon at about two when the phone rang. It was Clair. 'Listen, I just wanted to let you know as soon as possible that Rina and I held another workshop last night and saw another thirty women, and then we discussed who we wanted to work with on this project, and we narrowed it down to four people and you're one of them.'

I was stunned. 'Me? But I've never done anything like this before.'

'Oh that's OK. We think you'll be just great. See you tonight. Bye.' And she hung up.

'Uwe,' I called him in from the kitchen, 'they want me!'

'Fabulous.'

'It's not fabulous. I don't want to go, and I didn't have the guts to tell her.'

'Why don't you want to go? I think you should give it a chance. Just one meeting. Just one Sunday night. You can always change your mind, tell them something else came up. If it's awful, you just won't go again.'

I finally gave in and went. And I kept going to meeting after meeting. We sat on cushions on the floor of Clair's large airy room in her house in Kentish Town. The walls were hung with posters and spider plants, and pictures of Clair's family in Minnesota. We spent days just telling our stories, going back into our past and delving around, trying to find the first moments when food became a problem for us. Trying to remember the time, the year, the day when we first started to hate our thighs or our breasts or our whole bodies. There was Clair, who had been dieting and bingeing from the age of twelve. Janine, who was always trying to starve away her big bust. Shane, who had, during her teenage years, come close to anorexia nervosa. And Katina, for she was here too, whose addiction to chocolate had started with her father innocently popping a sweet into her baby mouth every time she cried. We shared our stories, we probed delicately but remorselessly into each other's backgrounds and slowly the patterns of our eating and self-loathing emerged.

And as we talked I began to understand just what all of the dieting and bingeing had been about for me. The women of Spare Tyre became my own compulsive eating group. I had come to the auditions looking for help and I was getting it. I began to learn how to break the connections between my emotions and my eating. I watched what I ate and when I ate it. This, of course, was nothing new for me. What was new is that now I began to ask myself why. Why was I reaching for the chocolate biscuits after that phone call? Why did I go through a box of Ritz crackers if Uwe was late home for dinner? Why did I continue eating well past the point of fullness whenever I had the chance?

The major eating triggers, the ones obviously related to anger, to loneliness, to deprivation, were easier for us to understand than the seemingly minor ones. Why, for instance, did I always have to have something to eat the second I got into a car? It had been like this for as long as I can remember. No kidding, Uwe and I would set out for a weekend trip or some Saturday shopping, and no sooner was the key in the ignition than the urge would hit. Chocolate. Or maybe some pistachio nuts or cashews. No matter that we'd just finished a terrific lunch or were on our way to friends for dinner, I had to have eatables within arm's length.

Why did travelling do this to me? Car travel in particular? What dark secret lay behind this compulsion? One night, sitting up late, working on a scene that I was writing for the show, it hit me, and I remembered.

I'm six years old. Or seven. Or twelve. Or sixteen or twenty-one, or any age up to twenty-four when I left New York to live in London. It's a Saturday morning and my family is preparing for the New York ritual known as 'going to the beach for the weekend'. We're not concerned here with the long, lazy summers on Fire Island, but with the many spring and autumn weekends when the whole family would pile into the car together and hit one of the various highways leading out of the city, and head for Bay Shore and the ferry to Ocean Beach.

Sounds like a fairly simple procedure, right?

'I'm going to wake Nancy' – this from my father in an already rather strained tone, wafts into my final moments of childish sleep.

'Nancy, Nancy, time to get up, darling, we have to make the ten o'clock boat.'

Anticipation creeps in. I love Fire Island. I get up quickly. I wash, dress, and pack my overnight bag, before heading for the kitchen.

My mother is already there, sitting at the breakfast counter in her nightgown, sipping her coffee and smoking a cigarette. She can't quite get to grips with being awake at this hour. She is surrounded by an assortment of large plastic 'cold bags' filled with food for the weekend; turkey and ham and cucumbers and frozen packages of meat and enormous jars of Hellmann's mayonnaise.

This tranquil scene is interrupted by my father who comes hurtling down the passageway fresh from his shower, rubbing vigorously at his hair with a towel.

'Norma, darling, are you almost ready?'

'I'll be ready, Kenneth, just give me a minute. I've been packing the food.'

'Well, I want to make the ten o'clock boat.' He rushes off, still towelling.

'He makes me crazy' – this to me. I commiserate, and glance up at the kitchen clock. It's 8.15. To be really sure of making the ten o'clock boat we have to leave by 8.30 – latest. Will she make it? Will we make it? Good, she's making a move.

'I guess I'd better get going. This makes me so crazy every weekend. If we miss one boat, we'll get the next one. What's the rush?' She sighs and shuffles off to the bathroom, her one sure place of refuge.

My father completes his own personal preparations in no time at all. He's already putting the bags together by the front door.

'You ready, Nancy, darling?'

'Yes, Dad.'

'Tony, are you ready?'

'Coming, Dad.'

'Where's your mother? I'm going to start taking these things down to the car. NORMA! I'm taking the bags down. Is everything here?'

Muffled irritation from the bedroom: 'Just a minute, Kenneth. I'm just closing this.' She comes struggling out, half dressed in jeans and bra, lugging a large canvas holdall.

'Here, let me take that, darling.' He relieves her of the bag. 'Be down in five minutes, or we'll miss the boat', and with a whoosh of the elevator doors he is gone, my brother bringing up the rear. This leaves my mother and me alone in the big apartment, to race around, turn off the lights, put the milk away, put the few breakfast dishes in the dishwasher. She is neat, even at moments like this. 'I hate to come back Sunday night to a messy house. Have you closed your windows? Check the living-room, please. Wouldn't you know it, your father's left the light on in his closet.'

I'm holding the front door open. I've already rung for the elevator. Its presence, I know, will spur her on. 'The elevator's here, Mom!'

'I'm coming, I'm coming.' She checks the door lock one last time, nods hello to the elevator man, who is used to our Saturday morning routine, and we've made it. Out of the apartment at least.

My father sits behind the wheel of the car, waiting. 'Come on, come on, come on, it's twenty to nine.'

'It's just twenty-five to. You know you're going to kill me, Kenneth. What's the rush? We can always make a later boat. You know I have to get the food ready, and the bags. I've got to turn off the lights and close the windows. What the hell's the difference if we get the 10.30 boat?'

'There is no 10.30 boat, just an eleven o'clock.'

'So, we'll get the eleven o'clock. My God, I can't stand this every weekend!'

We are not yet ten minutes away from home, heading north towards the Triboro Bridge, when we enter the second great area of Saturday morning conflict. Not really conflict between members of the family, more an agonizing decision-making process between my father and himself. 'Should we go the Expressway or the Major Deegan?' This spoken thoughtfully to himself.

'You know the Expressway is always terrible at this hour,' my mother reminds him.

'I don't know, Al Mendelsohn took it last week and he made it in an hour and ten minutes. Maybe we should try it.'

This is not my mother's department. 'Whatever you think.'

We pass another highway to our left that doesn't look so hot. My father decides we are better off where we are. At least we are moving. And so we are staying on the Major Deegan. For now.

That settled we enter the third stage of this marathon journey. My father is afraid we are going to miss the boat. And so he is driving very fast. And erratically. He crosses from lane to lane like some punchdrunk halfback, squeezing in wherever there is an opening, and cursing at anyone who dares to get in his way. We try to kid him out of this phase, but he is unreachable. 'I've never had an accident!' he proclaims proudly.

And so off we go, sweeping and rolling around in the back seat, the car radio blaring, the smoke from my mother's nineteenth cigarette of the morning all but blocking our vision of the road ahead.

'What time is it, Norma?'

'Kenneth, just relax, we can make the next boat.'

'Yeah, Dad, we can go into Porky's.' Porky's is the place of my dreams. It is the wonderful greasy-spoon at the ferry dock where everything they serve is guaranteed fattening. Sometimes we eat there and then I am in heaven. The few times in my life I can remember eating doughnuts with my mother, it was in Porky's.

But no, not today. Today my father is determined, and after a death-defying drive across the railway tracks in Bay Shore, where we barely miss being smacked on our collective head by the crossing gate, we screech to a halt at the dock. The last passengers are climbing aboard the 10 o'clock ferry.

'Wait, wait!' We all jump out of the car, virtually throwing the assorted shopping bags and suitcases out of the trunk, and my father leaps back behind the wheel and heads off the two hundred yards to the parking lot at ninety miles an hour, the wheels of the car screaming along the gravel.

The deckhand grabs our luggage, tosses it up to the top deck, and we hurry aboard, greeting familiar faces who smile sympathetically. My brother and I run to the back of the boat to look for my father. The engines have started, smoke is pouring out of the engine room, and the ferry is raring to go. Please wait for my Dad. We can't leave without him. He'll have to wait here all alone for the next boat.

But here he comes, flying across the parking lot, his trenchcoat flapping, his crocodile shoes glinting in the sunlight, he holds his hat on his head with one hand, his newspaper in the other, and he is laughing! My God, is it possible he actually enjoys this? He leaps on to the dock without a second to spare, and just as the grand old ferry *Fire Island Belle* slips away from her berth and, accompanied by a rapturous round of applause from his fellow passengers, he launches himself into the air and comes crashing down to land amidst the piles of cardboard grocery cartons and bulging canvas holdalls that blanket the ferry's lower deck.

And so another Saturday rush is over. We are all safe on board. We have made the boat, and all is right with the world. We can relax. Relax that is until Sunday night, at around 5 o'clock when it's time for the return journey to the city, and with a few minor variations, the whole thing starts all over again.

And for years I wondered why, whenever I got into a car, my anxiety would mount, the muscles at the back of my neck would tense up, my mouth would go dry, and I would be struck with the absolutely irresistible urge for something soothing, something comforting, something relaxing, something to EAT!

Because my own particular eating trigger turned out to be tension. Tension and anger. I had, of course, always *realized* this, but it was only then, in the days of working with Spare Tyre, that I began to really *understand* it, and that I

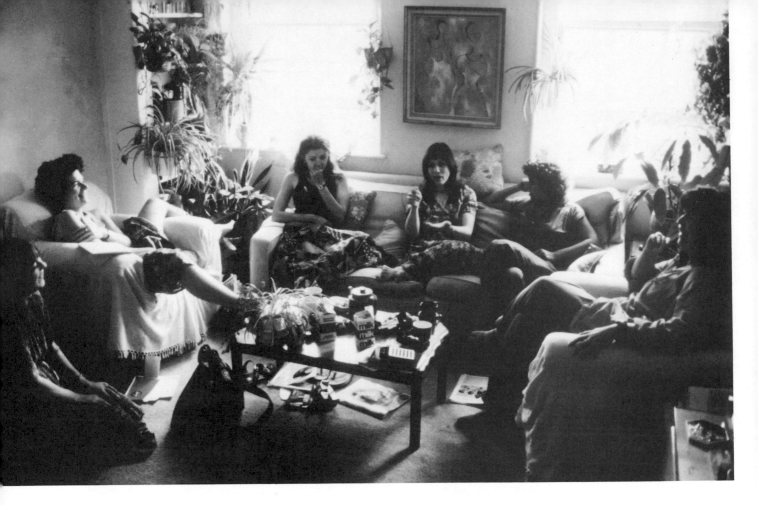

*The Spares writing. From the left:
Harriet Powell, Clair Chapman,
Adele Saleem, Katina Noble,
Janine Turkie and me.*

became capable of doing something about it. Because when I had unearthed the truth behind my car-eating, it simply stopped. Oh, there are still times when a chocolate bar during a long journey hits the spot, but there are other times when we will drive for hours, going somewhere on holiday, or for the weekend, when I will suddenly realize there's no food in the car – and I don't even miss it.

There were other variations of my own compulsive eating that were not so easy to cope with, that were a lot more difficult to understand and overcome, but even so, gradually during that summer of 1979, I realized that food was becoming something that I thought about less and less. When I did eat, I tried to eat just what I wanted, whether it was salad or spaghetti or tinned peas. And I struggled to be able to identify the feeling of fullness, because in much the same way that hunger had never been a reason for eating during all those years of weight watching, so fullness had never been a reason for stopping. Every day I asked myself, am I really hungry, do I really want that sandwich, or apple, or Mars Bar, or am I bored, angry, depressed? And if the answer was, 'Yes, cut out the psychological crap, I'm hungry!' then I ate it, and I enjoyed it, in a way that I had never enjoyed eating before.

At first, the idea of being allowed to eat whatever I wanted, whenever I wanted, was frightening. I alone was in control of my eating for the first time in my life. There was no diet sheet taped to the front of the fridge, no calorie counter in my handbag, no weekly meeting at which I would be weighed or measured. Waking up every morning and saying 'I can have anything in the world that I want for breakfast' at first resulted in a confusion of mixed tastes. First a bite of bacon, then a pancake, maybe a sausage, then some toast or maybe a cup of cocoa. But that period was shortlived, and I discovered very quickly the wonderful truth that if you can have, every day, at every meal, anything that you want, you don't want it all at once. You become selective. Just knowing that I could have it if I wanted it made it less appealing. When I was dieting, all foods were divided into two categories: the ones I could have and the ones I couldn't. The ones I couldn't have were irresistible, and every day that I managed to get through without having a forbidden food I congratulated myself. But now there were no forbidden foods and, as I soon found out, no desperate cravings and no binges either. I was eating, for the first time in my life, like a normal eater.

The excitement, the happiness, *the relief* that I felt had unleashed an energy in me that I had never known was there.

We began to write our play. In it we told the story of five women, all different, all somehow the same, some fat, some thin, all suffering from the same obsession with food and dieting. We did improvisation after improvisation. We wrote scenes alone at night and read them aloud to the group the next day, where they were dissected, rewritten, and put back together again. We worked till all hours, we laughed and we argued and we wrote. Scene after scene was completed, song after song was added. We were meeting every day now, in a disused shed at the back of a school in Islington. And then one night, at a meeting that had gone on later than usual, as we sat amidst the remains of our dinner of ham rolls and cardboard coffee, Clair said, 'I think it's time we started to think about a director.' We all nodded. 'And I also think it's time to talk about casting.' No arguments here either. 'I think it's pretty obvious that Nancy has to play Joanne.'

I sat bolt upright 'What? Obvious? Obvious to *who*? *Writing* this play is one thing, but I can't be *in* it. I'm not an actress!'

'Don't be silly,' Katina laughed, 'you're a natural.'

Later that night, sitting alone upstairs on the number 30 bus, looking out at the darkened streets, I saw nothing. All I knew was that I was going to be in a play. Me. I was going to act. To be up there on a stage with other people out front watching. I walked home from the bus stop in a daze and floated up the four flights to where Uwe was sitting watching television.

'Hi, are you hungry?' he asked.

'They want me to be in it. I'm going to be in it, Uwe…I'm going to be an actress!'

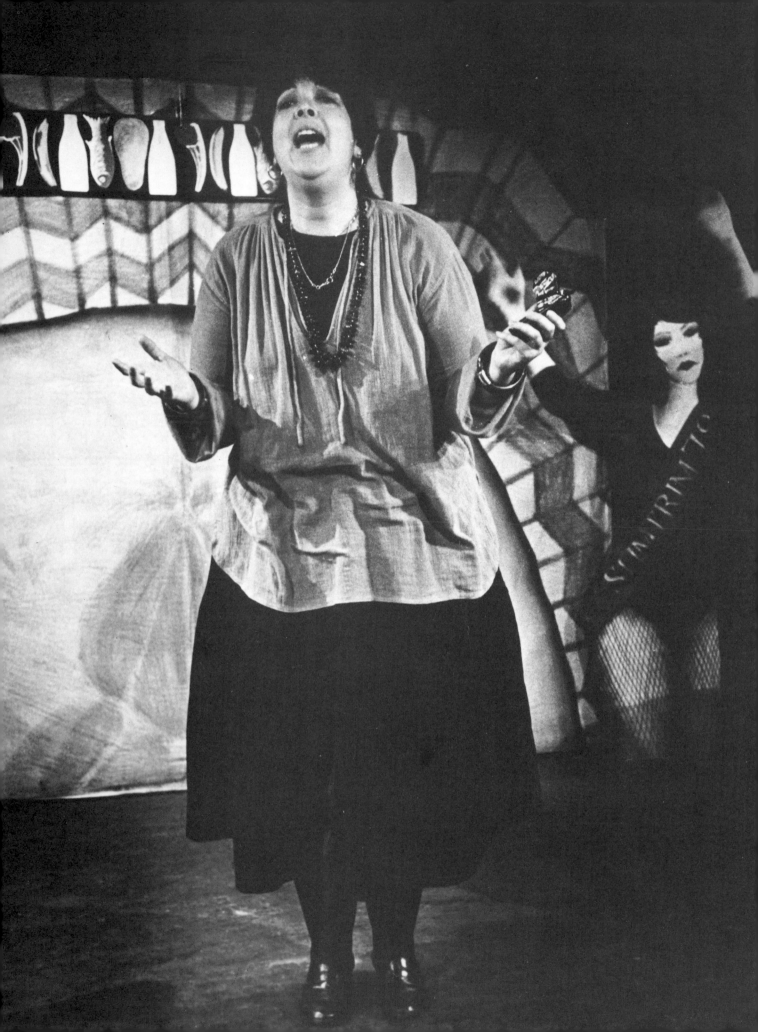

5

'BARING THE WEIGHT'

Rehearsals started soon after that night. We chose a director, Caroline Eves, and began with a read-through in the shed in Islington. I held the script in my hands and waited for my first line. I was afraid that when it got to my scene I wouldn't be able to speak. But even though the sound of my own voice sounded false and every word seemed to have the wrong emphasis, I managed to get through it without swallowing my tongue.

I lived through those weeks in a perpetual daze. I was, at every moment of every day, running my lines through my mind. I had a very long monologue about dieting that was difficult to learn. I walked to the bus stop in the morning with my lips moving furiously and my head dipping and swooping as I tried to get the expression just right. The people I passed on the street and sat opposite on the bus first looked at me blankly, and then turned their own heads away. I'm sure they thought I was crazy, and suddenly I thought that all the nuts I'd ever seen mumbling to themselves with such conviction on the city streets of London and New York must have been actors learning their lines.

Our show, *Baring the Weight*, was a cabaret made up of short scenes, comedy bits, monologues, and songs. And two of these songs had been written specifically for the character, Joanne, the fat, lonely, over-achieving journalist. I played Joanne. That meant that they expected me to sing. That's right, me. Little Miss Tone Deaf. I tried to tell them that this was out of the question. I actually gave them a demonstration. 'Listen, you're gonna hate this.' And out came the opening notes of 'Mars Bar', the first of Joanne's numbers. 'There,' I said, smiling with satisfaction, 'I told you.'

'Terrific,' said Clair, turning to our pianist, Sylvia, who had just done her best to accompany me. 'But I think she'd be better in a different key, don't you?'

'Try this,' said Sylvia, and she hit a note.

'Ah,' from me.

'No, no, a little lower,' and she sang the note herself. I joined her. 'How does that feel?' she asked.

'I don't know,' I answered. 'How's it supposed to feel?'

Sylvia looked at Clair. 'Why don't we just leave it there for now, and see how it goes? Nancy, why don't you try singing it all the way through?'

'Why is it every time my mother rings me on the phone I want a Mars Bar?' Singing in Baring the Weight, *1979*

I had certainly heard this song often enough. We had heard all the songs many times by now. Clair, who had written them, had brought each one in to us, like a gift, as soon as it was completed. We'd all sung them together, but never alone before. Now, haltingly and with fists clenched, nails digging into my palms, I followed Sylvia as she played the melody on the piano. We did it again and again, until finally I was singing at the same time as she was playing and, by the end of the day, I had learned my first song, in my own key.

During the weeks that followed, those women, Clair and Katina, Shane and Janine and Sylvia, gave me something that I had never even hoped would be mine. They gave me confidence. Confidence in myself as me, and confidence in myself as a performer. I loved those rehearsals with the fierce love of a woman of thirty-three finally doing what a child of five had dreamt of.

As our opening night approached I embarked on an intensive letter-writing campaign to the press. There was something staggering about a play that actually said, in these diet-obsessed days, that dieting was an obsession best forgotten. And the reporters poured into our rehearsal shed, expecting to see a bunch of enormous women leaping around on stage. Instead they found the Spare Tyres, all shapes, all sizes, and eager to talk and explain the serious message that we were trying to put across. In the week before we opened, stories appeared everywhere, from the *Express* and the *Observer* to *Spare Rib* and the *International Herald Tribune*. When the night of our preview arrived the shed was packed to the rafters, not only with friends but with the press and people from other fringe companies around London.

At last Caroline jumped up on to the makeshift stage to where we huddled behind our flimsy set. 'Is everyone ready? Then let's start.' She smiled broadly and gripped my arm: 'Enjoy it.' And she was gone, out front. The strains of the opening number sounded and we were off. I waited backstage, my hands and feet frozen, my mind a total blank. How would I get through this? I couldn't even remember my first line! In the next second Clair and Katina were rushing past me tearing off bits of costume as they went, and it was my turn to go on. I casually ambled out carrying the half-eaten bag of crisps that was my first prop and before I had even sat down at my desk and delivered my line, there was a ripple of laughter, of anticipation. 'They know they're going to have a good time,' I thought, and suddenly I wasn't afraid any more. My lines came into my head, and I got through my scene without even realizing it. Then came my first song. Sylvia played the now familiar introduction and after the first line, 'Why is it, every time my mother rings me on the phone I want a Mars Bar?', out there, in the dark, my first-ever audience erupted with laughter. I responded, and my voice was louder and surer and clearer than I had ever imagined it could be, and the notes didn't matter, and the key didn't matter. What mattered was the story that I was telling. I finished with a sad but defiant last bite of my Mars Bar, and I turned and walked off stage for the first time in my life to the indescribable sound of an audience applauding.

The show went without a hitch and soon we were all on stage together singing the last number and then bowing and grinning as the applause filled the ramshackle building. We were besieged by people wanting to know all about everything, how did we think to write it, had it really been our own experiences, had the other members of our group ever been fat themselves.

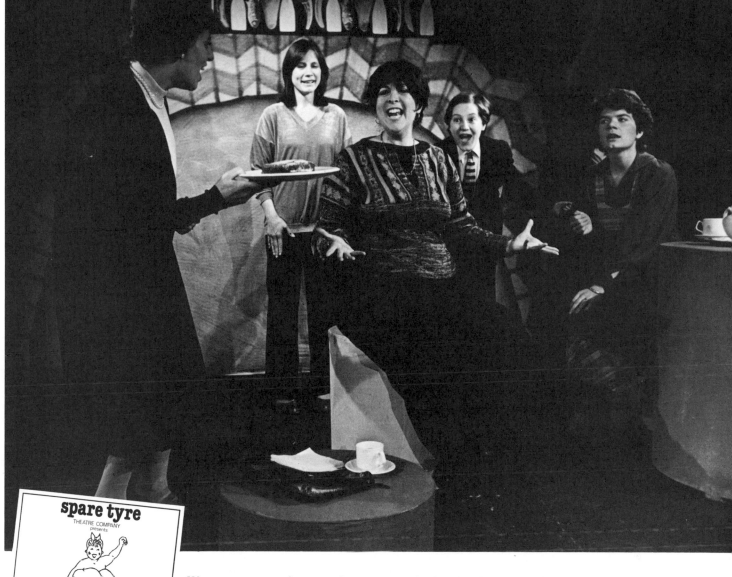

Baring the Weight – *the finale
with Janine, Katina, Shane and
Clair*

Inset: The first poster for Baring
the Weight

We were escorted across the street to the local pub, ensconced in a large booth
and plied with drinks. I sat between a journalist from *Time Out* and an admini-
strator of another fringe theatre company. 'Why haven't we seen you before?
What else have you been in recently?'

'Nothing,' I replied, 'this is the first thing I've ever done. You see, I'm not an
actress.'

They thought I was kidding around, but that didn't matter. I was sitting in a
grimy, cracked leather booth in a run-down London pub, yet to me it was the
best banquette in Sardis, and this was Broadway and my first opening night. I
could not have been any more excited than I was.

Baring the Weight opened the next night to the public in a tiny theatre in the
suburbs of deepest Croydon. It was a theatre that normally sat fifty, could at a
pinch fit in sixty and we squeezed in eighty. Even so, we turned away dozens.
And for every night of our two-week stay there the lines stretched around the
block and we always had to turn people away. Our audience was always made
up of the most varied mix of people. We had the usual aware Londoners who
regularly attend fringe theatre and the committed women who follow women's
theatre groups, but we also had the suburban housewife, the women from the
local council estate, and sometimes even their husbands. The publicity had
worked well, and all types of women were eager to see this show about a
problem that was common to us all, whatever our backgrounds.

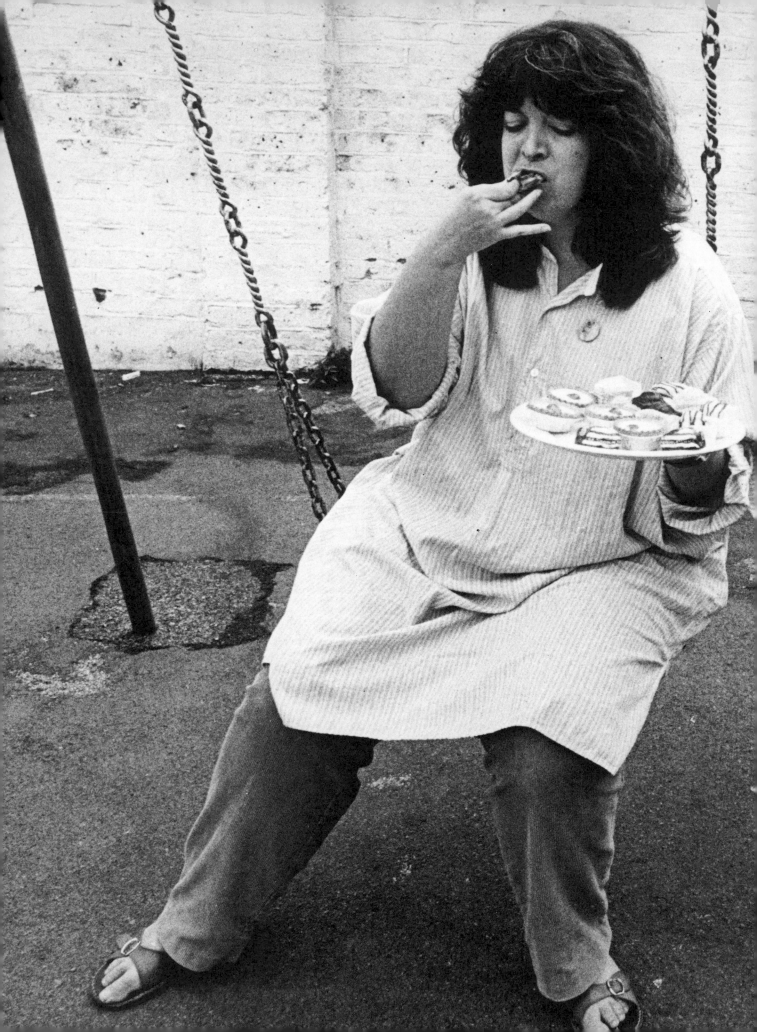

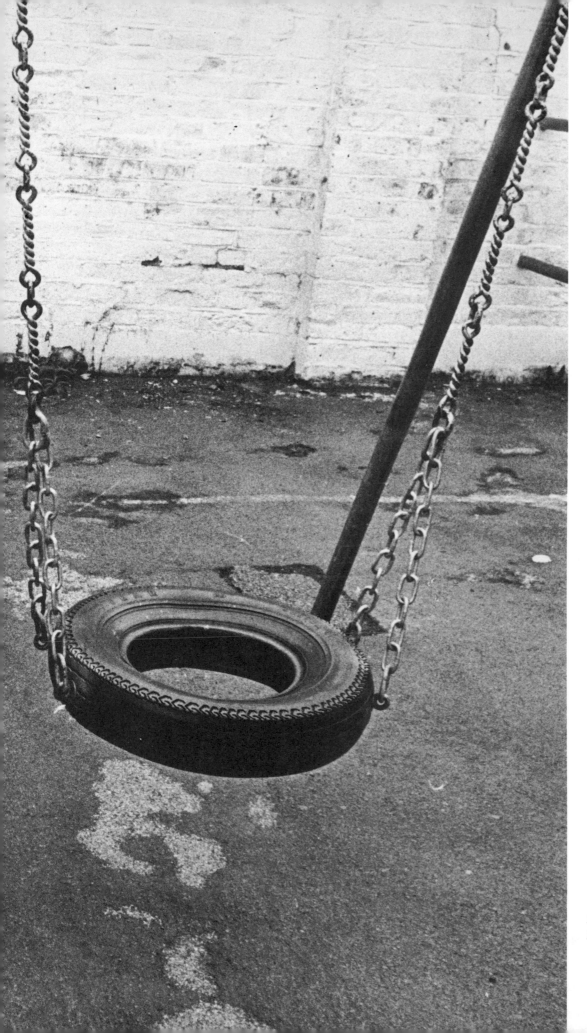

Early Spare Tyre
publicity photo, 1979

So many of these women came up to speak to us after the show, wanting information about how they could rid themselves of the agonies of compulsive eating, that after the first few performances, we decided to have audience discussions after each show. These sessions became as important as the show itself, as women told, sometimes for the first time, of their own dieting experiences, and their own pain. These stories were sometimes funny, always moving, and the feeling in the hall or theatre was one of understanding and relief at finally getting it all out in the open.

Then began the next phase of Spare Tyre's work. So many of these women wanted to join a compulsive eating group that we found ourselves taking down names and promising to put them in touch with other interested women in their area.

A compulsive eating group is basically a self-help group. There is, ideally, no leader, as most women who join one already have too much experience of giving up control of their eating patterns to an outside influence. But groups do usually need help getting started, so we devised a system whereby one member of Spare Tyre would go to the first one or two meetings of a new group and then provide the members with a series of notes and guidelines which would see them through the initial months of weekly meetings. We maintained contact with our own groups, once started, and because Spare Tyre toured our first show all over Britain, we soon had a network of women all over the country, running their own groups and setting up more locally.

The first group I ever set up myself was in a small terraced house in south London. There were six women. Among them were an ex 'Slimmer of the Year' who had sadly put back all the weight she had lost, a young woman with a dieting history which started when she had hit puberty, a middle-aged woman whose battle with her weight had started soon after the birth of her first child, and a very slim, beautiful young woman who at first appeared to have no problem at all, but who, it turned out, was addicted to weighing herself. She had three scales in her suburban home and would go from one to the other, checking her weight first thing in the morning and last thing at night, as well as after every meal in between.

I listened to these women's stories and then I gave them their 'homework' assignment for the first week, which consisted of the following instructions:

1. Keep a detailed food chart listing everything eaten during the week, along with the time eaten, whether or not you were physically hungry before eating, what feelings you had just before and after eating, and whether or not the food satisfied you. Analysing these charts was the first step in identifying the emotional triggers that lead to compulsive eating.

2. Stop weighing yourselves; throw away those scales.

3. Dispose of all of your clothes that are too small for you. Give them away, throw them away or put them away, out of sight.

These last two instructions were there for one reason, to begin to build up a positive self-image. We all know how wonderful it feels to jump on the scale in the morning and see a weight loss. We also know how demoralizing it is to see a gain. And the truth of it is, it doesn't matter, it makes no difference what the scale says.

Too many women evaluate themselves solely in terms of what that early-morning weighing reveals. And it's time to start 'measuring' ourselves in other terms, so 'out with the scales'.

Getting rid of all those 'thin clothes' is also there for a very good reason: the only thing worse than hopping on the scale to see the pointer head for the skies, is opening your wardrobe and being faced with hanger after hanger of clothes that don't fit, skirts that won't close, T-shirts that cling, jeans that won't slide above the hips. It makes you feel lousy. It's better to have one or two things that fit you as you are now, than dozens of glorious garments that are too small.

To start to feel good about yourself you have to begin to live for the present, right now. Compulsive eaters tend to live for the future. 'When I'm thin then I'll do all the things I've always dreamt of doing, but can't do fat.' 'When I'm thin, I'll find a better job, a better husband, a better way of life.' There is as wide a range of 'when I'm thin' dreams as there are women with this problem. But a popular and constantly recurring one is the 'when I'm thin, then I'll wear wonderful clothes' dream. And women who feel that they are fat, even if they are only a few pounds over what they would like to be, often hide themselves inside dark, drab, concealing garments, dreaming of the day when they will burst out of their cocoon and into the kind of clothes that they would prefer to be wearing, clothes that say to themselves and to the world, 'Look at me, I'm beautiful!'

Hiding within your clothes is a common syndrome for the compulsive eater, the woman who dislikes her body, and most of us know only too well what we mean when we speak of our 'thin clothes' and our 'fat clothes'. Just as one of the long-term aims of a compulsive eating group is to learn to 'live for now', one of the short-term aims which contributes to the achievement of that goal, is to 'dress for now'. Get rid of your 'thin clothes' and buy clothes that fit you now, as you are. Wear the kind of clothes that you've always liked, that you've always wanted to wear, but that you thought you could only wear if you lost weight first. If you've always dreamed of pretty frilly things, wear them. Jeans and a sweater? Wear them! Or maybe you've always longed for but never dared to wear shocking-pink dungarees. Go out and splurge. And if all of these changes seem too drastic, then begin gently with a bright scarf or a pair of socks in a loved colour that you've never had the guts to wear.

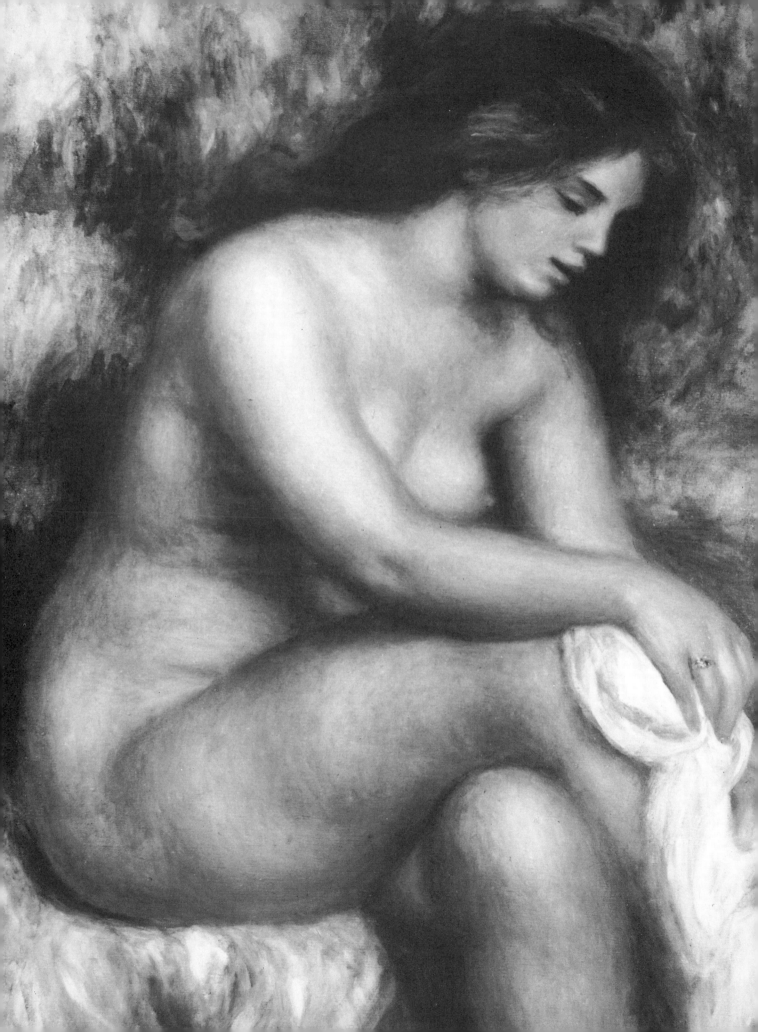

6

TRANSITION— BIG CAN BE BEAUTIFUL

In May of 1980, just before Spare Tyre started rehearsals for our second show, we gave ourselves a holiday. I went home to New York to visit my parents. It was the first time I'd seen them since the changes that had taken place in my life. They were thrilled with it all, and carried the Spare Tyre press clippings around with them in their wallets. My mother still had some trouble getting used to my new eating habits, which to her seemed highly erratic. Having a snack at 4.30 when dinner was at 6.30 was still something that grated, but she resisted the urge to protest, and, by the end of the first week, she had to admit that although I ate at rather unorthodox times, I didn't seem to be eating 'that much'.

During those days at home, I saw my mother's concern with food and with the family's eating in a new light. Through my work with other women with food problems, I had come to realize that for many women food, its purchase, preparation, and serving, is of vital significance. It is one of the traditional areas over which women have reigned through the centuries, and it is an area over which it is difficult to relinquish control. My own mother, like so many other mothers, had tried to maintain her control over my eating so fiercely that eventually I had rebelled.

I realized during that trip that it was of prime importance to be able to maintain my new eating habits while in my parents' house and that I had to find a way to do that while avoiding the kind of confrontation that we had always had where food was concerned. I talked to my mother a lot about food during that trip. About the battleground that it had become for her and me. About my own needs to free myself from my compulsive eating behaviour, about the suffering I had gone through as a dieter. We also talked about her need to watch what I ate, about her concern and unhappiness over the fact that I had always had a 'weight problem'. I tried to make her see that although I was still fat, I was feeling better than I ever had before. It was a difficult time for us, but a good one. As my own eating became less of an emotional issue for me, so it became less of an emotional issue between the two of us.

Renoir, Bather Drying Herself,
c. *1910*

During that short spring holiday in New York, I did all the usual things. I saw friends and family, went back to favourite haunts of my youth, movie houses and Chinese restaurants, and indulged in one of the favourite New York sports, shopping. Whenever I go home to New York I love to go to the big department stores. Wandering around the aisles, looking at the latest gadgets and clothes, always makes me feel back in touch with what's happening in my native city.

I didn't alway enjoy shopping, clothes shopping in particular. My ambivalent feelings began early when I first discovered the fashion pages of *Seventeen* magazine. As a pre-teen I spent hours gazing at those snub-nosed blond models with their perfect profiles and their shiny lips and their flawless skin. They were perfect in every way – how would I ever measure up? I had elaborate fantasies of these perfect girls going with their mothers on wonderful shopping expeditions to all the best New York stores, Saks and Bonwits, and Lord & Taylor, where everything that they tried on not only fitted, but looked gorgeous.

My own shopping expeditions with my mother were somewhat different. I always looked forward to them and woke up early Saturday morning full of anticipation. 'Today we'll get something wonderful, something that will make me look just like the girls in *Seventeen*.'

It's 11 o'clock and I've been waiting for three hours for my mother to wake up. I can't bear to wait any longer, and so, armed with a large cup of coffee, I tiptoe ever so gently into her room.

'Mom' – this very gently. 'Mom' – this time a little louder – and she stirs. My eyes are growing accustomed to the darkness and I can make out her slumbering shape. Maybe I should just go away and let her sleep until she wakes up. But she may not wake up in time and then we won't go. For I know my mother, and she is no speed freak when she actually does get up, so I persist.

'Mom, I brought you some coffee.'

'Aren't you sweet. What time is it?'

'Almost 11.30. We're going shopping, remember?'

'All right, I'm up.' And she really is, slipping on her robe and heading into the bathroom for the first of several visits that she will make, before, a full two hours later, rushed by me and already harassed, she is ready to leave. I, of course, have been ready to leave for ever, sitting in front of the TV, with my hat and coat on, watching cartoons.

Finally, with a last shuffle through her charge cards and a hurried search for gloves, we are off. We walk to the corner, my mother hails a cab, I slide with some difficulty across the seat, and as my mother announces our destination to the driver, my heart sinks. For now I know the awful truth. Today I am not destined to enjoy the heady pleasures of Altmans or Saks or Bonwits, or even Orbachs. Today we are heading for that one place on earth where it will be impossible for me to forget that I am overweight, obese, heavy, big-for-my-size, a little on the chubby side, and just plain fat! Yes, folks, today we are going to Lane Bryant! My mother has kept this from me; I guess she anticipated my reaction. For I am stunned and instantly miserable. Lane Bryant is for me, in the diet-ridden days of my childhood, the supreme torture, the store where everything, but everything, is specially designed, cut and manufactured for the true outcast of our society, the fat woman. And not just the adult fat woman, oh no, all the seven ages of fatness are served up by benevolent old Lane Bryant, from Baby Chub on the third floor to women's half-sizes on the second, everyone is catered for here, the soup to nuts of fat dressing.

'Oh, Mom, do we have to go there?' I plead.

'Yes, dear, I'm afraid we do.' She sounds genuinely sorry. She too, would prefer to be heading for one of the 'normal' stores with me, her daughter, her pride and joy. But she knows what lies in wait for us at a normal store – agonized sessions in the fitting room while I try on the largest size in everything, to no avail, and finally the hurtful advice that 'Perhaps the little lady would do better in the women's department upstairs.'

And so today it's Lane Bryant, and I grit my little teeth, always remembering not to chew through the rubber bands of my braces, and prepare myself for the ordeal ahead. There is actually one saving grace about the whole thing. At least in Lane Bryant some things will fit. Of course, they won't necessarily be the things I want, but I learned at a very young age the unalterable truths of 'fat shopping'; you don't ever go into a shop looking for something you like – no, you go into a shop with fingers crossed and eyes lowered, praying that you find something that fits. If it fits, you buy it; if you also happen not to hate it, you're ahead of the game.

As my mother and I got off the elevator at the children's floor, I would head eagerly for the rails from which I would make my choices. I always knew just what I wanted – what everybody else was wearing, that was what I wanted. Very few eight-year-olds are non-conformists. So why, oh why, didn't the designer at Lane Bryant understand this simple fact? Why did I have to hunt so carefully for a sweater or a dress that even vaguely resembled what my school friends were wearing? Surely it was awful enough to be big, without my clothes also signalling to the world that I was different?

And my mother and I would disagree. I wanted the shocking-pink organza number with the enormous tulle petticoat – she wanted me to have the black velvet princess-line with the white collar and cuffs. She was determined to slim me down, if not through dieting, then through the careful choice of a 'makes-me-look-so-much-thinner' wardrobe. And of course, she always won. It was her charge card, after all.

I must admit, that as I grew older my taste in clothes changed. I gradually saw the virtues of black velvet over shocking-pink organza. I also found out that there was more to life than *Seventeen*. There was *Glamour* and *Mademoiselle* and eventually even *Cosmopolitan* and *Vogue*, all carrying their monthly quotas of perfect bodies, decked out from head to toe in the latest mouth-watering offerings of the fashion business. But those sizes! Those 5-11s, those 6-14s! Even if I could have afforded the stuff, could I have gotten into it?

Strangely enough, the answer to that question is, 'Occasionally, yes'. There actually were periods in my life, during some particularly strenuous bouts of dieting, when I could and did venture into ordinary department stores, and there was even a very brief period during which I managed to buy a dress in a size 8. Two dresses, as a matter of fact.

It was during the Jackie Kennedy reign of fashion, and they were short, simple A-lines, one in pastel blue, and the other dark wine. I can still see myself in the mirror wearing them, turning and turning endlessly and gazing at the wonder of my new small self, during one particularly hot New York July.

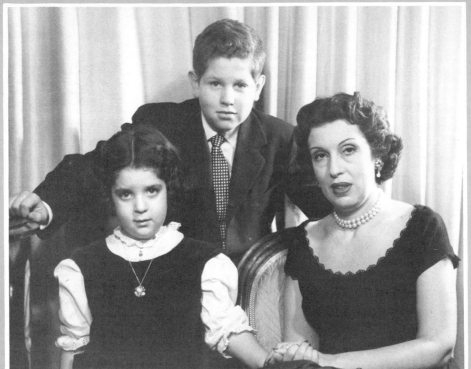

Several versions of the black velvet that helped me to look 'thinner'

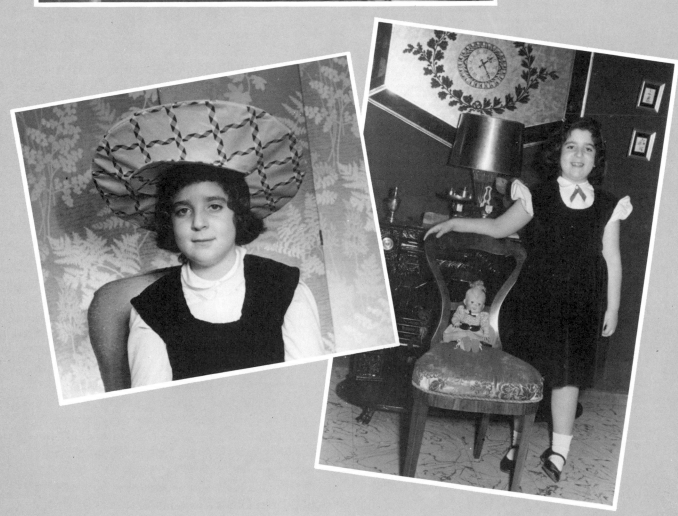

But by the next summer the dresses didn't fit any more. Neither did the black man-style suit that I had worn with such triumph to a party in New York, where all my friends had marvelled at the 'new me'. Didn't I look wonderful? I can only remember wearing that suit once. I have a vague recollection that it was too tight even on that one occasion – but in those days, and in all the days of my life until recently, things were always tight. New clothes were always bought just a bit too small to allow room for the inevitable human shrinkage that would take place thanks to the latest miracle diet.

My mother would sit in the dressing-room at Bonwits or Saks on a tiny satin chair, blithely ignoring the 'No smoking' notice, and contemplate me critically.

'Do you really want my opinion?' she'd ask.

'Sure,' I'd answer nervously.

'This one doesn't do a thing for you. I can see it from the back. The other one's much better.'

'But, Mom, the other one's too small!' I'd beseech.

'It may *feel* too small, but it doesn't *look* too small, and by next week it will be just fine. You're losing every day, your face looks thinner already, it always shows first in your face.'

And it was settled. For how could I not take the one she suggested, the 'small' one? To refuse was to admit that I was going to stay the same, that it was not going to fit next week, or next month, or next year, or ever. And we'd head tiredly home and in the taxi up Madison Avenue my mother would say, 'Well, I think we've done very well, don't you?' And I'd agree, all the time staring at the fancy box between us on the seat and calculating exactly how many pounds I'd have to lose and how many calories I would have to omit from my diet before I could actually wear the garment nestled within on its bed of tissue paper – no longer merely a dress, but a living, breathing, threatening challenge.

That balmy spring day in 1980 my mother wasn't with me. I was alone as I strolled through one store after another, not really looking for anything special, just looking. I wasn't out to buy, just to amuse myself. I went through Bloomingdales and Alexanders and Saks, and then headed downtown to Macy's, 'the largest department store in the world', which had recently enjoyed a highly publicized facelift and was bidding to join the chic uptown Fifth Avenue stores as one of their number.

I was just completing my inspection of the seventh-floor wig department, when a large hanging sign caught my attention. BIG CITY WOMAN. What does that mean? Was it perhaps some coy new way of identifying a department for large sizes – they had actually put *big* in the title but in a kind of roundabout way that made you think that it referred to the city and not the woman. Ummmmm. Whatever, I decided to continue my stroll and passed underneath that ambiguous sign and into a new world.

For there, in row after row of multi-coloured splendour, set up as if in some King's Road boutique for the young and slim and trendy, were thousands of pairs of jeans, jeans in every shape, every style, every colour – Levi jeans and Wrangler jeans, and 'designer' jeans – blue and black and emerald green and shocking pink and ruby red. But the true wonder of it was that the smallest size on display in this emporium of delights was an 18! Yes, ladies and gents, the *smallest*, not the largest, and the largest – what was that? Something they called a 42. Now, I had no idea what that referred to. Was it size of hips? I prayed that it was not, for then I was surely lost. Was it waist? Some hope there. Was it bust? No, why have bust measurements on jeans? But with the vagaries of the fashion world, one never knows. So I took those 42s, in every conceivable style and cut, and threw them over my arm, pair after pair, until I could barely struggle across the sales floor from the weight of blue denim, and I headed for the changing-room. Here there awaited another miracle – for it was not the dreaded communal changing-room, but private and curtained, and designed for looking at yourself and at yourself alone.

I gingerly stepped into the first pair. Now, there is a point beyond which no trousers will rise unless they are going to fit. Everyone has an instinct about where this point is on their own body. That knowledge comes from years of trial and error, and, as that first pair of jeans effortlessly slid past my own danger zone, I suddenly knew, with all the blinding insight of someone who has just discovered Jesus, that not only were they going to go all the way up, not only would the two rows of metal teeth that were the zipper meet in a sweet clenching over my stomach, but, and this realization came to me with all the wonder of Moses receiving the Ten Commandments – THEY WERE GOING TO BE TOO BIG!

How was this possible? Nothing, but nothing, had ever been too big. Not my brother's sweaters, not my father's cast-off shirts, not old flannel nightgowns, nothing. Not for me the baggy denim workshirts or the 'sloppy Joe' sweaters so popular during my youth. It's hard to remember anything that wasn't interrupted in its voyage up or down my body by the swell of my ample behind. There the biggest shirt, the sloppiest Joe, stopped dead and came to rest in accordion-like folds over my stubbornly unyielding posterior. No matter how large things looked on the hanger, I had always managed to fill them out.

Until now, now in this heavenly place called Macy's, my prayers have been answered, and as I try on pair after pair, and they slip off without even having to be unzipped, I realize that I will finally get to utter the words that have always haunted my dreams but until now have eluded me – and as I emerge hot and flushed with triumph from the dressing-room, the salesgirl looks at me inquiringly and I casually murmur, 'These are all too big, I need a smaller size.' Hallelujah!

And I left Macy's that day with three pairs of jeans, no elastic waistbands either, but zippers and studs and five pockets and all the other prerequisites, and as I headed up Sixth Avenue, I felt reborn, and alive, and *normal*. And I suddenly realized, really realized with my guts and not just my head, how much the tyranny of those size 5-11s, those 6-14s, had contributed to my feelings of unworthiness, of uselessness, and of ugliness.

I went back to Macy's the next day and went through every garment hanging on the rails in that vast Big City Woman Department. I then made a journey that I had never expected to make again. I went to Lane Bryant. But now, instead of feeling miserable and defeated, I went there full of anticipation. I couldn't wait for more of the positive charge of trying things on that would actually fit. I walked through the big front doors for the first time alone, without my mother by my side, and I thought of all those tortured times that we'd spent there together, when merely being there was the symbol of my defeat. Things couldn't have been more different. The ground floor was a sea of sportswear, jeans and pants, and wonderful cotton skirts and T-shirts for the coming summer. I spent hours there trying on everything I could get my hands on. It had been quite some time since I had been able to actually *choose* from several garments that I liked. Once you get above a certain size this choice element disappears completely from your shopping experience. I also was painfully aware that, although, here in New York, things had obviously started to improve vis-à-vis clothes for big women, in England, where I lived, things had stayed irritatingly the same. There was no store like this in London. I never bought anything in an 'outsize' shop in all the years I'd lived there. I'd tried. Many times I'd gone to the flagship branch of the only chain of shops catering for large sizes. After looking carefully through their merchandise I'd leave in despair, overwhelmed by the hideousness of the designs and the slimy feel of the fabrics. The department stores were no better, filled with floral polyester smocks and navy crimplene tents. So shopping for me had become a major challenge, only to be engaged in when the mood was absolutely right. I'd spend hours scouring the 'normal' shops, looking for that one baggy, shapeless, one-size-fits-all gem that I would pounce upon and buy in all available colours.

During the rest of my stay in New York, I made the rounds of every store that sold big sizes. There was a bit of everything, from cheap casual to expensive party clothes. Compared to the standard sizes that were available, the bigger sizes were a drop in the ocean, but compared to what we had in England, it was paradise.

Back in London, I met with the Spares. 'It's so much easier there,' I enthused; 'you can actually find things that fit. We keep telling women, "wear what you like, don't wait until you're thin", but it's impossible to find what they like here. How can we go on encouraging them to wear shocking-pink dungarees if they're a size 22 and the dungarees stop at size 14? We've got to do something about it.'

I began to talk with some of the larger women in our groups, and discovered that we shared the same frustrations where clothes were concerned. It's hard to start to feel better about yourself, to build a more positive self-image, if you can't find anything decent to wear.

But how could we change things? We realized that we had to get women involved. We had to get the message across and make them see that it's easier for clothing manufacturers to make things in our size than it is for us to spend the rest of our lives on diets, trying to get down to a size 12.

I now embarked on my second major letter-writing campaign, and also appeared on 'Woman's Hour' talking about our new 'Big and Beautiful Campaign for Real Clothes'; and was besieged by letters and phone calls. It was at this time that I discovered the startling fact that 47 per cent of British women are a size 16 or above. This added fuel to our fire and made me even more determined to get other women angry, to encourage them to fight for a better deal.

Now, whenever I was interviewed about Spare Tyre and the issues of compulsive eating and self-image, I made it a point to discuss 'Big and Beautiful' too. It was, I had discovered, impossible to divorce the problems of obsessive dieting and negative self-image from the injustices foisted upon big women by the fashion industry.

We in Spare Tyre had become so involved in our work with compulsive eating groups that we decided to base our second show on the actual goings-on in a group. We created five characters who were composites of the women we had worked with and wrote *How Do I Look?*, a show which followed them into their

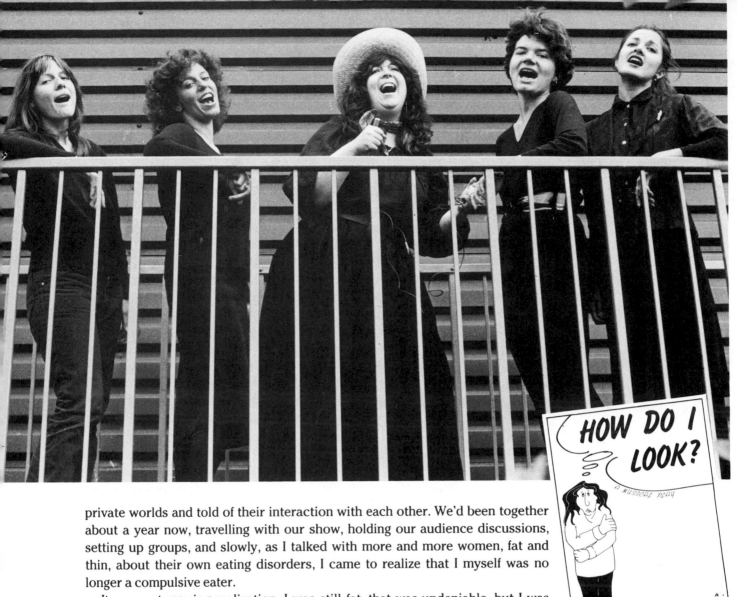

private worlds and told of their interaction with each other. We'd been together about a year now, travelling with our show, holding our audience discussions, setting up groups, and slowly, as I talked with more and more women, fat and thin, about their own eating disorders, I came to realize that I myself was no longer a compulsive eater.

It was a staggering realization. I was still fat, that was undeniable, but I was OK. I had stopped indulging in all the behaviour that we were, night after night, describing as compulsive. I no longer binged, I no long weighed myself. Most of the time I ate only when physically hungry. I had even begun to stop when I was full, to leave food on my plate, because gone was the fear, bred by many years of dieting, that this meal might be my last. And I was feeling good about myself, good in a way that I had only before associated with being thin. Yet, here I was, at just about the same weight I'd been when I first joined Spare Tyre. I guessed I weighed about fourteen or fifteen stone. I didn't know exactly because I practised what we preached and I hadn't weighed myself in a year and a half. But whatever my exact weight was, it was without doubt in the upper reaches of fat. Yet I was finally doing the one thing that I had wanted to do all my life, performing, and I hadn't had to lose a single pound to do it.

Me as Candy Cotton at a rehearsal of How Do I Look?, *1980. From the left: Katina, Janine, me, Clair and Adele*

Inset: Poster for How Do I Look?

I had wasted a lot of time waiting to get thin, waiting for the dial on the scale to say the right thing, to register the numbers that would signify that I was thin enough, acceptable enough, to go out into the world and grab what it had to offer.

Well, midway into my thirties I stopped waiting. I was always going to be the same person, no matter what my weight, and whatever I wanted to do, I could do just as easily at fifteen stone as at eight.

And side by side with that realization was the completely unbelievable but undeniable fact that I was, at the age of thirty-four, eating normally for the first time since I was a toddler.

I was so excited, so filled with optimism, that I could hardly come to grips with this new discovery, with the fact that it hadn't been my weight that had been the problem all those years, it had been my obsession with it.

I was so enthusiastic that at first I was able to brush off the sceptical questions of journalists and friends alike... 'But surely you'd rather be thin?' they persisted. 'I really don't care,' I replied; 'it's such a relief to be rid of that awful guilt, of that all-consuming obsession with food and eating, that still being fat doesn't seem to matter...' This was greeted by a series of polite nods and raised eyebrows. 'It's true!' I insisted.

And I gradually became aware, that although I felt better than I had ever felt in my life, the world still looked at me and saw FAT. And no matter how good I was feeling inside, in our society fat means ugly, unhealthy, lazy, self-indulgent, lacking in willpower, neurotic, greedy; above all, fat means failure.

It was all these terrible connotations of fat that had led my parents, so many years ago, to take me, their young daughter, to that first diet doctor. For they were worried. They wanted me to be happy, to feel accepted and confident like everyone else, and they believed that as long as I was fat, this would never be possible.

Now, almost thirty years later, even my colleagues at Spare Tyre were sceptical. They had overcome their own compulsive eating behaviour and were now thin. So surely, if I were really eating normally, if I had successfully dealt with my problems, then I would be getting thinner too. Right, I thought, I'll keep an even closer watch on my eating patterns.

Compulsive eating has subtle variations for each of us who suffer from it, but there is a general checklist of 'symptoms' that we were using in our groups:
- eating when you are not physically hungry
- feeling out of control around food – either dieting or gorging
- spending a lot of time thinking and worrying about food and fatness
- searching the latest diet for vital information
- feeling awful about yourself as someone who is out of control
- feeling awful about your body

(See Susie Orbach, *Fat is a Feminist Issue*, Hamlyn.)

I went through this list carefully, trying to be honest. There were still times when I ate although I wasn't hungry – going out to dinner, for example – but the emotional eating had stopped almost completely. I no longer felt out of control around food, and therefore I no longer suffered those dreadful feelings of guilt, self-loathing and helplessness that had been a part of my life for so long.

This gaining of control over my compulsive eating had given me an unaccustomed sense of being in control of other aspects of my life. There was no way, fat or no fat, that I was ever again going to give up these feelings of being in charge of myself.

So far, so good. Everything that had happened to me, all my progress, all my feelings were those that I could expect to experience as a cured compulsive eater. There was just one problem – I was still fat.

Now all compulsive eaters believe they are fat. A distorted sense of body image is one of the prime symptoms of the disorder. Thin compulsive eaters think they are fat. Anorexics think they are fat. For much of my early life, when I can now clearly see from my photographs that I was thin, I believed myself to be enormous.

But, at the moment of realizing that I was no longer a compulsive eater, I also had to face up to the fact that I didn't just *think* I was fat...I *was* fat.

It was at this point that I had to take a quantum leap beyond the theories that had so influenced me. I was doing everything right eating-wise, and yet my weight had not, as was expected, stabilized within the range of what might be considered 'normal'. It had stabilized, but at a much higher level.

If dieting didn't keep me thin, and abandoning my compulsive eating didn't get me thin, then it seemed that I had to accept my fatness as a permanent condition. And, as a fat person, I was doomed to be treated as over-indulgent and unappealing, not only by the ignorant of this world, but also by those who consider themselves to be enlightened and generally sympathetic to all the other physical nuances within the human condition.

I was left with two alternatives. I could accept this unjust stereotyping, or I could try and do something about it. I could somehow try and alter the way our society views fat.

I had already seen the relief and happiness that challenging the all-pervading diet-gospel of our times could bring to women who were compulsive eaters. Just learning the facts, just sharing their problems, brought understanding and with it relief. Maybe this same process of education and discussion could work for us, for those of us bigger than 'normal'.

To change the way the world looks at fat isn't easy. To try and change the way fat people think about themselves is equally difficult.

We live in a time and a culture where fat is one of the great taboos, where millions of people spend an inordinate proportion of their time, their energy, and their money trying to lose weight, where even those who are naturally slim become miserable and depressed if they gain a pound or two.

Until now, I've done all the talking in this book, but now it's time to bring in the other women whom I spoke about in the introduction. And who better to discuss contemporary problems than the author and advice columnist to millions, Claire Rayner.

> ❛ I give the same advice to women who are unhappy about their weight as I give to all people who are obsessed about their appearance. I get letters from blokes who are obsessed because they are too thin or because their penis is too small. I get letters from women who are obsessed because their breasts are the wrong shape, or they have pimples, or whatever... You change what can be changed and what you can't change, you leave alone and live with it. If there are things you can change, change them, but only if you can change them comfortably and you really want to. If it's very difficult, then you don't want to, so leave it alone. Get on with something else.
>
> Anyway, whoever told you what beautiful was? This year thin is beautiful, but if you'd been an Edwardian, then you'd have grizzled if you were thin, because you had to be busty and big. ❜
>
> *Claire Rayner*

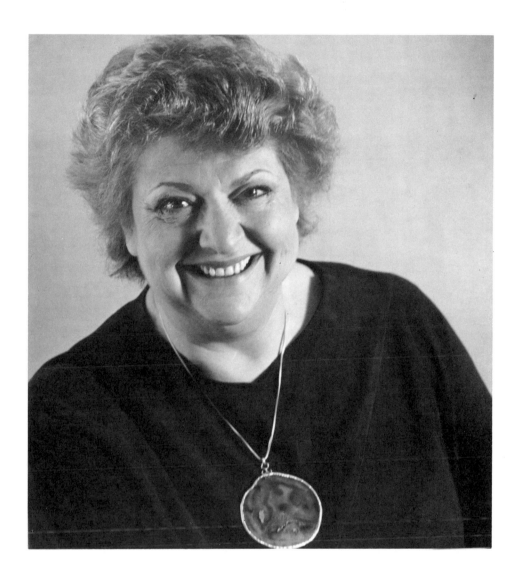

Claire Rayner

It may help us to get our current obsession with slimness into the proper perspective if we view it in a historical context. Because it hasn't always been like this. The hard, pared-down, lean-muscled torso of the latest Hollywood exercise goddess that has become the ideal in this last quarter of the twentieth century would not always have been greeted with such rapture. She is very much an image of our time and should be viewed as such.

The ideal body shape for women has fluctuated constantly over the centuries. There are certain elements of this ideal that we take for granted. We know that thin is in during times of affluence and fat is a symbol of wealth and prosperity in times and places where hunger and starvation are a real threat. We are also aware, even during the present time, of the way that criteria of beauty differ in various parts of the world. Many of us have been surprised and delighted to discover while travelling abroad that the body that is the butt of insulting humour at home is greeted with real delight and appreciation by the people of a different culture. It is important to bear these cultural preferences in mind when evaluating ourselves.

It may be helpful to think in terms of an eternal ideal. Is there one? And if so, what are its defining characteristics, and how relevant are they to the body shape considered to be ideal in our Western culture at the moment?

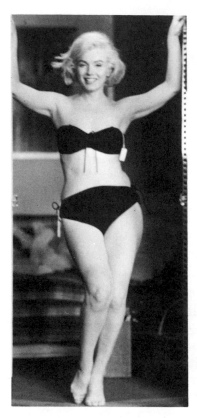 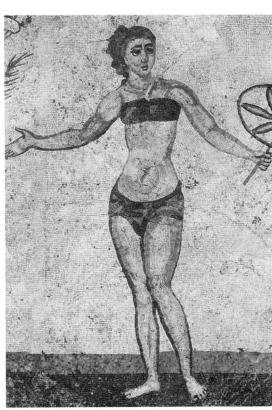

Marilyn Monroe wearing a bikini (left) and a Sicilian mosaic of the fourth century BC (right). Is this the eternal ideal? Far from it!

If you look at the illustrations above you could be forgiven for thinking that things haven't changed much in the past twenty-four centuries. In one we have Marilyn Monroe, wearing a bikini. In the other, a Sicilian mosaic of the fourth century BC, we have a woman wearing – a bikini? Even the pose is almost identical. Is this then the eternal ideal of woman? The shape and size that women through the ages have striven to attain? Far from it. Marilyn Monroe was soft and full and rounded and every man's dream of perfection, but just a few years after this picture was taken, a woman of her measurements would have been considered too fat to be a model, and she'd now be considered 'out-of-shape' by the latest Hollywood standards of sinewy, close-to-the-bone tautness.

Some 2,400 years separate the Sicilian bather and the idealized shape of Marilyn Monroe. And the supreme irony is that for much of the time in between they would both have been considered too thin.

We can get a more well-rounded (forgive me, I couldn't resist the pun) view of the eternal ideal if we trace the images that artists have created of their ideal through the centuries.

How many times have you thought to yourself, 'I should have been born during the time of Rubens – big women were appreciated then!' But how seriously have you ever really thought about this statement and the implications of it? The historical reality of the current vogue for thinness is worth closer scrutiny and more of our attention than the casual Rubenesque joke thrown in between the diet meals and the disheartening shopping expeditions. Looking at artists' ideals can actually make us feel better about ourselves, can help us to see our size in a different light.

The carving from the Ice Age (possibly as much as 500,000 years ago) shows a naked woman carrying a drinking horn. She might be mother, goddess, sex-symbol, or all three – but the image is clear. Not only the delineation of her sexual features, but also the fat around her waist, stomach, hips and thighs. (It's not too hard to work out that fat might have been useful during the Ice Age!)

> ‹ The 'if you stop worrying about food, then you'll get thin' attitude is a cop-out that annoys me. It's aimed at people who are genetically small, but some of us are just not made that way. We're winter survivors, descendants of people who were able to put enough fat on them to last through the freezing winters in the hard north. Your fat stores were what you lived on when times were hard. It was eat now, live later. People who, genetically, had great difficulty storing fat were less likely to reproduce themselves. I always think it's a great joke: 'I come from a long line of winter survivors!' ›
>
> *Claire Rayner*

It is the Ice Age carving and not the bikini 'pin-ups' that shows the essential elements of the female image – woman as fertility symbol – that have been repeated down the centuries, changing subtly but with the essentials the same.

The women in the pictures on pp. 72-3 have several things in common. They have rounded stomachs, voluptuous bottoms, and comfortable, well-padded thighs. When I look at these paintings, I feel an enormous sense of relief. Relief that at another time, in another place, an artist has chosen female forms akin to my own as his idea of perfection. Forget for a moment the *risqué* seaside postcards of our own time with fat women portrayed as bulbous, hen-pecking harridans, and allow yourself instead the pleasure of seeing something of yourself in the images in these paintings. Do your arms and thighs resemble those of the revellers in Ingres's *Turkish Bath*? Are your stomach and hips like those of Leonardo's *Leda*? Does the shape of your face have more in common with Seurat's woman than with the face on the cover of the latest copy of *Vogue*?

It is essential to keep reminding ourselves that today's craze for thinness can be seen in historical terms as just that – a craze. All of the paintings in this section are of beautiful women, women whose bodies were the ideal. They were not considered fat, or obese, or overweight, just beautiful. Most of us look more like an Ingres or a Renoir than a contemporary fashion model. But we're living here and now, and it's hard not to want, more than anything, to conform to the contemporary ideal. We can, however, look to the ideal shapes of the past to help us get our contemporary situation into the proper perspective. And we must keep reminding ourselves that one thing is undoubtedly true: the ideal presented by the stick-thin models of the late sixties onwards is the most extreme image of thinness – and therefore possibly the most difficult ideal to attain – that has ever existed. (In some ways, we women have never had it so bad.)

It is interesting to note that in the past different ideals of beauty coexisted at the same time. In the late nineteenth century it was fashionable to be wan and frail but at the same time a more voluptuous type of woman was also in vogue as was a third type of popular beauty, the athletic, natural type. Today we have no such luck. We have one sanctioned 'look' and if you don't happen to conform naturally, or unnaturally, to this 'look', then it's just too bad for you.

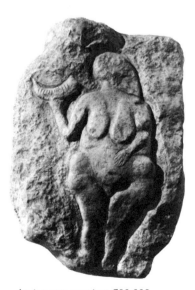

An ice-age carving, 500,000 years old

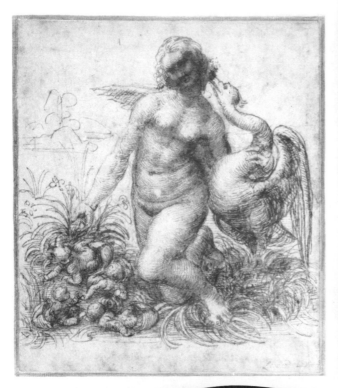

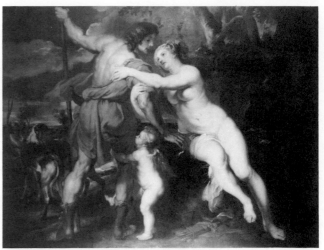

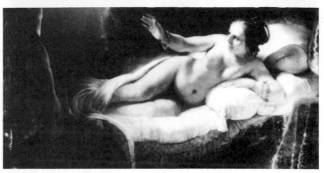

Above left: Leonardo da Vinci, Leda and the Swan, *1504*

Above top: Rubens, Venus and Adonis, *first half of seventeenth century*

Above: Rembrandt, Danaë *(detail), 1636*

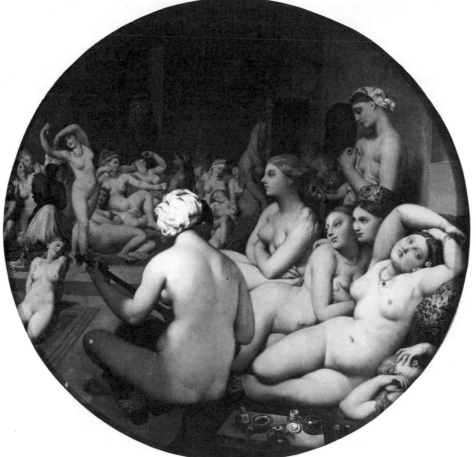

Left: Ingres, The Turkish Bath, *1859-60*

Right: Gauguin, Women of Tahiti, *1891*

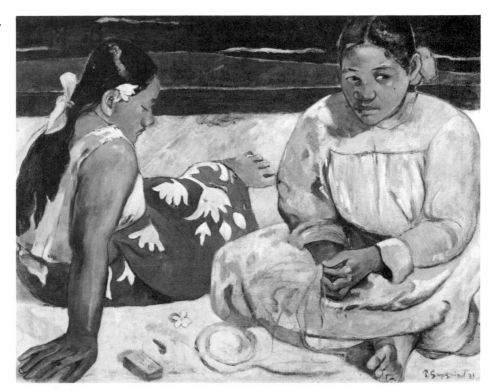

Below left: Seurat, Woman Powdering Herself, *c. 1889-90*

Below right: Modern sculpture displayed at the Athens Biennale in 1964

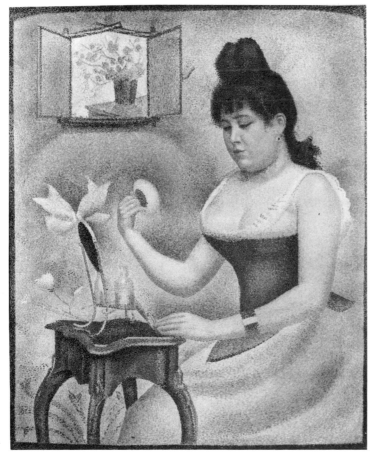

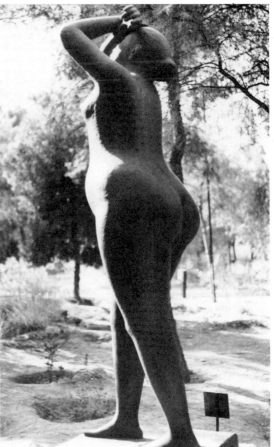

The mass media reach out into every area of our lives, guiding us, instructing us, influencing us and providing us with an endless diet of ideal images. It's impossible to get through a single day without being reminded of the shape that we're supposed to be in, a shape that seems to grow slimmer every day.

> ❛ There's a lot of propaganda aimed at us and it makes me angry. It's funny that I should believe the media more than I believe the people who love me. I've never been told I was ugly or undesirable by anybody who mattered, but I thought it was just because they knew me and I had such a wonderful personality that it superseded all other problems – quite arrogant of me really! ❜
> *Elizabeth Osborne*
>
> ❛ TV doesn't use enough fat people in plays and series. It's as if we don't exist. The fat woman disappears as she gets bigger. The bigger she gets the less important she becomes. It's because people assume that if you're fat you've got some massive problem; you can't cope with life and therefore you eat. ❜
> *Mandy Crane*

A recent article in a popular women's magazine told the story of a young girl who had just won their annual modelling competition. She was described by one of the judges as still needing to lose a 'few inches' off her waist, but she wasn't going to do any fad diets, she promised, just eat 1,200 calories a day, and, of course, no alcohol! She had just won a modelling competition, for God's sake, so surely she looked all right. Why was she dieting? Is it because in our society not to diet is somehow immoral?

Another recent article analysed the diets of six famous thin beauties, three of them 'exercise queens'. The expert nutritionist who had been called in to comment ticked them off mildly for the lack of calcium in their heavily fruit-and-vegetable-based regimes. He advised them to try and follow a better-balanced diet. Then he added a few lines about diets in general: 'Most of the time they [diets] are unbalanced and dangerous, not only for your health, but also to your figure. People who go on fancy diets always put on weight as soon as they go back to their normal eating habits, and this becomes more and more difficult to deal with as you grow older.'

So far so good. You would assume from this analysis that this particular magazine was getting to grips with the reality behind the dieting myth. But now we get to the schizophrenia that permeates most women's magazines. The same issue of the same magazine was running all the usual slimming ads for products which encouraged exactly the kind of behaviour that their nutritionist had warned against. And this was no isolated case. There has been a spate of articles lately about anorexia nervosa, and bulimia nervosa, warning of these two disastrous results of the current slimming craze. Flip over the page and you're more than likely to find the latest diet, illustrated with pictures of models who look as if they themselves are suffering from these sad conditions.

I remember the first slimming food that I saw advertised when I was an adolescent. It was a diet salad dressing. It wasn't bad, and I used it religiously. The slimming industry was in its infancy then. That was just over twenty years

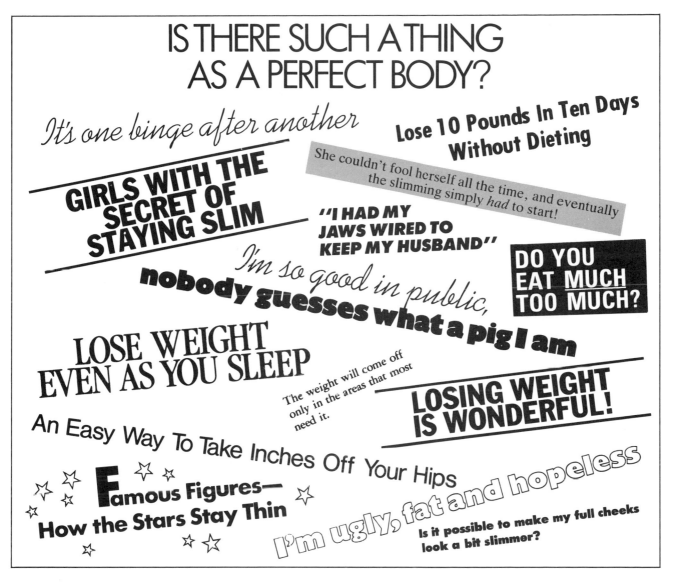

ago. That same industry is now a business that turns over billions of pounds a year. Slimming books and slimming clubs and slimming magazines and slimming foods, all out there pitching at us, trying to do one simple thing and doing it supremely well – making us feel terrible about ourselves. For that is what the slimming industry must do if it is to remain profitable.

It always used to amaze me that the guinea pigs the slimming industry chose for their products were always women who seemed thin to me. You know the kind of advertisement. A bedraggled, depressed looking woman steps on to a scale. She faces the camera forlornly. 'Look at me,' she sighs, 'I weigh 9 st 9lb/135 lb/61 kg.' 9 st 9, I silently scream, what's she on about, I'd cut off my head to weigh 9 st 9! The next we see of her, she's smiling, made-up, beautifully coiffed, she stands tall and proud, her stylish new clothes freshly pressed. 'In just three weeks on the Slimmette diet, I've lost 12 lb/5 kg,' she grins. Well hoop-de-doo. Good for her, but if she's fat at 9 st 9, then what about old slobbo here, at home in front of my TV, who weighs at least fourteen stone, or thirteen, or twelve or

❛ I wasn't aware of being big as a child. What really brought it to my attention was the Twiggy era. I was sixteen years old and weighed about 10½ st/147 lb/67 kg and I thought I was enormous. People who were 20 st/280 lb/127 kg couldn't have felt bigger than I did. Looking back I could cry, because it's really sad that I felt I was so big when I was probably the thinnest I've ever been.

When I was twenty-one I got married for the first time and my husband used to say when I was at my thinnest (because I always yo-yoed a bit) 'You look so good – why don't you cut out a few things, don't eat so much.' I started seriously dieting then, and my weight just zoomed *up*. Then when I was twenty-two I had my son. Afterwards I weighed about 10 st 10lb [150 lb/68 kg] and I went to work for some American doctors who told me I should weigh 7½ st [105 lb/48 kg]. They put me on a diet of boiled eggs and prawns and I lost 2 st [28 lb/13 kg] in five weeks – ridiculous. From that point on I was on a continual diet, up and down; my metabolism went haywire. I reckon if I'd stuck with what I used to eat I would still be 10½ st. ❜

Janis Townes

❛ I don't think I was ever small, but I wasn't conscious of being fat when I was very young. People started calling me names in junior school and then I realized I was different.

I once overheard a doctor saying to my mother, 'Watch what she eats', so of course I ate in secret. Then when I got to the age of eleven or twelve I discovered boys. It was around the time of Twiggy and Biba; everybody was exaggeratedly thin, and I couldn't get the miniskirts that everybody was wearing. I developed a fat mentality. I wouldn't eat chocolates in the street because I was sure everyone was thinking, 'Look at her, no wonder.' It always remained, that sense of being wrong. There are two layers, first a sort of guilt, you think 'It's my fault, I'm making myself like this', but underneath that layer you know that it's not your fault, and you think, 'Well, I don't really behave any differently from anybody else.'

From the age of about thirteen or fourteen I would diet occasionally. I never followed specific diets because I was a vegetarian and there weren't any specific vegetarian diets. Vegetarian books always start by saying, 'vegetarianism is a very healthy way of life, you never see a fat vegetarian'. I wanted to send them a picture and say, 'Here's one!' ❜

Elizabeth Osborne

even 9 st 10 for that matter? What about me? And then I realized, and I understood. The thinner that happy dieter is on TV, the smaller she is to begin with, the more of us they can scoop into their insidious dieting web. Because if she, at 9 st 9 lb, needs to diet then so do all of us who weigh more than that.

But the promise of the latest diet is never merely a weight loss. It is always also a promise of a different life. A whole new world will open up to you when you lose that unsightly midriff bulge. Friends, lovers, husbands will all appreciate you in ways never before possible. Your life will be full of excitement, and glamour, and success.

Slim with the stars, with the rich, with the privileged, and, the implication is, you will become a star yourself. Apart from this snob appeal of being thin, with its underside, the withering belief that to be fat is to be somehow 'lower class', big women face a multitude of other pressures to lose weight.

The pressures on men to slim are not nearly so fierce. Although the agonies of compulsive eating remain just as painful for the male sufferer as for the female, and men too have recently begun to become enmeshed in the slimming web, there's no denying that things are different.

No matter how successful a woman may be she is still, unfortunately, evaluated by many people first and foremost in terms of her looks – the sad but true legacy of centuries of being regarded as a decorative accessory to 'her man'. Men, on the other hand, have always had so many other criteria by which they measure themselves, with their careers usually heading this list, that their physical attributes take a back seat to their other accomplishments. We used to say in Spare Tyre that a fat man can be a bank manager or a politician, but a 'fat lady' is just a joke on a seaside postcard.

This is not to say that men are not also concerned about their weight, but it's rare to find a man who is only a few pounds 'overweight' despising himself because of it, and feeling that he is totally worthless if he fails to stick to a business lunch of yoghurt and an apple. Most slimming propaganda is still aimed at women, and at slim women at that. But as soon as the scions of the slimming industry wake up to the potential profit to be gained from making men as insecure about their weight as women already are, then I have no doubt that they will rush in to rectify this 'oversight'.

> ❛ I'm a television costume designer and most of the women I dress have got a bit of a hang-up. They either think they're too thick around the middle, or their hips are too big, or their arms are too fat. They're just not completely happy with their bodies. I don't find men particularly hung up about their shapes. They might say, 'I'm ever so big', or be concerned that one arm is a bit longer than the other, but they are usually apologetic about it because it could be a problem for the costume, rather than bothered about it because of their looks. ❜
>
> *Sue Formston*

> ❛ Fat men have a much easier time. They are allowed to get fat without it diminishing their economic or sexual power. But, if you're a woman over a size 16, then you are no longer viewed as viably sexual. You are not a person whom anybody will admit to wanting to take to bed. ❜
>
> *Jan Murphy*

Whether they admit it or not, is it any wonder that many men would prefer their women to be thin? Men are, after all, subjected to the same barrage of media hype as women are. They see the same advertising, the same films, the same television programmes. They see the same stereotyped fat women, portrayed always as strident, overbearing, henpecking, to be avoided at all costs. To be a fat actress is to be constantly offered this type of part.

> ❛ I don't get the type of roles that I would really like to play. I'm always somebody's mother or somebody's sister. I'm never the one that gets the guy! People are so accustomed to thinking of desirable women as being small, it's hard to change that way of thinking. ❜
>
> *Kathy Beard*

Opposite: Annette Badland

❝ I was actually once booked to do a comedy show because of my size. They wanted me to look as big as I could and as old as I could, but really they just wanted as much tonnage as they could possibly get to come and sit next to the star and squash his transistor radio. Although the people were very nice and charming to me I would never do that again. I was utterly humiliated and loathed it.

Being a big woman and an actress can be painful. The Royal Shakespeare Company was where I had always wanted to be and three months out of drama school, there I was, playing Audrey in a modern dress production of *As You Like It*. Opening night came and went, and one of the reviewers said that he saw no reason why they should cast a cute ten-ton truck as Audrey. I don't read reviews any more.

People always assume a particular character goes with the size. It's either a depressed failure, someone who's terribly unhappy with themselves, or someone dominating. I'm always attempting to break the mould. If there's enough scope to create something other than the stereotype, then I'll do it. Sometimes people may give me a part *because* of my size, but then I'll see something else in the part and start pushing it into another dimension. I refuse to just be seen as a certain-sized piece of flesh. In some ways I've been fortunate, because I've had a large range of roles. But never the successful young wife, lover or executive. Those battles are yet to be won. ❞

Annette Badland

When I was offered my first acting work after Spare Tyre, in the film *Superman III*, I was so suspicious of the director's motives for even *considering* me, a fat actress for the part, that I almost didn't go to meet him for the interview. I was then, and am now, constantly wary of being cast because of my size. If the 'fat lady as awful joke' syndrome is to be broken, we must first acknowledge that it is there, that it is wrong, and that it is dangerous. Dangerous because it perpetuates the myth of the fat loser, and reinforces the negative self-image from which so many of us suffer.

Subtle pressures can be the most insidious. The casual remark made by a television personality or journalist is the one which reaches millions and goes sharp and fast into the Achilles' heel that most of us possess as far as our weight is concerned. Several years ago I saw, on a popular afternoon television programme, an eminent fashion editor about to present a fashion show featuring the new season's look. She opened with the words, 'This spring sees the return of the wide, tight belt, so it's diets for most of us!' I was incensed. I know that her remark was made in all innocence, that remarks like this have become part of the currency of our language. I know that she would be loath to cause unhappiness or suffering to the viewers. And yet I also know just what it's like to be a woman, unhappy and depressed about her size, who hears or reads this type of casual quip. It doesn't feel casual, it feels enormously important and true. Guilt flows over us and we turn for help to the latest diet book, or enrol in the local slimming club. We plunge headfirst yet again on to that long and mostly futile slimming road. 'Why not just make bigger belts?' I wanted to scream at the television screen!

In Superman III

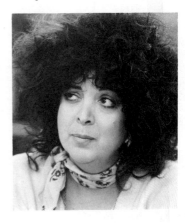

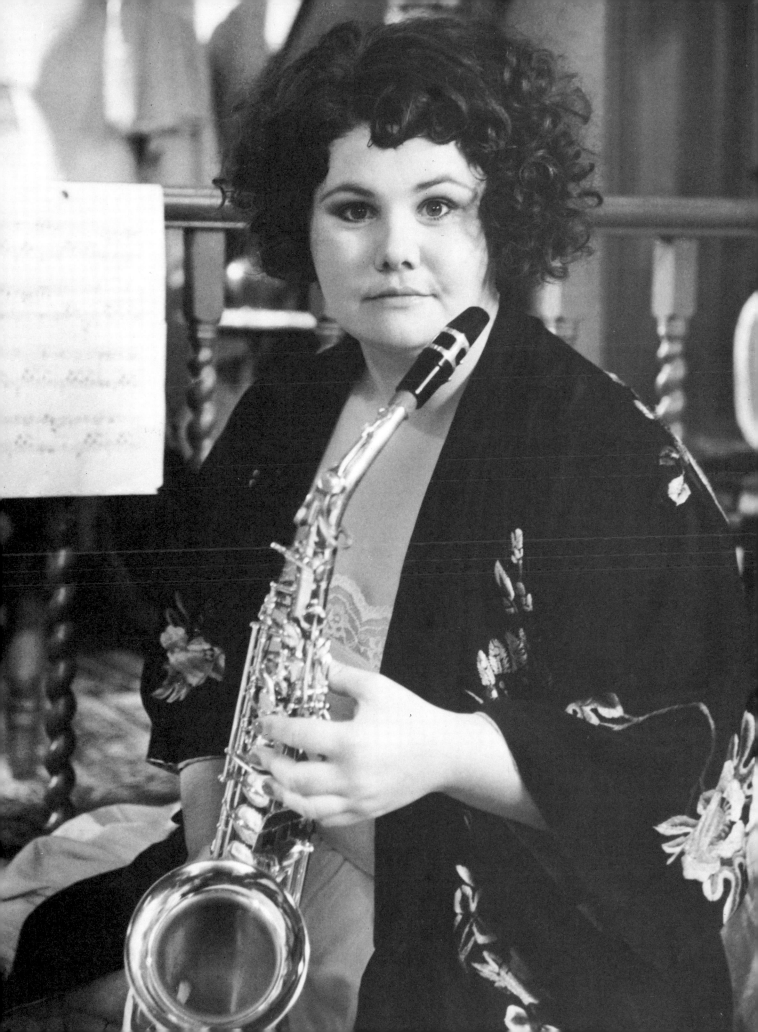

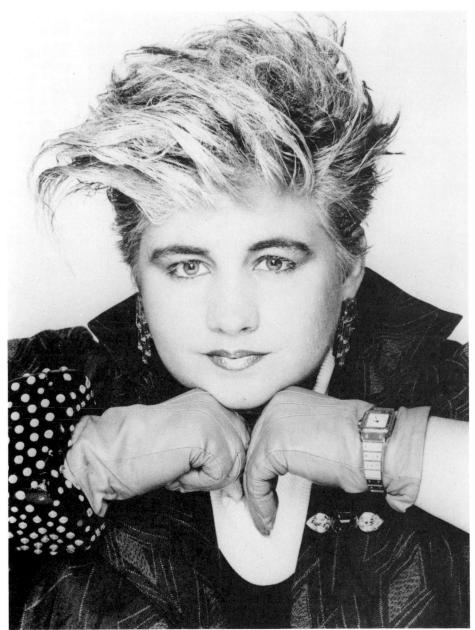

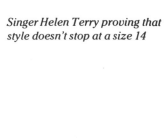

❛ I remember reading a review of one of Culture Club's records that said, 'why on earth George has this big fat screaming tart in the background, one will never know'. It hurt me because I don't think my size has anything to do with the way I sing. I don't like my size being used against me in terms of somehow diminishing whatever talents I've got. They frequently do use it in that way, as if to say somehow that because you've got extra body weight, then you should have slightly less talent.

My record company and my management don't put any pressure on me to diet. As long as I don't drop dead, they don't mind. As long as their investment doesn't peg out on them. ❜

Helen Terry

Why not indeed? Perhaps because to make it easier to be big would eliminate one very important element of the whole slimming business. And that is the competition between women that the dieting and the weighing and the measuring encourage. Although women are now making their presence felt in the traditionally male-dominated working spheres, many people still consider it unacceptable for women to compete in the same way as men. Where a man is seen as ambitious, a woman is viewed as 'ball-breaking, pushy'. Where it *is* seen as perfectly acceptable to compete, and this applies to all women, whether we work out of the home or in it as mothers and wives, is in the area of our physical appearance.

It starts in adolescence, when our need for acceptance is strongest and our self-esteem so easily destroyed. We need so much to feel as good as our friends. We constantly measure ourselves against our peers to reassure ourselves that we are OK. Is she prettier than me, we ask ourselves fearfully, as we stare at our rapidly changing faces in the bathroom mirror. As we grow up the comparisons become more sophisticated. Is her hair shinier, better cut? Are her clothes more fashionable, more expensive? And last but certainly not least, is she thinner than me? Does she look better in her Lycra leotard, do her ribs stick out further than mine? Is she really thinner, and therefore better?

What a terrible, expensive game we play with each other. And what a colossal waste of our resources.

> **❛ I was swimming a while ago and something I saw really put things into perspective. There was a little fat girl in a funny little swimming costume. She was there with a thin friend who had a really lovely swimming costume and who preened and pranced and drew attention to herself in front of her little fat friend. It took all my efforts not to go up to her and say 'Please don't do that.' It was clear to me that the little thin one's ego was being built up on the back of her fat friend. They were about ten, sort of pubescent, getting to that age, and as I stood in the changing-room watching it I went back to being a kid again. I felt so much for that little fat girl, she looked so helpless. ❜**
>
> *Jan Murphy*

> **❛ Round about thirty-five women are starting to worry about their looks going off. It's the beginning of the mid-life crisis, the time when husbands start straying, whatever. So they begin to diet because they equate being sexy with being thin, which is not true.**
>
> **I went to a cocktail party and met the most smashing guy and a thin woman said to me afterwards, 'I don't understand it, you're so large, why did he take you out to dinner?' That's a very neurotic comment – made by someone who trades on being thin. I've never traded on being thin or fat, I actually traded on being amusing more than anything else, and I've never really had a problem. But the thing is, I wasn't going to let it be a problem. It's self-determination really, isn't it? ❜**
>
> *Meredith Etherington-Smith*

> ❝ People resent that you've got a handsome husband, a happy family life, that you go out, wear zany clothes. The hostility is incredible. Why aren't you hiding from life? I think they're hostile because women are supposed to conform to a certain image. We're supposed to have everything the same, eyes, mouth, tits, legs.
>
> The way we look is tied up with our behaviour. If you say, 'I'm going to be big, because this is the way I am', you're saying, 'I'm not going to do everything you say.' Therefore, I think, that to men especially, big women can be very threatening. There are still a lot of women who go along with the traditional physical stereotype. But if you persist and keep telling them, 'I actually *like* myself like this', it gives them food for thought. ❞　　*Janis Townes*

The quest for thinness can become so important, so all-encompassing, that any inference that it may be unnecessary can terrify the dieter. For the past few years as I've talked to audiences and read letters from viewers of my TV programmes, I've been struck by one thing that comes across again and again. The only women who ever get angry about the anti-diet stance are those women who have themselves recently been through a long and difficult stint of dieting and who are hanging on tenuously to their 'goal weight'. They don't want to hear that other women are coming to terms with being bigger. It is too threatening. It can be compared to hearing that your job, the one you have spent a lifetime

On the Thames TV series 'Large as Life' with my guests: A. E. Pitcher, Dorothy Genn and Annette Badland

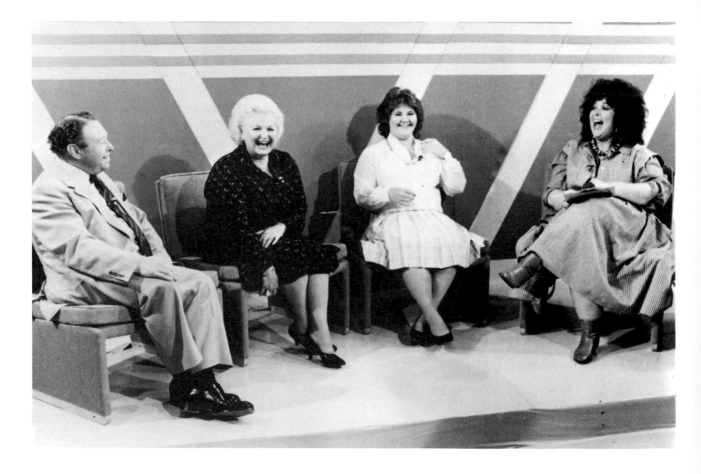

training for, is about to be replaced by a computer, that everything you do will no longer be necessary. And these women fight back and hold on to their slim waists and their miracle diets with a vengeance.

Many of the day-to-day problems of being fat came up again and again when I was interviewing women for my television series 'Large as Life'. In these programmes I set out to defuse the 'fat' issue, to show other fat people and thin ones alike that we are not just ugly stereotypes.

I was joined on the series by guests who had themselves overcome the stigma of being large and had become successful in their chosen careers. We discussed the emotional and psychological pressures that we felt 'living fat' in a thin world. We also dealt with some of the more practical difficulties that we faced: where to find decent clothes, how to be healthy, how to deal with doctors, parents, well-meaning friends. My audience of large women, who contributed their views and experiences, were of all different ages and from all different backgrounds. I received many letters as a result of these programmes. Some of the women who wrote to me were 'dieters' like myself. They had been through the mill, calorie-counting, low-fat, high-fibre, Stillman, Scarsdale, Atkins, they'd had their jaws wired, they'd been hospitalized and put on starvation regimes under doctor's supervision, and they all, without exception, had put back every pound that they had lost. I also had letters from women who had never been on a diet, who thought, 'the hell with it, this is me'. These non-dieters shared one very significant, crucial experience with the dieters. Both these groups of women knew only too well the pain and humiliation of being treated as second-class citizens, as outcasts, by a society which idolizes slimness.

❛ People patronize you. They think you're funny. They say, 'Oh, Jan. Oh, Jan!' You're never taken seriously. You can't possibly be intelligent, because you're fat; you can't possibly have a sexual life. One dancer I used to work with, who was all of twenty-three and weighed 8 st/112 lb/51kg, said to me, 'Oh, Jan, does someone fancy *you*?' A man said to me three weeks ago, 'If you lose two stone [28 lb/13 kg] I'll marry you.' I was so stunned I actually didn't say anything, but afterwards I wished I'd said I didn't want to marry *him*. But you know, I just couldn't believe anyone had actually said that to me. The relationship finished that night. ❜
Jan Murphy

❛ My friends say to me, 'Look, you are what you are, we love you, why can't you just acccept it, why get hung up when you hear people saying, "Wow, what a pair," when you walk past a building site, why do you care what they think?' But I know what it feels like to be twelve years old with a big bust and have people look at you in a way you don't even understand properly, and feel that you must walk around with your shoulders hunched. ❜   *Elizabeth Osborne*

❛ Recently a man walked right up to me in the street and said 'You're obviously a fat woman, that's what I want to talk to you about. I'm selling a diet.' I said 'Wait a minute, what makes you think that just because I'm fat I want to lose weight. As it happens, I don't.' He looked at me like 'What! You're kidding! You don't want to be normal?' ❜   *Kathy Beard*

❛ I'm twenty. I've never been on a diet. I started at stage school at the age of eleven. I wanted to be a dancer, a choreographer, I wanted to be everything. I did tap and modern jazz and my dance teachers always told me how talented I was. They never said, 'You're so good *but* you're overweight', they just used to say how good I was. Then when I was about fifteen, ordinary maths and English teachers used to come up to me and say, 'I can see a bit of a belly growing on you, Liz,' or 'I was watching you earlier on, it's such a pity you're overweight.' They used to weigh me and say 'I can pinch more than an inch.' They never told me I was good, just drummed into me how fat I was. I never let it get to me though, because I had this thing that it didn't matter, because I was going to be famous anyway.

Then when I was seventeen I had to re-audition to get into the next stage at school. I went in that day thinking, 'I'll flip through this, no bother.' But the teachers sat in a row, and they just ran me down, till I felt like nothing. They expected me to burst into tears and say 'All right, lock me up in a room and I'll diet for a year, two years, whatever it takes.' What I did say was 'If you don't want me here I'll go somewhere else. I'm not going to diet, because I feel that if I do, I'll lose my talent…this is me.'

They were shocked that I didn't cry. They all looked at me as if to say, 'Don't you feel in the least bit ashamed of yourself?' Then they said, 'You can go now.' But I said, 'No, I'll still do the pieces that I've prepared for you.' And I got up, did my song and dance, said 'Thank you very much', and walked out.

I didn't bother with teachers after that. I entered myself for my own degree in teaching, taught myself, and passed. Then I tried to get a teaching job. I tried dancing schools and dance studios, but no way. I'd show them all my certificates and qualifications, but they'd just look me up and down, and say 'No.' You have to be tall, blond, really skinny. ❜
Liz Birru

The women who wrote to me had been subjected to all forms of discrimination because of their size. They'd found it difficult to get jobs, they'd found themselves relegated to some dingy back-room office although their skills were superior to their workmates' who sat out front.

My correspondents had all encountered strangers who assumed that because they were fat they were also deaf and made cruel remarks about them within earshot.

They'd all learned to strike first, to make a joke about themselves before someone else could make it. Many felt that this was the truth behind the cliché of the jolly fat person.

They'd learned to protect themselves from the embarrassment of simply being too big to fit into many public places. They avoided walking through turnstiles, sitting down on buses, and going into any establishment where the seats are secured to the floor.

And they all knew what it felt like to be viewed as greedy. A particularly poignant story came from one young woman who had been seated on a train opposite a man and his young son. The child, who must have been about five, pointed across at the woman, asking, 'Daddy, why is that lady so fat?' 'Because she eats too much,' replied the father without hesitation. It's thus that misconceptions are born and stereotypes perpetuated.

In fact this woman, like many of the other women whom I met, did not eat too much. She had in the past been a compulsive eater, but she had long ago come to grips with that and her weight had been the same for some time. Thank goodness recent reports and books, among them Geoffrey Cannon's *Dieting Makes You Fat*, are finally beginning to challenge the fat-equals-greedy stereotype. The latest studies reveal that regular dieting actually lowers the metabolism, so that with each successive diet the body needs less and less food to function successfully, and to maintain its present weight.

❝ It's odd, I should be a beanpole. I don't eat very much, I drink a bit. And I burn up a tremendous amount of energy. The amount of neurotic energy I burn up running around like a chicken without a head is incredible. It makes me angry when people equate being big with eating too much, because I don't eat much at all. My flat-mate eats more than I do and she's a size 10. ❞

Helen Terry

❝ I went to the doctor with sore tonsils and he gave me a diet sheet saying no potatoes, no pastry. I remember my mother saying 'Maybe it's her glands,' and him saying, 'No, she just eats too much, put her on this diet.' And my mother said, 'She doesn't eat a lot.' In the last few years I have actually discovered that my thyroid doesn't work properly and I do have a very slow metabolism. But I always had this feeling that it was my fault, that I was naughty and a pig, I was made to feel greedy. That still happens now. In a jokey way. All this last week I've been working mainly with men, and at lunchtime I'll have a salad, because that's what I enjoy, and they've got meat and three veg and spuds and a pudding and all the rest of it, and they'll say 'Oh God, Badland's eating again.' It *is* lunchtime, and we're all going for lunch like normal people, but for them it's an easy and obvious joke. ❞

Annette Badland

❝ I used to think I ate more than my thin friends, but now I know that I don't. In fact I know that I eat a lot less than some of them. People always say to me, 'But Jan, you don't really eat that much!' as if they expected me to stuff my face with Mars Bars all day long. A lot of people equate being big with being greedy, being lazy, being slothful. When they see that you're not, they don't know how to categorize you and it confuses them. ❞

Jan Murphy

Many other ex-compulsive eaters wrote to me. They felt that they had achieved a major victory and whether or not they had lost weight was incidental. The relief and sense of accomplishment came from getting to grips with their eating problem. Meeting these women, reading their letters, hearing their stories, reinforced my belief that the real problem we face today is not fat, but compulsive eating.

Just as being fat does not necessarily mean that one is a compulsive eater, so being slim does not necessarily mean that one is eating normally. There are millions of slim women who are weighed down by the terrible symptoms of compulsive eating. About 60 per cent of the women in the compulsive eating self-help groups started by Spare Tyre were within the range of standard weights. These women, who appear perfectly acceptable to the outside world, diet and binge and dislike their bodies. Their lives and social obligations revolve around their latest diets, they hate themselves when they eat something 'naughty' and congratulate themselves for being 'good' when they don't. In extreme cases they develop anorexia nervosa and bulimia nervosa, the binge/vomit syndrome now so frighteningly common.

There are many reasons why women develop eating disorders, but one of them is undeniably the fear of fat. And yet who is really 'sick' here? The big woman who eats normally, leads a healthy existence, and who treats food the way any other normal eater does, something to be taken for nourishment and pleasure when hungry, and then forgotten about till the next time hunger strikes? Or the eight-stone dieter, whose life is a never-ending round of self-denial and self-loathing, and who puts off many of the pleasurable pursuits of life because she's 'just too fat', and whose first and last thought every day is of food and her figure? I've been both of these women and to me the answer is clear.

If you are a compulsive eater, whether fat or thin, of course you will want to deal with that problem. Sometimes joining a compulsive eating group or forming one in your area can be a help. Sometimes, just taking the big plunge and giving up dieting can be the solution. I know it sounds terrifying, but in spite of our worst fears, most women do not blow up like balloons when they stop dieting. They gradually begin to discover that when they can eat anything they want, they don't want everything all at once. It is a sublime moment when you first realize that, although there is nothing stopping you, you just don't *feel* like eating that once-forbidden piece of chocolate cake or bag of peanuts.

If you're not a compulsive eater, then whatever you do, don't be tempted by the barrage of dieting propaganda to become one. As anyone who has suffered from this painful syndrome can tell you, it can all start the moment you go on your first diet. Any temporary weight loss is just not worth the struggle and loss of self-esteem that you will be letting yourself in for. I must stress here that I am not against weight loss, just against dieting. If you are a compulsive eater who begins to normalize her eating habits and thereby starts to lose weight as well, then that's terrific, but the sane, unneurotic eating should always be your first aim, not the weight loss.

> ❛ I think compulsive eating is just one of many reasons why women are big. Fat *can* be a weapon against society for women who have no other weapon, saying 'I will not conform', but that's only one of many variations. There are so many different reasons; sometimes it's just that that's the way you are. We're all individuals, and we must stop worrying about *why* we're fat. Be concerned that you're eating a healthy diet, getting all your vitamins and minerals and stop worrying. Some people are just big, and society has got to accept that. There isn't always a reason underneath. It can come down to the simple fact that I am big because I am big because I am big, and so I am going to forget about it. ❜
>
> *Janis Townes*

‘ I don't diet any more. I gave up because diets don't work. They make you miserable and they make you boring. Boring in as much as you interfere with your friends' lives because you become so obsessed with what you're eating that you ignore other things in life that are more important. When you stop dieting you stop thinking constantly about food. Eating becomes a pleasurable necessity, something you must do in order to live. ’

Jan Murphy

‘ I did hesitate about talking to you about this because I get so bored by people who will try and define other people by their size. There's a great risk of defining people totally by their appearance. 'She's a dear little thing, so petite and charming', 'What a large woman', 'Isn't he a little fellow?' What the hell's it got to do with anything? You should be saying, 'Isn't he a clever fellow?', 'Isn't she a funny woman?', 'Isn't he enjoyable?', 'Isn't he gentle?', 'Isn't he a bully?', 'Isn't he a whatever?' I think it's very important to say that you cannot get your head right about your own appearance until you stop defining other people by what they look like. That's where it starts. If you'd learn to define people by their qualities rather than by their mere appearance, you will stop getting your knickers in a twist about your own appearance, won't you?

I don't diet any more. I don't reckon it. Life is too short to spend it thinking about something so unimportant. I did in the past, I got bullied into it. When you're younger you haven't quite the self-confidence you've got when you're older. It was only because of a certain amount of peer pressure, I suppose, and even then I was never that interested, never for more than a couple of days. I'd think 'Oh, I really must do something', and I'd go for one of those crackpot things that people do. Then I discovered the truth that we all know, which is that dieting enlarges you. If you start mucking around with your eating patterns, you may lose weight for a little while, but then after that it all goes back on – only more so. Dieting really does make you fat. ’

Claire Rayner

7

WHY CLOTHES?

Breaking the stereotype

There are so many areas of fat discrimination that you may wonder why I have chosen to devote a large part of this book to clothes. You may say that trying to better our lot clothing-wise is a very simplistic solution to the problems of being 'overweight'. However, as I travelled around the country and met and talked with more and more big women, I was impressed by how many of them told me the same thing…that much of the agony and despair they suffered from being big would disappear if only they could find the same kind of clothes that their slimmer friends wear.

On one of my 'Large as Life' programmes I took the opportunity of dressing several of the women in my audience in the type of clothes they had never worn before. They also had new hairstyles and make-up designed for them. These were 'makeovers', but not of the usual 'before and after the diet' type so popular in women's magazines.

The reactions of my models and my audience and the piles of mail from viewers made me realize just how important this clothing issue is. All the women stressed what a difference it made to them when they were given the chance to dress 'normally', to wear something they really liked, something with style.

For me the turning-point came shortly after my Macy's trip in the spring of 1981. I was asked to do an interview with the women's page of the *Daily Mirror*. They wanted to do a feature about 'Big and Beautiful' with a picture of me wearing the kind of clothes that I wanted to see made for big women.

I was thrown into a panic. What was I going to wear? I went frantically through my closet. I somehow didn't think that jeans, albeit wonderful ones, were the right thing for this picture, but I had nothing else, nothing beautiful enough to make the point that I was trying to make. I realized that my choice of clothes for this picture was crucial to the impact the whole article would make. It was essential that they be fabulous, as fabulous as anything currently on view on any size 10 model in any fashion magazine you'd care to name.

I was into my second week of searching when, one day, flipping through the latest issue of *Company* magazine, I saw it. The perfect outfit. It was cotton and

Bold, oversized tops, clingy, fluted skirt, hair wrapped and twisted for a young exuberant feeling. Don't be afraid to try new fashion ideas. Size is no barrier to style

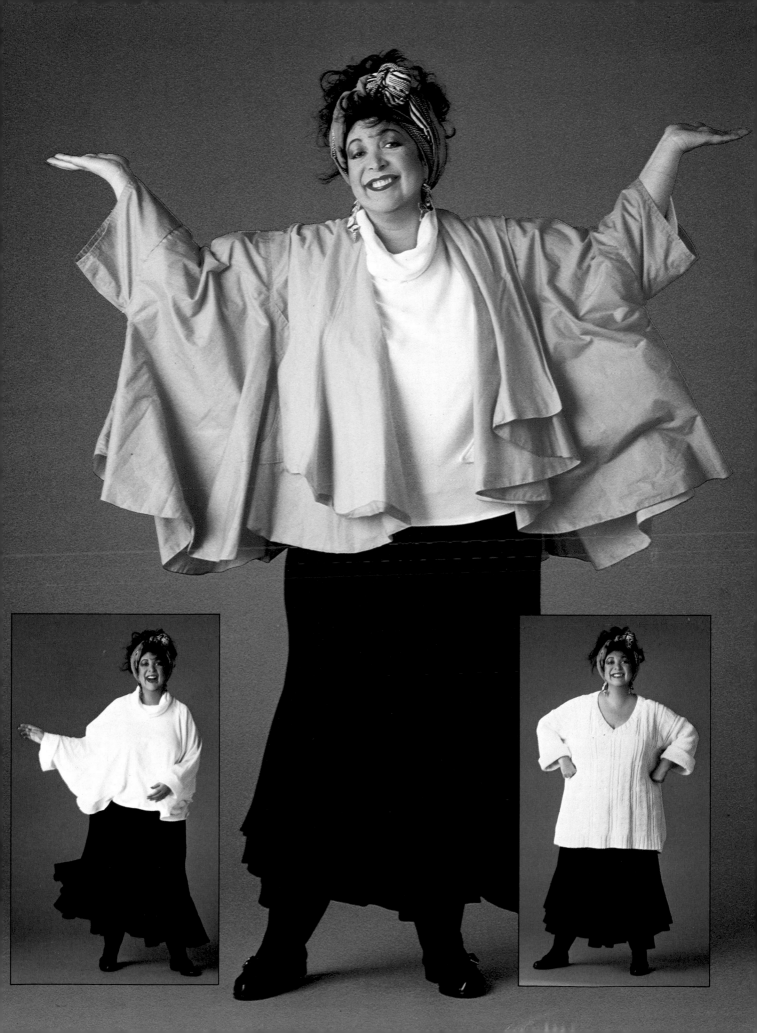

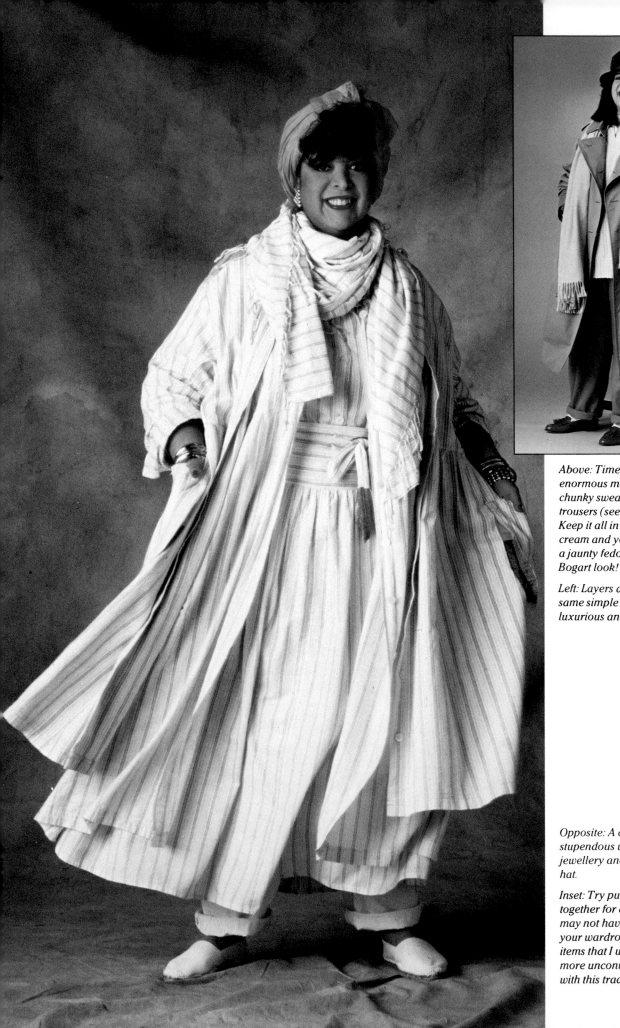

Above: Timeless and chic – an enormous man's trenchcoat over chunky sweater and home-made trousers (see p. 158 for the pattern). Keep it all in shades of beige and cream and you can't go wrong. Add a jaunty fedora for that Humphrey Bogart look!

Left: Layers and more layers of the same simple fabric creates a rich, luxurious and highly individual look.

Opposite: A classic black suit made stupendous with satin gloves, glitzy jewellery and the most magnificent hat.

Inset: Try putting your clothes together for a different look that you may not have even guessed was in your wardrobe. By putting together items that I usually wear in a crazier, more unconventional way, I came up with this traditional elegant style

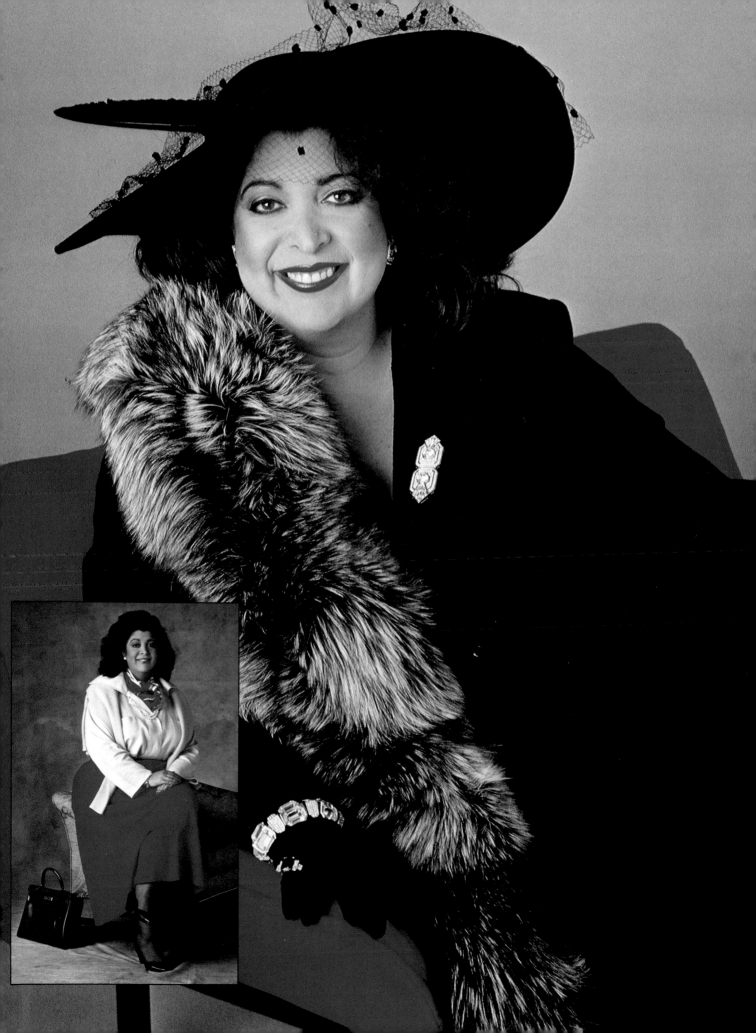

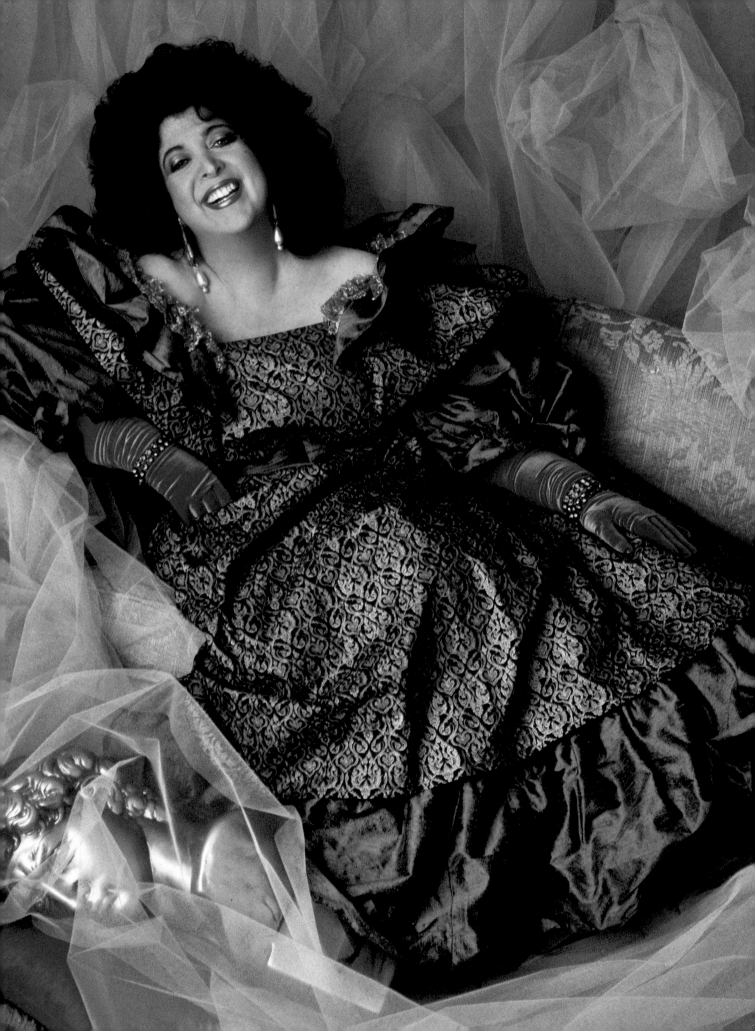

multi-striped in beautiful muted colours and the model who wore it also wore an enormous turban, armfuls of bangles and several chunky necklaces. I loved it. It was designed by Wendy Dagworthy and came in the inevitable sizes, 10 through 14. I knew that it would never fit, because it wasn't some shapeless, voluminous tent of the kind that I had seen in my shopping expeditions, but a skirt with a waistband and a skinny camisole top under a straight jacket. I put the magazine aside, but I kept going back to that picture over the next few days. Nothing I could find in any of the many stores I searched through came anywhere near this outfit. I had to, at least, try to get it.

Five years earlier I had spent a brief spell as a fashion buyer. I had been introduced to several young designers at that time, among them Wendy Dagworthy. But would she remember me? And even if she did, would she be prepared to consider the proposal that I was planning to make? For I had decided to ask her if she could make the outfit that I had seen in *Company* especially for me, in my size. I called her. She remembered me. I asked her to lunch. I told her about 'Big and Beautiful' and my desperate search for something to wear for the *Daily Mirror* pictures. She agreed to make the *Company* outfit for me.

In her tiny workrooms in Poland Street, Wendy's assistant Barbara measured my waist and my hips and my bust and my arms and other bits of me that I didn't even know existed. Wendy then painstakingly worked out just how to size up her original pattern so that it would fit. I was nervous and did a lot of talking and we all did a lot of laughing. Wendy was patient and enthusiastic and when the three pieces were finally finished they fitted perfectly, hung beautifully and had lost none of the pizazz of the original.

On the day that the outfit was completed I went to the workrooms with my own jewellery and various shoes. We experimented and tried on one thing after another until we got it just right. Wendy then threw a matching scarf over my shoulders and gave me a lasting devotion to big scarves with the immortal words, 'Put on a big scarf and the right jewellery and you can make anything look good!' Not that my new outfit needed any help – it was beautiful, perfect.

I was amazed at how good I felt in that Wendy Dagworthy outfit. Sure, I felt great in my jeans from Macy's, but this was different. I'd had jeans that fitted me before, at thinner times, but I'd never had anything like this skirt and jacket with the matching scarf and all the chunky jewellery. I felt I could go anywhere in it, that I would always look right. I felt stunning, chic, comfortable, all of those. Of course, it fitted, but there was more than that. Something about the pattern, the flow of the skirt, the way the collar turned up made me feel right, and gave me confidence. It just seemed to be me. A me that I liked. And that feeling of liking myself made me feel remarkably strong. It wasn't the first time that the right clothes had made me react like this. There had been some times during my life-long yo-yoing, weight-wise, when I had felt like this, but always when I had been thin. In fact one of the major rewards of getting thin was always the clothes that waited for me at the end of the latest diet. But now, I had not just my collection of jeans from New York, but this wonderful new high-fashion number that was as good, if not better than, anything I had worn when I was thin, and I felt great.

The importance to big women of feeling great in our clothes is something that cannot be overestimated. We live in a visual society. All around us are

Most people assume that a fat woman could never look glamorous and romantic. Here we've set out to prove them wrong

billboards and television and magazines and movies screaming out at us that there is only one right way to look and that way is thin. We have a fashion industry that, for the most part, ignores us, treating us as second-class citizens, and providing us with the kind of shoddy inferior merchandise that is an insult to our intelligence. We are stereotyped as self-indulgent, lazy, lacking in willpower, and downright ugly. To break through this stereotype, to begin to create positive images of big women must be our goal.

The easiest, most direct way of doing this in a society that cares above all about the way we look is through our appearance. When I see a big woman walking down the street who has really gotten herself together, whose clothes and hair show that she cares about herself, my immediate reaction is that she must be very strong, a very powerful woman. I know what she has had to overcome, in terms of prejudices and mere practicalities, just to get herself to look like that. And I admire her and respect her for it. Don't get me wrong, I love to slob around in old white pants and fraying men's shirts, in fact most of my time working at home and at the weekends is spent like this. But to be able to put together a look for yourself that you like and that makes you feel terrific, whether you do it every day or once a month, is essential. It's essential if we are to rid ourselves of our own inhibitions about being big, and it is essential if we are to challenge the way that we are viewed and treated by the rest of the world.

Because there's no denying that people treat us differently when we look good. I'm not the only one who's impressed with the powerful-looking, well-dressed big woman whom I see in the street. She demands a different kind of attention, better treatment than does the embarrassed-looking, shy, sadly dressed woman in the navy crimplene tent.

And of course, being treated better feeds our self-confidence. It allows us to demand more out of life, and out of our interactions with others. This new, more assertive behaviour increases our self-confidence yet again in an ever-ascending spiral.

So looking good, wearing clothes that we like and feel confident in, is just the beginning. It's the beginning of saying to ourselves and to the world, 'We're OK. We're not going to hide any more. We're going to go out there and grab what the world has to offer. We're entitled to the same choices that smaller women have, not only in respect of our clothes, but ultimately in respect of our lives as well.'

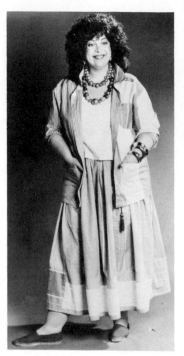

My first Wendy Dagworthy outfit – bold stripes, big comfortable pockets, a turned-up collar, and lots of chunky jewellery – a far cry from navy crimplene

> ❛ It's just as important for large ladies to have fun with their clothes as it is for anybody else. I don't think I'm any different from Jane Fonda, I am just larger and younger! It's just that you've got to put more spadework into finding the stuff to have fun with if you're larger. I remember once going into the *New York Times* office to do some work and I was dressed in my Vita Sackville-West look. I was wearing a wonderful huge panama which came down to my eyebrows, a sensational man's Christian Dior cream-coloured broadcloth silk evening shirt, really enormous with frills down the front, jodhpurs from an army surplus shop, and riding boots. As I went up in the lift one of the subs turned to me and said, 'Hey, lady, where do you stable your horse?' Now that's what I call having fun. It's a sort of conspiracy if you like, – other people can enjoy you as well. ❜
> *Meredith Etherington-Smith*

❛ I began to sort things out when I read *Fat is a Feminist Issue* and then started to see a lot of media coverage about the fight for better clothes for big women. That helped a lot because the main problem had always been clothes. That was what always set you apart from other people. I could cope with everything else – I had a lot of friends and boyfriends – but when I was at college I wanted to look like everyone else, I wanted to wear jeans and I couldn't. Going shopping was a horrendous experience.

Something that really annoys me is the hard-line feminist argument that says it's superficial for big women to care about their clothes, about their appearance. This really irritates me because the women who say this have usually had a choice about what to wear. I never have. I consider myself a feminist and I don't think that wearing make-up (which I always do), wearing frills, and wanting to look pretty interferes with my feminist thinking. These are silly distinctions that take away from the essence of feminism. The argument that I shouldn't worry about what I look like comes from thin feminists. I've yet to meet a very large feminist who talks to me in that way.

It's all about having a choice and I want the choice. ❜

Elizabeth Osborne

❛ I'm very fussy about what I wear. I do spend a lot of time and attention on what I look like, because the way I figure it – if you're going to get slagged off, if you don't look good, you're going to get slagged off double, so if you look OK, sort of glamorous, then you can pass. When you're big you've got to spend more time on yourself. When you're feeling down it's easy to just not wash your hair for two weeks and go into a slump, but then you can just turn into a parody of what everyone assumes fat people are like – miserable. ❜

Helen Terry

Finding your own style

I've been talking a lot about 'looking good'. What is good? What's 'good' for me might be poison for you. I've seen many women for this book. Some wore classic, timeless clothes, and natural-looking make-up or no make-up at all. Others were dressed in the most outrageous examples of modern fashion, with layers and layers of flamboyantly coloured garments, spiky hair and over-the-top make-up to go with it. But they all had something in common. They all had a sense of their own personal style. I've asked many people, friends and fashion experts, to define style. Some of them have had a ready definition at their fingertips, others have moaned when I've asked them, saying it's impossible to define such an elusive quality.

❛ Style is a word that's around a hell of a lot these days – it used to be chic, now it's style. You've also now got to be 'individual'. Have you ever noticed that people trying to be individual look deeply similar? The essence of true style is a total disregard of what anybody else is doing. It's doing your own thing, the thing that relates to your own life and your own interests. Clothes should be a reflection of one's person. ❜
Meredith Etherington-Smith

> ❛ I'm quite a noisy person and I tend to reflect that in how I dress. I wear lots of colours and flamboyant shapes. 'Elegance' is not something that comes naturally to me. Even if I was thin, I don't think I'd reflect elegance terribly well, because it's just not part of my character. My style is fairly flashy, a 'bright colours and I'm going to be noticed if it kills me' sort of style. ❜ *Denise Smith*

> ❛ You have style when you know how you want to present yourself to the world and to do it, you break fashion rules. When a woman goes to a designer and gets dressed from top to bottom in a designer look, that isn't style, that's just slavish insecurity. The man or woman who will wear what they want to wear in a way that adds to their confidence, that's style. ❜ *Kate Franklin*

> ❛ Style is more important than fashion. Fashion can be set by people with style, but not by people who only know 'fashionability'. You have to be inventive. Good style like good anything else is an amalgamation of experience, honesty, a certain amount of fantasy, and tremendous confidence in saying, 'I love that.' It helps to read, look at pictures, go to the theatre and observe other people very carefully, because then you know what to avoid.
>
> I'm going to bring up a terribly old-fashioned word: grooming. For instance, you see girls today with very bizarre hairstyles. Never mind whether you like them or not: it still takes a lot of care, a lot of thought and attention to achieve this look. This is what it's all about. It's care and thought and pleasure.
>
> Style has nothing to do with age or with size. Big women can have just as much style as anyone else. There is absolutely no difference at all on that score. But one must have the courage to develop an appreciation of oneself as a large woman. ❜ *Joanne Brogden*

To me style is that unique combination of confidence and comfort that I feel when I'm wearing something that's right for me. It's how I felt in that first Wendy Dagworthy outfit. It's wearing something that highlights the aspects of myself that I like the most. So how can we, as big women, begin to develop an appreciation for and a look of 'ourself'? By looking around us, as Joanne Brogden says, by observing, but most of all by forgetting the notion that we can only wear something if we are thin.

If you've spent a lifetime hiding in the kind of clothes that you hate, waiting till that magical day when you will be thin enough to wear what you really want, starting to develop a style of your own can be daunting. It needn't be. Think of it as a new adventure, a creative enterprise upon which you are embarking. You are going to begin to have fun with yourself, to decorate and embellish your body so that it will be pleasurable to view yourself in your bedroom mirror or to catch an unexpected glimpse of yourself in a shop window as you pass by.

A good way to start to find out the kind of things you like is to go through magazines. That's right, those dreaded fashion magazines. But forget about those unattainable sizes and just look at the clothes, the hair, the make-up. Is there something there you like? A look, an idea that can be adapted to things you already have in your wardrobe? Treat a fashion spread the same way as slim women do, as inspiration. Very few women, even if they are a size 10, can afford the clothes they see in these magazines anyway, so don't worry if the things you

> ❛ The smile on her face is what gives a woman style ❜
> *Vicky Pepys*

Professor Joanne Brogden of the Royal College of Art

see there are not available in your size. I know that that is frustrating, but for now, let's just look for ideas. It's amazing how just tying a scarf in a new and different way can alter the look of a dress you may have had for years and make it feel new. I am a great one for wrapping my head up in any available scrap of fabric and I get a lot of ideas from the latest copy of *Vogue*. The model there may be a size 8 and I am a 26, but the effect can work just as well for me.

You can even keep a file of pictures that you've collected and that you like the look of. Go through your closets and experiment with what you've got and see how it can be adapted to these looks. When I was preparing the pictures for this book, my husband was amazed at some of the outfits that I came up with. He couldn't believe that they were sometimes made up of things that I had had for years. But I was coming up with new ways of putting them together that made them look completely different…for example, just adding a new pair of loafers and some chunky socks to my much-worn man's trenchcoat gave it a new, preppy look that it had never had before.

There are many different kinds of clothes in this book, and many different 'looks'. They are all photographed on big women. My 'models' ranged from size 18 to size 30. One of my major complaints against manufacturers and catalogues who cater for larger sizes is that most of them photograph their clothes on small women. When I've asked them why, they inevitably tell me that it is a question of aspiration. Big women, they say, need to aspire to something, and so they want to see their clothes shown on slimmer models. Rubbish! This is another one of these insults to us as big women that we must protest against.

There are three main categories into which the clothes in this book fall. The first of these are those clothes which can be found in most urban centres, no matter where you live. These clothes come from chain stores, men's departments, stores selling work clothes, ethnic clothes shops, second-hand clothes shops, thrift shops and markets.

The second category are those clothes that belong to the 'models' themselves. In most cases these clothes are things that they have had for years and that they have acquired through the painstaking searching that is familiar to big women the world over. Whether these clothes were bought in London or Leeds, in Chicago or Nashville, in Sydney or Toronto, is irrelevant. What is relevant, and the reason why they are included, is to show you that if you persevere, if you look in ordinary shops, *any* ordinary shops, you can find lovely things.

The third category, which includes many of the clothes by top British designers, are those clothes that have been specifically made as one-offs in a large size. These clothes have been made by *British* designers simply because Britain is where I now live, but don't think for a moment that if only you could take a trip to London these clothes would be available in large sizes. Sadly, that is not yet true.

Some people may think it wrong to include clothes that are specially made and are not on the market, but I do this for two reasons.

The first is practical and has to do with the hierarchy that exists within the fashion industry. High-fashion looks, shown on the catwalks of London, Paris, Rome and New York, eventually become diluted by the mass manufacturers and filter down to high-street level where they are available at prices that are accessible to most people. The influences of top designers are felt all through the 'slim' fashion world. There has never existed a similar hierarchy for bigger clothes. For some reason the manufacturers of 'fat fashions' ignore the prevailing styles and offer us the same things year after year. It is my intention to show that big women *can* look good in high-fashion gear. I hope that will encourage outsize manufacturers to get off their backsides and start making better things.

The second reason I make it a point to show these kinds of clothes, is to serve as an inspiration to you, to all of my fellow 'bigger' ladies, who like me have yearned for so long to see other big women looking terrific. I show them to prove to us and to the rest of the world that we can look as good as anyone if we have the opportunity to wear the same kind of clothes, to which those size 6–14s have always had access.

Breaking all the rules

> ❝ Fat women feel that thay want to fade into the wallpaper, and all you do then is look fat and boring! My mother does sometimes say 'Are you going out in that pink thing? You look like a big pink blob!' but I'd rather look like a pink blob than a boring big blob in black. People know what size you are. You aren't going to hide anything by wearing all those vertical stripes, you're not fooling anybody, so if you like horizontal stripes in green and purple then wear them, because people will be so knocked out by the outfit and you as a person that they won't even notice your size. ❞
> *Janis Townes*

There has been so much nonsense written about what big women should and should not wear that I hardly know where to start. All of the so-called rules of 'fat dressing' are based on the premise that we should be trying to make ourselves look slimmer. I am always infuriated when I read some article aimed at big women or see in some catalogue for outsize clothes, descriptions of clothes that tell you how much thinner they make your arms look or how they flatter you by fitting loosely and covering up a 'protruding tum'.

We all know the obvious rules, like never wear horizontal stripes, stick to darker colours, stay away from belts, patterns, ruffles, etc., etc., etc. But how many of you have heard of these outrageous no-nos that I have collected from various books and articles over the years?

Never wear:
- round necklines
- short necklaces
- heavily gathered sleeves
- double-breasted jackets
- tops with broad shoulders
- large round clip-on earrings or hoops
- billowy sleeves, bows or flounces
- satin (it reflects light in all the wrong places)

And last but not least, my favourite piece of 'advice': Never wear linen – it creases and creases spell F-A-T.

I hope that, like me, you have reached the point where this kind of advice makes you angry. If we were to follow all the guidelines laid down by so-called fashion experts, we'd be left with absolutely nothing to wear.

One of the worst excesses of the fashion world seems to be this tendency to generalize. Big women shouldn't wear this, short women shouldn't wear that, tall women should be careful about so-and-so. What nonsense. Each woman is an individual and she will look and feel good in some things, bad in others. Big women are no different from our thinner sisters in this respect. A big or round earring may look terrific on you, awful on me. I may leave the house swathed in the kinds of ruffles and flounces that you would only wear in your worst night-mare, and a certain double-breasted, huge-shouldered forties jacket might be just what you've been looking for to make you feel like a film star. Don't let these crazy 'rules' inhibit you from letting your imagination run riot.

Throughout this book you will see examples of these rules being broken. Sometimes it's obvious, as in the use of horizontal stripes or gathered skirts.

Other times it won't be so clear because, frankly, I never think of the fashion rules when I'm putting together an outfit either for myself or for another woman. What I do think of is 'How does this look on me? Does it look as good as I thought it would, or does it need "fixing" in some way? Would it be better with different accessories, with my hair up and not down, with different shoes or tights, with a contrasting scarf or shirt and not the obvious matching one that I bought to go with it?' But always ask yourself, 'How does this make me feel, do I *enjoy* wearing it, do I feel proud in it, self-confident, beautiful?' If the answer is yes, then that's it. It works, and to hell with the rules!

Same woman – different looks

If you've no idea in which direction your own personal style lies, the pictures in this section should give you some ideas. You may love some of the looks, hate others. You may wish to try them out yourself. You may find that you enjoy alternating the image you present; cool and businesslike during the day, romantic or sultry at night. Let fantasy come into your wardrobe. Fantasy is an important element of style, fantasy and an element of courage. Don't be afraid to experiment. Try something on, stand in front of a full-length mirror and look. Sometimes, it's worth pausing for a moment to give yourself time to get used to something new. Sometimes a new shape may seem all wrong but when your eye gets used to it it can seem fabulous. That's just how I felt when I first tried on the selection of street-wise, youthful, Bodymap clothes *(facing p. 88)*. The clingy black skirt was an entirely new experience for me. I'd been so used to shying away from any kind of straight skirt, in fact I hadn't worn one since my teenage days when I was heavily girdled to smooth out any offending lumps. When I first tried on this black knit skirt that clung to my every generous curve I was convinced that it was too tight. I tried it on in front of the designers, Stevie Stewart and David Holah, to prove to them that it was too small. 'It's supposed to be like that,' Stevie calmly said. 'It fits perfectly.' I was still sceptical. But gradually I got used to the shape and to the idea. After years of seeing myself in full, gathered skirts, my eye needed time to adjust to the new contour. Now I love it.

The nautical look *(opposite)* is a completely different style. It's casual and crisp and classic, and it's easy to do. You simply pull together navy blue, white and red. In this picture I've used a horizontally striped T-shirt, against all the rules of fat dressing, over a pair of white trousers that I made myself. The pattern for these trousers is one that I made from a pair of army- surplus 'gas pants' that I bought five years ago, the drawstring baggy kind. On me they don't bag, but they fit rather well. So I copied them, added pockets, and made them a bit longer and narrower at the bottom. I make them up in a heavy drill cotton which is comfortable summer or winter, and they have become one of the mainstays of my wardrobe.

The jacket is another story. A couple of years ago, I saw the designer Calvin Klein on a chat show. Someone asked him why his clothes only went up to a size 12. 'Because it's easier for a woman to lose weight than it is for me to make my clothes look good on a fat body' was what he replied. I was, as you can imagine, incensed.

A brilliant red jumpsuit – don't listen to fashion pundits who tell you to hide yourself away in 'slenderizing' dark colours – why should you!

Inset: The 'nautical' look – all it takes is red, white and blue. Splash out with horizontal stripes, bright colours, white trousers

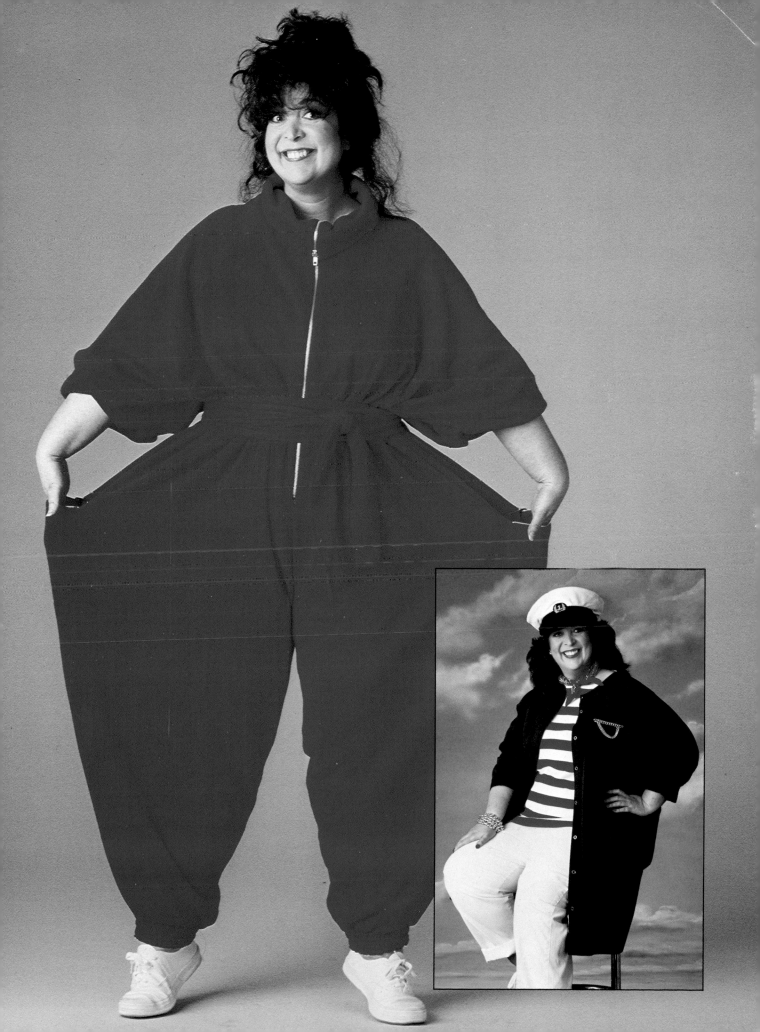

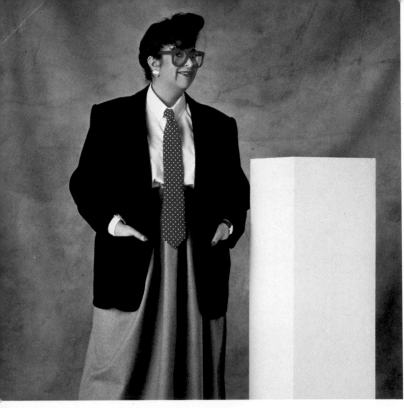

Two very different looks show just how wide is the range of possibilities open to you – one severe and businesslike, softened with red glasses and warm colours for the shirt and tie, the other an ethnic extravaganza of vibrant colour and sensuous fabrics. Clothes are, after all, an excellent form of self-expression and a marvellous way of having fun

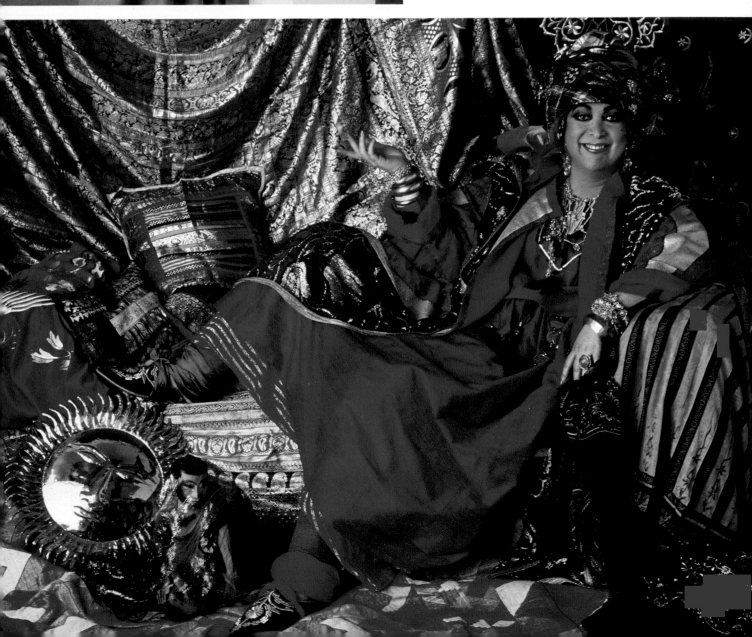

However, on a recent trip to New York, I saw this jacket hanging among hundreds of others just like it in a department store. It was a size 12. I tried it on. It fitted and I liked it, but it was too expensive. The sales started the next week, and I looked at it again. OK, I thought, this I can afford. From the look of the bulging rails, it seemed that I was the only taker. But I bought it and here it is, a Calvin Klein jacket in a size 12, on my undieted body.

The traditional British Sloane Ranger look *(between pp. 88 and 89)*, that mix of classic cut and fine fabrics, was enormous fun to put together because it is so different from what I usually wear. It was made up entirely from things in my own wardrobe, with the exception of the Hermès scarf and bag, which added the finishing touches. So, don't despair if you can't go out and buy new things; try putting together what you've got in a new way – you'll be surprised what you can come up with.

The beige-and-cream trenchcoat picture *(between pp. 88 and 89)* didn't end up exactly as planned. We were going for an Ingrid Bergman, Casablanca look, but somehow I ended up looking more like Humphrey Bogart. No matter, it's a very wearable, easy look, once again put together out of elements that I've owned for years. We started with an enormous man's raincoat. It's worth shopping around for this, because many I've tried on have been too slimly cut in spite of the fact that they were the biggest size I could find, or they were too narrow over the hips and enormous across the shoulders. This is an especially full-cut, old-fashioned version, that's as roomy as you could hope for. I found it at Burberry's years ago. It was expensive, but a great investment. I wear it constantly till it's ratty and filthy. When it's cleaned it looks brand new.

It can be very hard for us as big women to allow ourselves the luxury of what's known in the fashion world as 'Investment dressing'. This is the approach that says, 'Buy something good, really good, that's well-cut, in a quality fabric and even though it may not be cheap, it will last you for years.' Well for years I stayed away from this way of clothes-buying. After all, I reasoned, I'm going to lose ten pounds by next week, so anything I buy now will be too big by then – why spend any more than I have to? I'll just buy this cheapie for now and save the good stuff for later when I'm thin. Wrong, wrong, wrong! This is another variation of the 'I'm fat and awful, so I don't deserve' syndrome that we are trying to eradicate completely. You do deserve and you deserve now, so if you want a good coat or a pair of boots or a cashmere sweater, and you can afford it, buy it! I've bought more cheap garbage in my day than I care to remember, all because I thought it would be too big by next week. I think it's our willingness to settle for shoddy, badly made clothes, just because we feel that they are all we're entitled to, that makes outsize manufacturers continue to push these kinds of goods our way.

Here I've teamed my trenchcoat with a second-hand silk shirt bought for a couple of pounds in a street market, a big cotton knit sweater, and again, my home-made pants. The hat comes from a market too.

The tracksuit *(facing p. 96)* says a lot about colour, but I can sum it up in one sentence, 'Don't be afraid of it.' The thought of a fifteen-stone woman like myself in a fire-engine red boiler suit made of thick sweatshirting, goes against every rule I can think of, except my own: if it feels good, wear it! And this certainly did. It's great for exercising, going to the movies, lazing around at home in front of the TV. I've even worn it to a party.

The silk taffeta ballgown *(facing p. 89)* is slightly less flexible in terms of wearability! It was made for me by designer Ken Smith, who specializes in designing for big women. Ken made it from fabric that my brother brought back from a student trip to the Far East in 1968. The material had been waiting all this time for somebody in the family to be in a position to have something made out of it. I think it was intended for shirts, if you can believe that! I'm happy to say that I got to it first. This shot fulfils all my romantic fantasies – I feel like a bon-bon emerging from a chocolate box – and though I really have very little call for this kind of thing in my private life, I wanted you to see how successful it can be on a big woman. A lot of traditional no-nos here, including enormous sleeves, ruffles, flounces and all that reflecting taffeta.

For a complete change of pace I chose a 'dress for success' look *(facing p. 97)*. This is for the serious lady executive or just for the fun of looking like one. It can be a stark, rather cold look, but we've softened it up with a red tie and huge red specs. The grey flannel of the skirt and jacket add the right touch of respectability, and the man's pink cotton shirt is a comfortable fit.

Black doesn't have to be dowdy. After years of wearing only dark colours because I thought they made me look thinner, I made a concerted effort over the past few years to eliminate them from my wardrobe. It may seem odd to talk about my discoveries about colour when discussing black, but what happened was this. While reading an excellent book about using colour effectively, I began to experiment in the way that was suggested. I stood in front of my mirror in a good light, and because I didn't have the different coloured sheets of paper that the book suggested I use for this exercise, I held up various bits of different coloured clothing and other household goods, such as cushions and tablecloths and placemats. It was during this experiment that I made two surprising discoveries. The first was that blue and purple, colours that I had never worn in my life, did wonderful things for me. They seemed to alter my skin tone, making me look healthy and amazingly awake. Much more so than the camels and beiges that I had always preferred which, I could now see, tended to make me look washed out and sallow. The next 'colour' discovery I made was that both black and white looked sensational – particularly black. Once again it made my skin look bright and clear, my eyes large and sparkling. Not one to ignore this kind of discovery for long, I gradually and surreptitiously started to add bits of black to my wardrobe again, first in the shape of a large man's muffler which I wrapped up high around my chin to frame my face, then a black cowl-neck sweater, and finally this rather wonderful black suit *(between pp. 88 and 89)*. This is my Hollywood glamour, high-gloss, fantasy look. Try it yourself, with fake diamonds, a second-hand or artificial fur and a great hat. This marvellous saucer-shaped affair makes all the difference. I felt like I'd walked right off a film set. I now wear a lot of black, not, as in the past, because I'm hoping it will make me look thinner, but simply because I think it suits me.

Now for my 'white' look. This chic, opulent outfit *(between pp. 88 and 89)* uses several garments in the same pattern, piled one on top of the other. I love looking layered and wrapped up, and this is the epitome of them both. I started with lightweight trousers, added a skirt, shirt and overdress all in a floaty striped cotton lawn, then topped that off with a heavier cotton coat. In case that wasn't enough, I draped a shawl of the same lightweight cotton around my neck for that muffled-up look. This is an incredibly comfortable way of dressing. You get the freedom of pants with the floaty feminine feel of a dress. I finish it off with espadrilles, which are without question my favourite summer footwear. They're cheap and comfortable and come in any number of colours to match or add an accent of colour to anything you're wearing. I particularly like wearing pure white trousers and top with bright green or pink espadrilles. It's a clean, cool, simple and always classy look.

And now, come into my tent and I'll tell you a tale of a thousand and one Arabian nights. My Rudolph Valentino, Arabian Prince look is a fine example of what can happen if you let your imagination loose *(facing p. 97)*. This is a strong, dramatic look that starts out with a caftan, easy to make, but also available in markets which sell ethnic clothes. We then kept adding bits and pieces: a beautifully encrusted evening jacket, a long shawl around the shoulders, a second caftan tied as a skirt under the first, blue trousers, chiffon scarves tied around the ankles, and Moroccan slippers. We then wrapped my head in four different scarves, added a liberal dose of heavy brass jewellery and a chain belt made of old coins that I've had since I was sixteen years old – and *voilà*! This is a terrific thing to put together for a party, and you can be sure of one thing, nobody else will be wearing the same outfit.

The pictures in this chapter were taken not because I wear all these different styles myself – but as an experiment to show you how wide a range of styles is possible, how many various ways you can choose to look.

The looks that I don't normally wear – the Sloane Ranger, the Arabian extravaganza – were the most exciting to do. I felt like a kid dressing up, and why not? That is surely what clothes should be about no matter what our age – enjoyment.

Believe me, I know how difficult it can be to put together a look that you feel happy with when you have to work so hard at simply finding things that fit. But it can also be fun. Look at it as a challenge, something that you are doing for yourself. It can be tremendously rewarding, and if you use your imagination, adding a scarf here, an armful of bangles there, you'll find that gradually you'll get there. You'll find *your* style!

---

6 No matter what I'm wearing, I hold my head up and walk very straight and look people straight in the eye. It's not always easy to do, but your posture and the way you're holding yourself is so important. It's all part of dressing, it isn't just putting clothes on, it's standing right and sitting right. People notice and it makes a difference. 9

Carole Burton

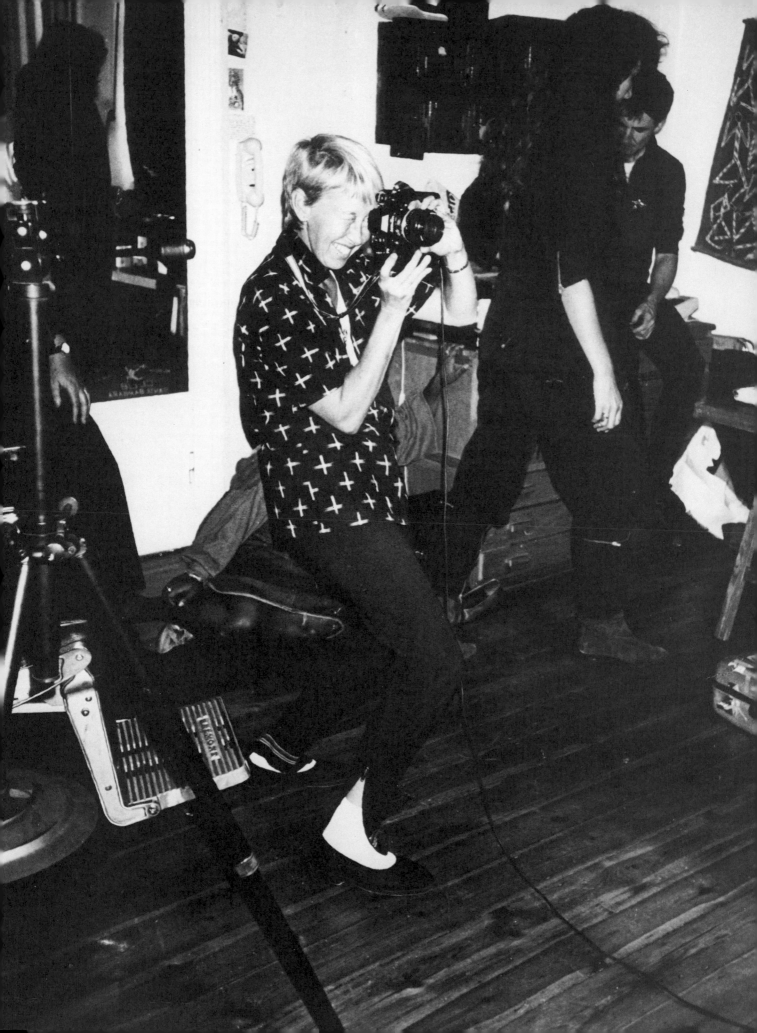

8

THE PHOTOGRAPHIC SESSIONS

Doing the pictures for this book was one of the most enjoyable experiences I've ever had. A fashion 'shoot' can be an intimidating experience for the woman who is not a professional model. The atmosphere at the studio, the feeling of familiarity among the other people taking part, the hairdresser, the make-up artist, the stylist, the photographer and his assistants, most of whom will have worked together before, can make the outsider feel nervous and intimidated.

It can also be fantastic fun. To wear beautiful clothes, have your make-up and hair done by the best people in the business, to be the centre of so much attention can do a lot to brighten up a dreary morning.

I did my own first 'session' for the London fashion trade paper *Fashion Weekly* in 1981. I had already given an extensive interview about 'Big and Beautiful' to their fashion editor, Bonnie Spencer, when I had this excited phone call.

'Hi, Nancy? Bonnie. Listen. I want to do some pictures to go with the interview! I'm afraid we wouldn't be able to pay you, but we'd do the whole fashion layout thing, you know, with a top photographer and hairdresser and make-up man, and we'd use that wonderful mohair jumper you were wearing when we met, and I think it would be a very good way of getting to the trade with your ideas. What do you think?'

What do I think? I am stunned. I am ecstatic. She can't pay me! Is she crazy? Doesn't she know that *I* would pay *her*?

It's 9 o'clock. A cold rainy morning in March. Uwe and I park the car on the kerb and gaze bleary-eyed at the old warehouse. Barbican Studios – third floor. Why is it always the third floor? We're lugging heavy bags of clothes. At the entrance to the building we meet a youngish man carrying a large metal toolbox.

'Hi, I'm Mark, make-up.'

'I'm Nancy, model.' Me, model? Who am I kidding? I'm Nancy, fat! Surely he thinks I'm pulling his leg. But, no, he's not laughing or even snickering. HE BELIEVES ME! Someone must have told him. Of course, Bonnie, when she booked him, must have said, 'Now, Mark, this one's a little unusual for a fashion shoot...'

And now here we are, face to face, me and my Professor Higgins of the maquillage. He looks nice. I look terrible. My still damp hair is half frizzy and sticking to

Robyn Beeche at work

my head. My face wears a shiny oil slick of unabsorbed Equalia, and under my eyes is a healthy mix of black lack-of-sleep shadow and last night's mascara. I am also not exactly 'dressed to kill'. Stretched out jeans, an ancient T-shirt, and a seven-year-old men's cardigan which I love, but let's face it, has had it.

We climb the stairs and arrive at the studio. There's already a lot of action here. Bonnie, the only familiar face I can expect to see, has not arrived yet, but the photographer and his two assistants are hard at work. He's bearded and gentle, they look like they've just been flown in from the set of *Peter Pan* – Captain Hook's pirate ship, to be more precise. They are young and female, and festooned from ear to ear with a motley assortment of twisted scarves and leather thongs. Earrings and bangles dangle from every available inch of skin. To top it all, they are mini-skirted and display the kind of legs guaranteed to make most normal mortals slit their throats. How in the world am I going to get undressed in front of these two?

Thank God, here's Bonnie. She knows I'm not a slob.

'Hello, hello, hello.' Kisses all round. 'Where's Dar? Isn't he here yet? Oh, he is naughty.'

Enter Gianni, carrying large leather holdall and apologies from Dar. He'll be here in ten minutes. Gianni, it turns out, is there to 'assist' Dar. Dar will be there, we hope, to do my hair.

I'm sitting in an uncomfortable little chair in the dressing-room. My limp fringe is pinned back, exposing the full wonder of my early-morning sleepless eyes. Perched over me and examining my face intently in the large mirror opposite is Mark.

'Have you got anything on your face?'

'A little Equalia.'

'It's fabulous stuff. I think it's the best moisturizer around.'

Hey, maybe this isn't going to be so bad after all. We agree about moisturizers. Not a bad beginning to our particular relationship. He opens his case, removes several trays containing more make-up than the perfume hall of Harrod's and sets to work. Unfortunately the top of his case is now blocking my view of myself in the mirror. I can see his face still reading mine like a map, and I can, of course, feel what he is doing to me. This consists of gently dabbing and stroking my face with an awe-inspiring assortment of sponges, puffs and brushes. I strain to see what he's doing and after an interminable 45 minutes I finally get up the courage to ask him to lower the lid of the box so I can see myself in the mirror. Wow! My skin is smooth and white. My cheekbones have suddenly appeared as if from nowhere, and my eyes! Well, my eyes are enormous. They're kind of swept up at the outside corners with orange shadow and my eyelashes seem to have grown about six inches. 'You have wonderful lashes.' He must be talking to me, there's nobody else in here.

'They're my best feature.' We chuckle conspiratorially. I really like this guy. Not only is he gentle, not only does he love my moisturizer *and* my eyelashes, but he is making me look gorgeous. Next my lips.

'I've always wanted big, pouty lips, you know, the kind like models have,' I venture.

He pulls a magazine over and quickly finds a shot of the most incredible, pouting, sex-object lips that I've ever seen. 'You mean like this? No problem.'

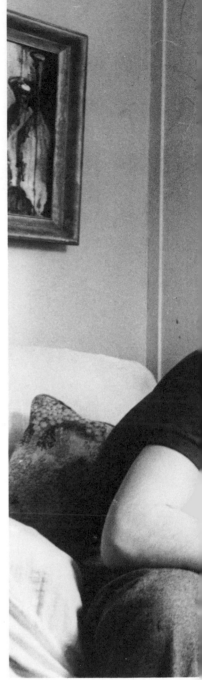

Uwe watches as Lyn Easton makes me up!

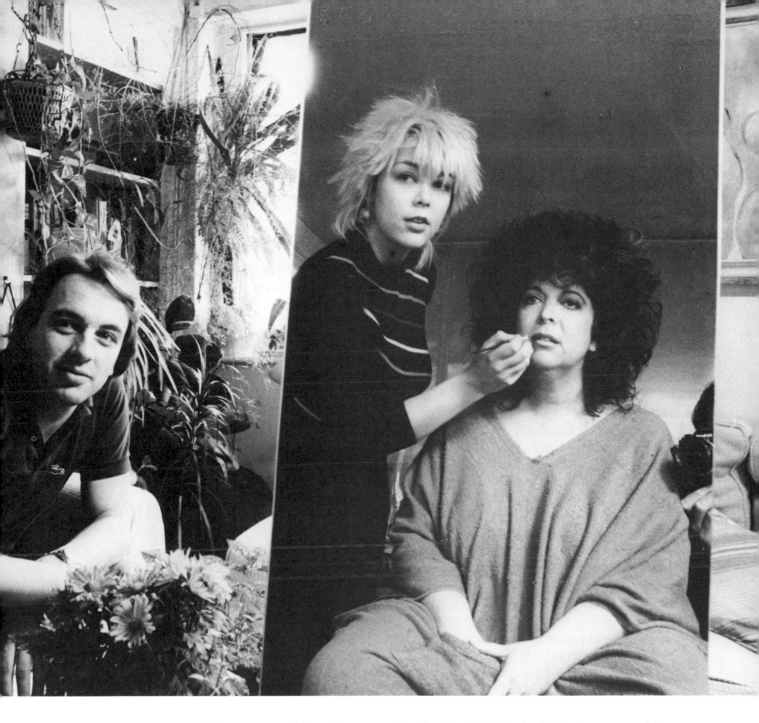

What are you doing, Nancy, wanting lips like that? You're betraying your public, your feminist fans around the country. Forgive me Germaine Greer, forgive me Spare Tyre, for I have always coveted pouting, sex-kitten lips, and now, after thirty-five years of going without, they are about to be created for me by this wonderful nimble-fingered Svengali. A little gold eyeshadow on the upper lip (*eyeshadow* on the lip?), a smooth glide of the pencil, a quick fill-in with the brush, and here they come – lips you could chew on for hours, and never get bored. And they're all mine.

By this time Dar has arrived. He and Gianni look approvingly at Mark's handiwork. Maybe there is hope after all. A multitude of electric gadgetry appears, roller and tongs and brushes and clips, and they start in on my hair like two master chefs preparing a rare and delicate dish. Clip, brush, curl, clip, brush, curl, over and over again all round the sides and the top and the front. And then brushing and pulling and tugging with knowing fingers, and then contemplative silence as they examine me. Bonnie and the pirates come in to stare in wonder at this divinity. The hair is big – fluffy and curly and wispy, and, miracle of miracles, my face is small. Yes, all this big floaty hair has made my face shrink and my eyes enlarge, and my lips – well, maybe enough said already about my lips. The person who gazes out at me bears little resemblance to the exhausted wreck who arrived two hours earlier. Still fat, still triple-chinned, but, dare I say it, beautiful. What an ego-trip. How do models survive without nervous break-downs? Don't they get crazy? Hey, all you women out there, you too can look like a cover girl. Just a couple of hours with the right sort of people around to work on you, and – Zowie! The face you've always wanted. I'm feeling a lot better now. It's going to be OK. They think I look almost as good as I think I look. They're all smiling and laughing, and the tension is washing away.

I put on my sweater. We confer about earrings, scarf, 'no, too busy', and shoes. The photographer, Roger, rejects my bronze loafers in favour of my white sneak-ers that I had arrived in – these fashion people, what will they come up with next? So, there I am, in front of the white paper in my new face, my new hair, my fabulous clothes…and my sneakers. Now the fun starts. They put on music. My God, it's just like *Blow-Up* which, luckily, was on the box just the week before. Will Roger crawl around on the floor at my feet clicking away and moaning, 'Give me more, more, baby. Oh yes, beautiful, beautiful'? No, he stays behind his tripod and instructs me to relax, just feel good, and look happy. How can I relax with all these people looking at me? So I start to sing along with the blaring sixties music that fills the studio and soon I'm dancing around in my own personal imitation of Veruska, and what's that, Roger is snapping away and saying, 'Good, good, wave the scarf around some more, darling,' and I am gone, well and truly gone.

Things are going well. So well, in fact, that Bonnie has an inspiration.

'I'd love to get shots of you in a ball-gown!'

A ball-gown! That sure fits in with my lifestyle. For evenings at her favourite Chinese restaurant Nancy favours this off-the-shoulder taffeta number. But, what the hell? Who am I to argue? And before you can say Christian Dior, she is on the phone to that arbiter of British ball-gown style, Belville Sassoon.

I listen to her side of this conversation in amazement. It seems they are actually agreeing to send some wonderful dress over here, by taxi, within the next fifteen minutes. Wonders will never cease. But will it fit? I have my doubts.

It is at this point that I drift off for a moment and, somehow, get an overview of this scene, and of all these people running around fixing lights, fixing cameras, fixing coffee and basically spending their whole day in the pursuit of the perfect picture of me.

The arrival of the ball-gown brings me back to reality. It's fabulous! But it's *tiny*. And strapless. But wait, there's hope. It seems there is a scarf, a sort of ruffled shawl affair that goes with it. Can we do something with it? Can we make it work?

'We must,' says Bonnie. 'It's divine.'

So back into the dressing-room, just us girls now, and it is here I learn the secret of fashion photography. You can make anything fit anyone. Using my bra as a kind of armature, we manage to pin the minuscule bodice – it must be a size 8 – to my front. There is no question of it going around the back, or even the

In my favourite sweater and jeans and clearly enjoying my first-ever moments in front of the professional fashion lens. My first fashion 'shoot' for Fashion Weekly

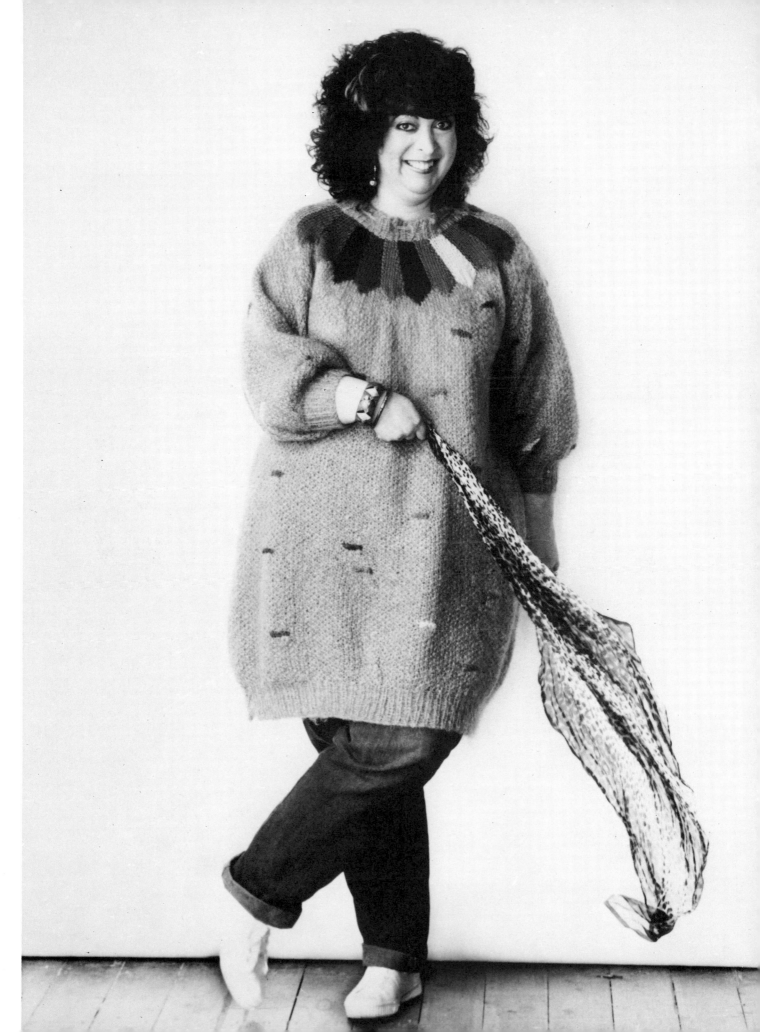

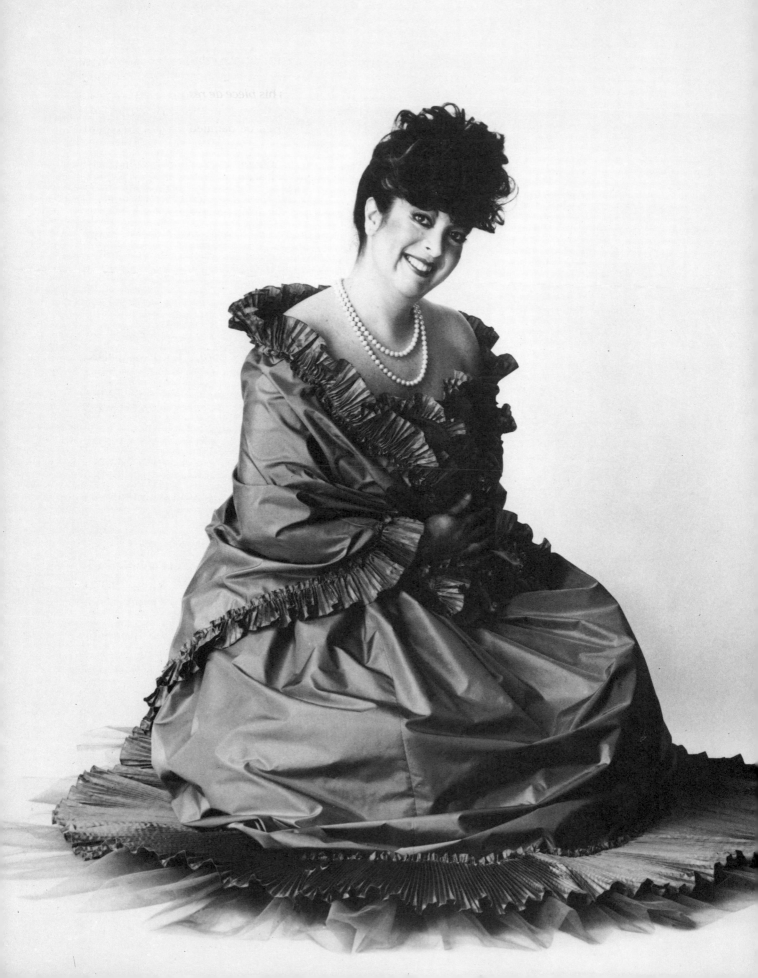

sides, for that matter. And here is the magic. By cleverly holding the shawl around my shoulders, it looks right. You can't tell it doesn't fit. Only the wind rushing up my back gives it away. And now, as his *pièce de résistance*, Dar comes in, orders me to hang my head between my knees, and in about ten seconds he has piled all my hair on top of my head, and I'll be damned if I'm not Scarlett O'Hara reincarnated.

This time the walk back into the studio is more reserved. It's a combination, I think, of the elegance of the dress, and the fact that if I so much as breathe, the whole thing will fall off and spoil this once-in-a-lifetime opportunity to have a picture of myself looking like this to go on top of my parents' piano.

All too soon it's finished. The last shot is done. Bonnie helps me out of the dress. I do my best not to put my heavy foot through the miles of billowing skirt, for this dress has turned out to be not merely beautiful, but an exact replica, in all ways, including price, of the famous black strapless 'nipple' dress worn by Lady Diana Spencer for her first official appearance as fiancée of the Prince of Wales. Quite a step away from my usual army surplus, I can tell you.

T he pictures appeared in *Fashion Weekly* in early April, 1981. I was accustomed by now to seeing myself in print, even to seeing myself on television. But to see myself like this, in a fashion photograph, was another thing entirely. Deep down, I guess I'd always really believed the experts who decreed that big could never look good, that big was ugly.

But now, looking at these pictures of me, I knew all those magazines, all those fashion editors who'd tormented me, were wrong. Oh, I was big all right, there's no denying that, but so what? I looked good…even to my own highly critical eyes. And if I could look and feel like this, then so could other big women, so could you!

W hen the oportunity arose to do this book, what excited me most about it was the chance to create beautiful pictures using other big women as models. I had so enjoyed the makeovers that I had done on my TV programmes that I wanted the chance to do it over again, to see more women having the simple fun that all this pampering can be.

The women in these pictures come from all different backgrounds and have different careers; some are married, some single, some are mothers, one is a grandmother. I don't think you could find a richer cross-section. But we are joined together by the common experience of being bigger than what is deemed acceptable in our culture.

P lanning the shots and choosing the clothes took up a great amount of time, every second of it a pleasure. Although it was a tremendous challenge just to find things that would fit, everyone pitched in and between my clothes, everyone else's clothes and the things that we managed to borrow from shops and designers, we got it together. We had such a good time doing the things that other women take for granted. We exchanged tips about where to shop, who had the best big sweaters, the best belts, the best everything. And trying on each other's clothes was a rare treat. To know that someone else's dress or trousers were actually going to fit was a sensational feeling.

Me in size 10 ball-gown – the deception that is fashion photography! My first 'shoot' for Fashion Weekly

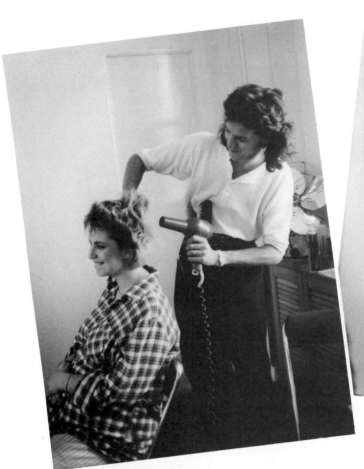

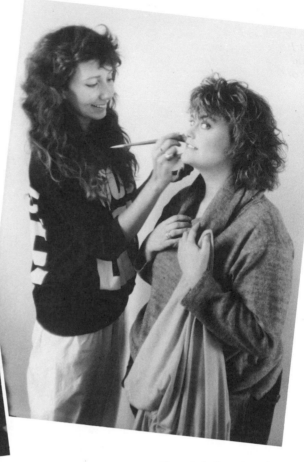

Above left: Greg does the coiffuring. Hair is wet, blown dry, even trimmed

Above right: Denise getting some finishing touches from make-up artist Paula Owen

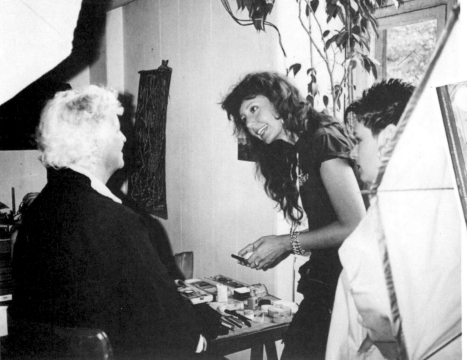

Above: In the dressing room at Robyn Beeche's studio

Left: The first step is make-up

Right: Her palette of colours spread out before her, Kim goes to work on Sue

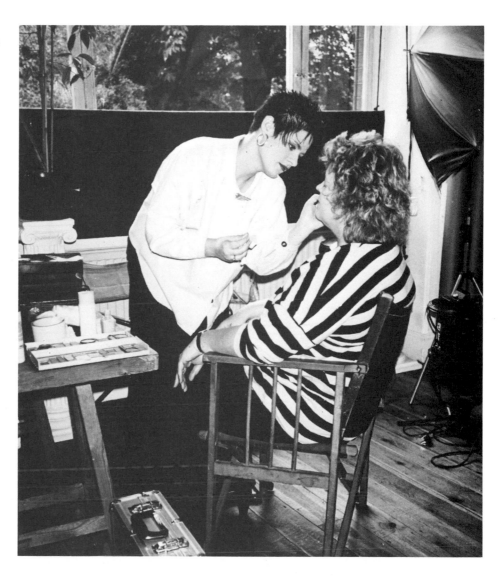

Below: 'Let's just get this jacket right'

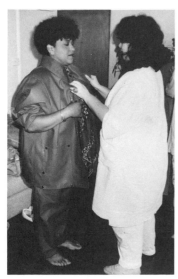

As each batch of new pictures arrived at my apartment I rushed into my kitchen and eagerly spread them out on the table. Again and again the first thought that hit me as I scrutinized that week's shots was, 'But they don't look "big".' They just look normal. They look beautiful and stylish and well-put-together and perfectly all right. Maybe they haven't been telling me the truth about their size, maybe they've all been on diets! The last thing I wanted was to be accused of that one thing that most angers big women, showing big clothes on women who are slim. And I even insisted that one model, Elizabeth Osborne, measure herself. She came out at 44-33-46/112-89-117 or, in her own words, 'a perfect 22'. Officially outsize. Another who looked tiny to me in the photos weighed thirteen and a half stone, another was a size 20.

When you look at the pictures of the 'smaller' big women in this book, remind yourself that women of this size are everywhere on diets. It is not only women who are as big as I am (I last measured in at 47-40-55/119-102-140), but women who are closer in size to these 'smaller' women who are making their lives a misery through constant dieting and bingeing.

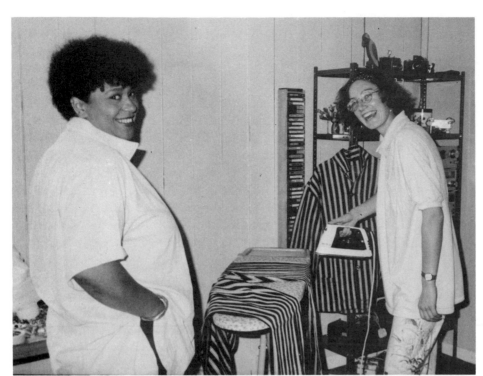

Left: Ironing – one of the less glamorous aspects of being a stylist!

Below left: Liz waits for her turn in front of the camera in Robyn's studio

Below right: Behind the scenes – it's not all glamour. Stylist Julia Fletcher takes up a last-minute hem on Jan's pyjamas

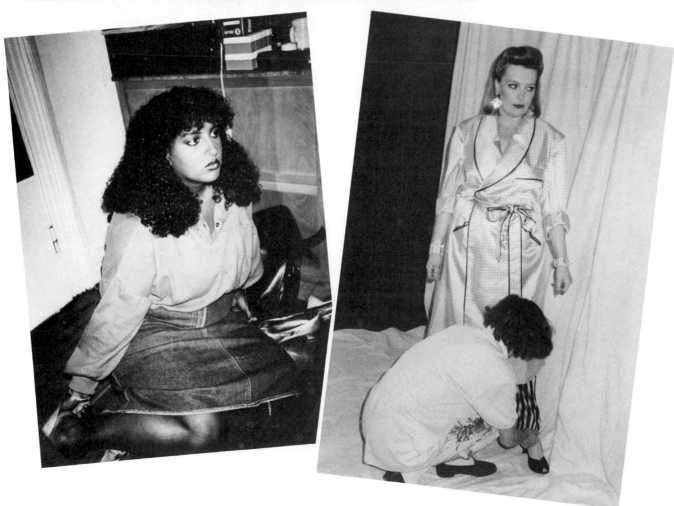

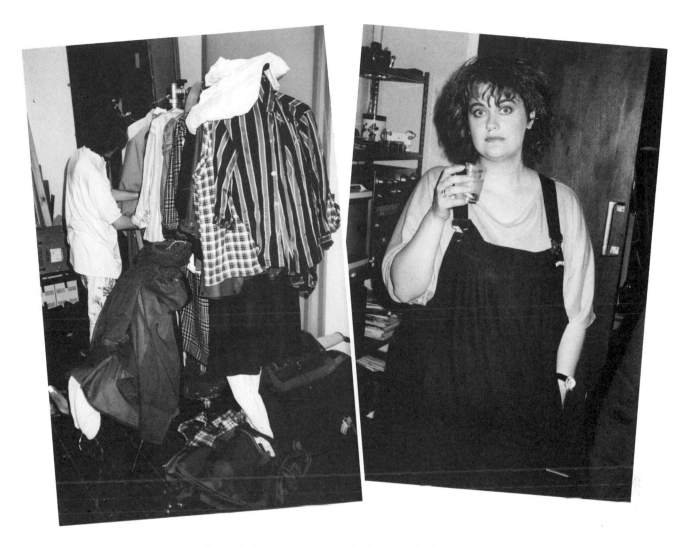

Above left: Andy Lane's studio – clothes waiting to be photographed. Julia tries to make order out of the chaos

Above right: Denise exhausted after her pictures

I've tried to represent all sizes of 'big' in these pages because women of all sizes feel bad about their bodies, feel guilty about their eating habits, and are caught up in the dieting trap. I could have taken pictures of even smaller women, of women sized 6-14 as well, because many of them would have known the same feelings of obsession with food, of discontent with their bodies. But women of this size can go out to a news-stand any day of the week and buy magazines that cater for them. We larger women can't.

Looking at our pictures, it seems crazy to me that my models should have trouble finding clothes to fit them. What kind of madness has brought us to this situation where we have to hunt and search for things to wear? For that was another common aspect to our lives, the difficulty of finding the kinds of things that we wanted in our size. And yet every woman in this book has persisted, has refused to wear the usual outsize rubbish and has insisted instead on holding out for clothes that suit her own particular style.

I hope you get as much pleasure from looking at the pictures as we had taking them. I also hope that they make you angry – angry that conventional newspapers and magazines regularly refuse to show bigger women looking as great as these women do.

9

GETTING IT ALL TOGETHER

You don't have to spend a lot of money to look terrific. It's not the budget you have but the imagination you use putting things together that counts. Some of my favourite things have been picked up for next to nothing in army-surplus stores, at street-markets, and in sales. My favourite evening outfit of all time is a second-hand man's tailcoat.

I've always loved the way men's tuxedos look on women. Every winter the fashion magazines feature the latest designer dinner suits on sylph-like, glossy models. Once, many years ago when I was going through a particularly skinny period, I bought a cheap copy of an Yves Saint Laurent tuxedo. It fitted me for about a week, and I only remember wearing it once. I never thought I'd have another one unless I somehow got rich enough to have one made.

And then a couple of years ago I was out shopping with a very thin friend. We were just about to stop for lunch when we passed by a men's clothes hire company that was having a huge closing-down sale. She, like me, had always yearned for a man's tuxedo and so in we went.

Never dreaming that there would be anything in my size, I sat on a stool in the corner and watched as my friend tried on dozens of tuxedo jackets, looking for the perfect fit. We'd been there almost an hour when the salesman took pity on me.

'What about you, honey, can't I fix you up with something?'

'Oh, you'll never have anything in my size,' I replied.

'Come on,' he laughed, 'we get them bigger than you every day.' With that he disappeared into the stock room and emerged several minutes later struggling under the weight of a huge pile of tailcoats, which he unceremoniously dropped on the floor in front of me.

'Start with those, and if they don't fit, I'll get some more!'

The first one I tried on actually did fit. I would have taken it there and then, but not my salesman. He thought we could do better, and he was right. I tried on at least a dozen jackets until he was satisfied with the lay of the shoulders, the hang of the back. We then proceeded to the trousers. No problem there either. The ones eventually selected were a bit big around the waist but a pair of braces/ suspenders soon remedied that. I bought this wonderful suit for only £19. Pretty

Carole Burton – proof yet again that bright bold colours and strong shapes can look sensational on a big woman. The leopard-print scarf adds just the right accent

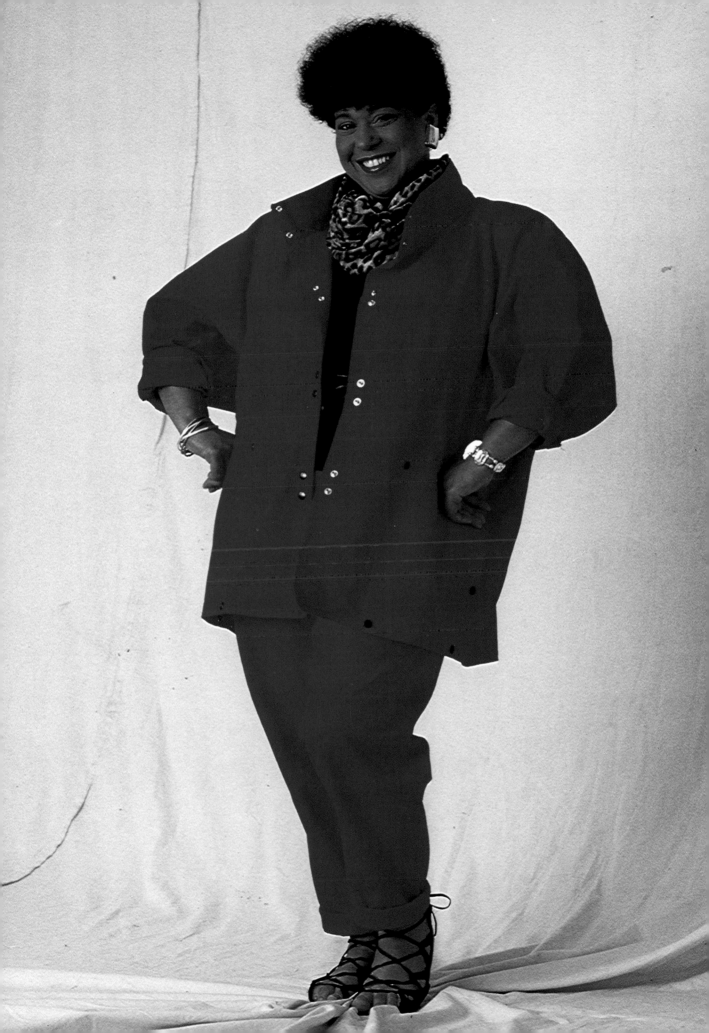

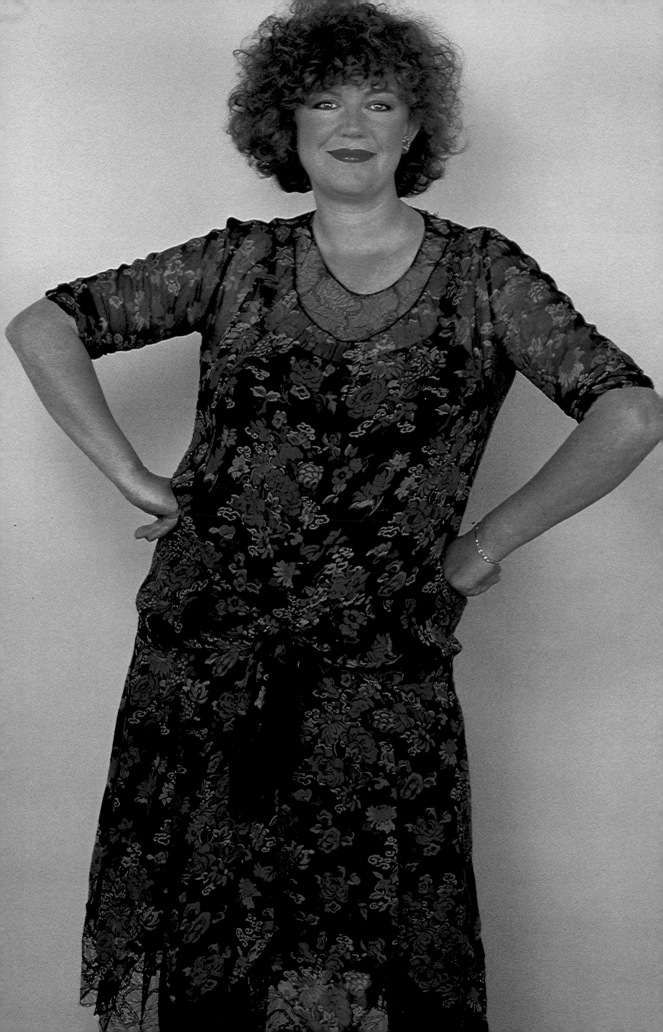

cheap for a 'dream come true'. I've worn it dozens of times since then. It always seems just right. What's particularly good about it is that I can wear it to any kind of party; no matter how dressed up or down anyone else is, I always feel good in my tailcoat, good and slightly zany, a combination that I like.

For the picture *(facing p. 145)* I've put it together with a second-hand man's dress shirt from a street-market and an old waistcoat. It makes no difference that the three pieces of the suit were not made to go together, they look great like this. I've added a pink cummerbund from an old dress and some earrings that I bought when I was fifteen years old. I do tend to keep things for a long time, and it usually pays off. A lot of the jewellery in these pictures is stuff I've had for ages. I just keep pulling it out year after year. I particularly like mixing very flashy, feminine jewellery with men's clothes. I think it makes for an unexpected and rather sexy look. You can't see my feet but if you could, you'd see that I'm wearing black lace socks and flat black satin bedroom slippers from the slipper department of Saks Fifth Avenue. They cost only $12, look just like men's evening pumps and are sublimely comfortable.

Men's clothes

Men's clothes are terrific on big women. Men's sweaters, shirts, T-shirts all form a mainstay of my wardrobe. You can buy wonderful men's cotton undershirts and dye them any colour. When I find a T-shirt that I like I buy it in multiples. There has been a vogue over the past couple of years for big, baggy T-shirts. When they're around, buy as many as you can afford in different colours, because you can be sure of one thing, if they're big this year, they'll be skimpy the next.

Army-surplus stores are a favourite haunt. I first discovered them when I was in high school and men's safari jackets were the 'in' thing. You can always find interesting sweaters, shirts, and coats. They're always well made in wonderful pure natural fibres, heavy cotton, gaberdine, wool. The many types of trousers you can find in these shops are great on big women, and they come in enormous sizes. I like my trousers really loose and baggy down the leg, so I always get the biggest size and take the waist in.

For our group picture *(pp 114–15)* I've mixed a lot of things from the army-surplus store with some other cheap bargains, some second-hand, some home-made. All the clothes in the pictures are in shades of khaki and olive green. These are such classic colours, they never go out of style and they always look chic. You can pay a fortune for the latest pair of designer khaki trousers at a fancy boutique or you can stop off at your nearest army-surplus store and buy some that are even better for a tenth of the price. And of course you can find the cheap ones in big sizes.

In our picture Mandy on the left is wearing stunning khaki trousers, a green cotton trenchcoat (both army surplus) with a man's second-hand seersucker jacket and an old chain-store sweater. It's the careful layering of all these different elements that makes this a smashing outfit.

Carole is wearing her own home-made culottes, topped by a man's T-shirt and khaki shirt. All her clothes are in heavy cotton and here we've put them with Carole's own sturdy lace-up boots, but you could just as easily wear this with

Meredith Etherington-Smith in flowered silk chiffon twenties frock from her collection of antique clothes

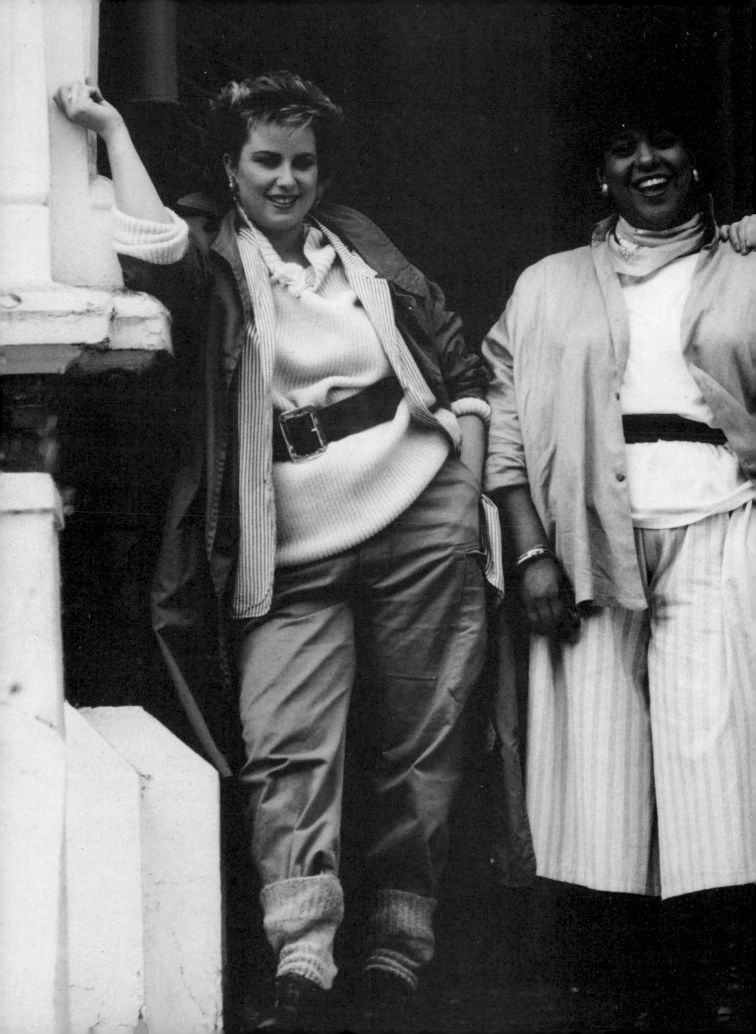

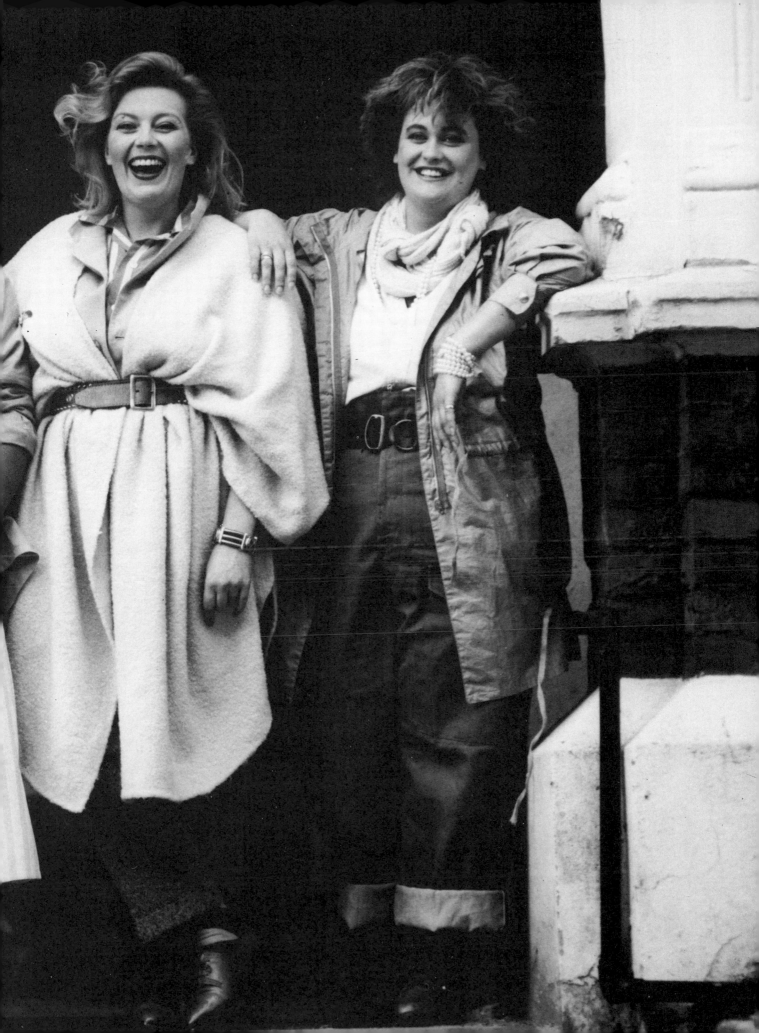

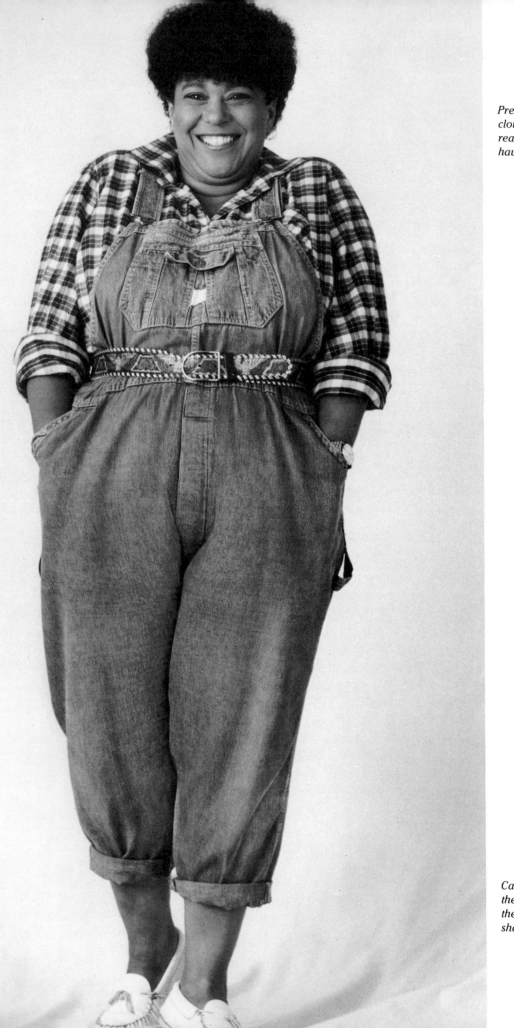

Previous page: Relaxed casual clothes like these needn't be out of reach for bigger women – you just have to know where to look

Carole Burton tapered the legs of these mens' dungarees and belts them in tight to give them the shape she likes

lighter shoes, or sandals when the weather gets warmer. Cotton layers are a great solution for those between the seasons times when you're not sure what to wear. Cotton needn't look too summery as long as you pick good strong colours and, by substituting a sweater for the T-shirt, this could take you through even the cooler autumn days.

Jan is wearing her own oatmeal tweed home-made poncho which we belted to give it a more casual look, over some well-tailored second-hand men's trousers with cuffs. These cost next to nothing but are beautifully made in the most luxurious woollen tweed. Take note of her sensational Argyll socks. It's little touches like this that make you look really pulled together.

Denise is wearing another version of the layered look – men's khaki T-shirt under second-hand silk shirt and waterproof parka. Her heavy green denim trousers are army-surplus camouflage gear and are meant to be worn over other trousers. They had a long slit at the side for getting into the pockets underneath, but we simply stitched that up. We've rolled them up to show her hiking boots, but you can ring the changes in other ways with pants – stuff them inside your boots, or tuck them under a pair of heavy woollen socks.

We've added tough leather belts and chunky brown leather shoes and boots to complete the picture. This army-surplus look is one that you can leave pure and simple or, by adding something unexpected like Denise's pearl necklace and bracelet (actually another necklace that we wrapped around her wrist), you can give it your own personal stamp.

Stores selling uniforms are also a good place to find cheap, fun things in big sizes. Chefs' pants, waiters' jackets, doctors' coats, all come big, and all can be mixed with other things in your wardrobe. A lot of these clothes come in white, which is always great in the summer. A cool crisp waiter's jacket can be buttoned up and belted over a skirt or you can wear it loose as a jacket over your jeans. As most of these clothes are made in pure cotton you can even dye them to mix or match with other things in your wardrobe.

When I'm on holiday abroad I always look for stores that sell work clothes. In most seaside towns there are shops where the fishermen and sailors kit themselves out. There you'll find unusual heavy-weather gear and sweaters. My own favourite is a navy-blue Breton fisherman's sweater that I bought on holiday in France, the kind that buttons on one shoulder. It was amazingly cheap and is the warmest thing I own.

Another good idea from the men's department are their pyjamas. Jan Murphy, whose picture you can see facing p. 144, lives in them. They're made in pure cotton, come in wonderful colour combinations, and she dresses them up with outrageous jewellery. We added a magnificent man's dressing-gown and diamanté jewellery to complete the picture.

‘ My favourite clothes are ones I don't have to iron! In the summer I wear men's white V-neck T-shirts. They are so cheap, you can buy a dozen at a time and wash them every day so they're nice and clean and fresh. My day clothes are really quite nothingy and laid back. Then for evening I wear a lot of twenties clothes which I have collected for years. ’

Meredith Etherington-Smith

Antique clothes and ethnic clothes

Antique and second-hand clothes can lend a highly individual dimension to your wardrobe and they needn't cost the earth. Of course, you can pay a fortune for certain rare pieces, but you can also be rewarded by regular visits to street-markets and jumble sales. Old collarless shirts come in wonderful striped cotton and are terrific belted over trousers or as cover-ups over bathing suits. Keep an eye out for the more formal dress shirts with pleats down the front. If you're really lucky you may even find one in heavy old silk.

Victorian and Edwardian lace-trimmed clothes are beautiful and incredibly versatile. You should look out for old petticoats, especially those with draw-string waists, camisoles and nightgowns. You can wear these clothes to parties, dressing them up with delicate evening shoes, old jewellery and perhaps a velvet ribbon at your neck. They are just as wonderful worn casually for those hot summer days. They look especially good with heavy belts, sandals or boots in rugged brown leather, and chunky silver jewellery. You can belt the nightgowns and blouse them over for a short summer dress or a great top over jeans. And you can, of course, always sleep in them. I have a silk nightgown from the thirties which is the slinkiest, sexiest thing I own; and nothing makes you feel more feminine than the ruffle of old lace around the edge of your Victorian camisole.

As with all clothes, it is essential that you try before you buy. Some things, especially the old nightgowns, look deceptively big on the hanger. But beware, the shoulders and armholes may in reality be tiny. Always check and be sure. The magnificent long nightgown in our Victorian picnic picture on pp. 120-21 is in fact a man's nightshirt. When you're buying old clothes, always check for tears and holes. Most things can be repaired but watch out for damage in the actual fabric at stress points and also check underarms and necklines, where you will find the worst signs of wear, including stains which can rarely be removed.

In the picture of Ozzie, Angela and Janis lounging on the grass *(pp. 120–21)*, I must confess I cheated. Everything they're wearing, the Victorian man's night-shirt, the Edwardian camisole and petticoat, is very old. Everything that is, with the exception of Janis's white off-the-shoulder sun dress which is only a little bit old. I bought it ten years ago and it's one of my favourite summer standbys. I usually wear it over trousers or a swimsuit, but I've shown it here over an antique petticoat to prove just how successful the mix of old and new can be.

Ethnic clothes can be another great find. Most large cities have shops selling native clothes from various countries. Often you can be lucky and find things in large sizes. Look out for roomy Japanese kimonos (men's are best), Chinese cotton or silk pyjamas, loose floaty Indian dresses and skirts, oversized African shirts in vivid prints, and beautifully coloured Peruvian sweaters.

My own particular favourites are a lacy Mexican wedding dress that I've had since I was a teenager, and a more recently acquired airy white Algerian caftan that I wear around the house or on the beach.

I also love jeans. There's something about them that makes me feel as if I'm on holiday. Maybe that's because when I was a child people had separate clothes for the city and the country, and when I put on my jeans it meant 'week-end'. Now, of course, people wear jeans just about everywhere. You can dress

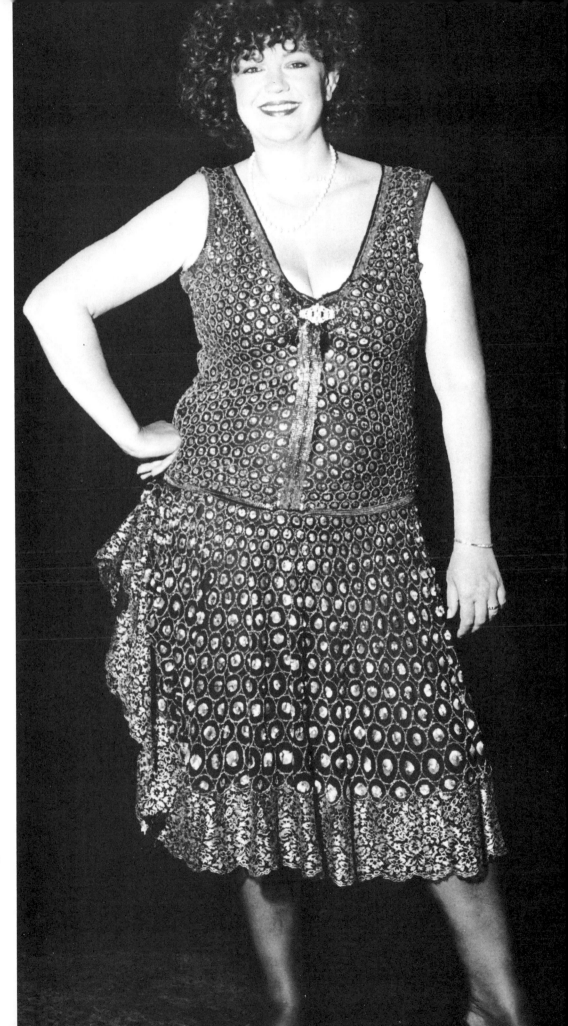

You can find wonderful dresses in large sizes in antique clothes shops and markets. Meredith Etherington-Smith in an original Paquin dress of 1926-7

Overleaf: These present-day picnickers on the grass, dressed in antique Victorian clothes, could have stepped right out of a nineteenth-century painting. From the left: Elizabeth Osborne, Angela Troak, Janis Townes

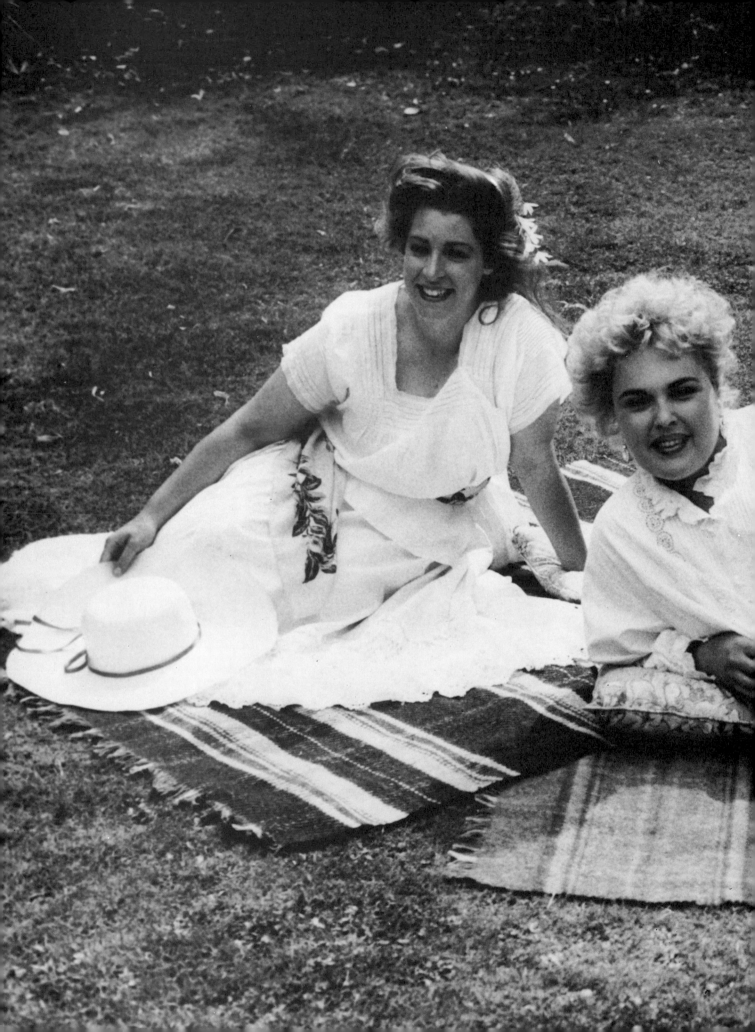

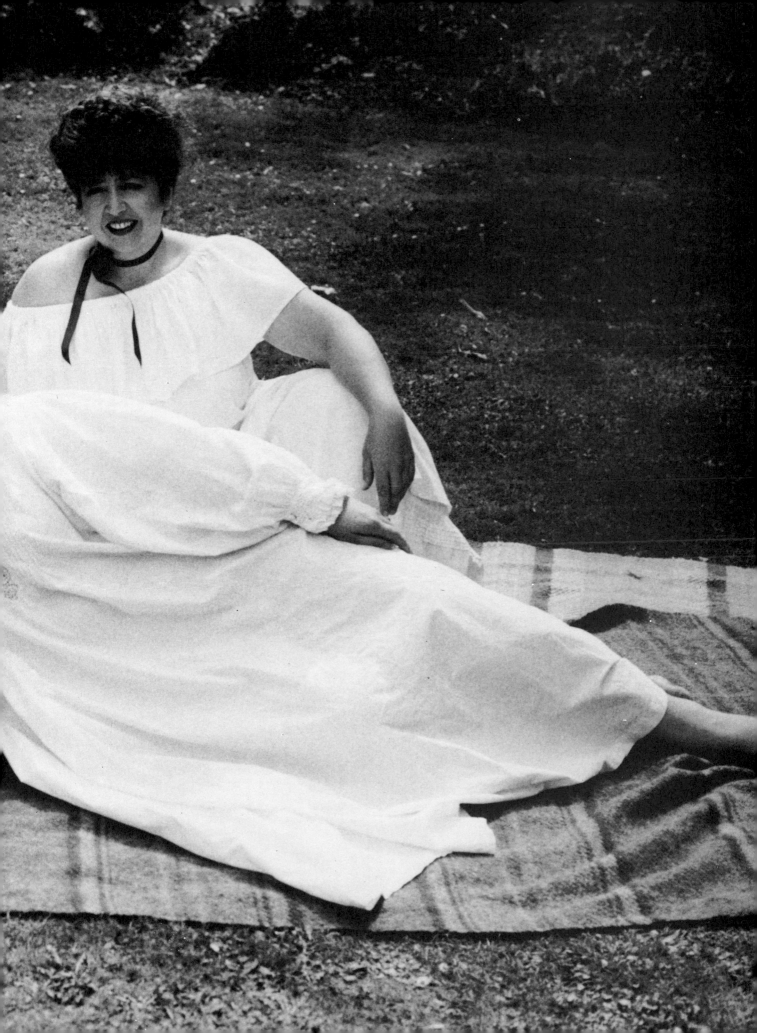

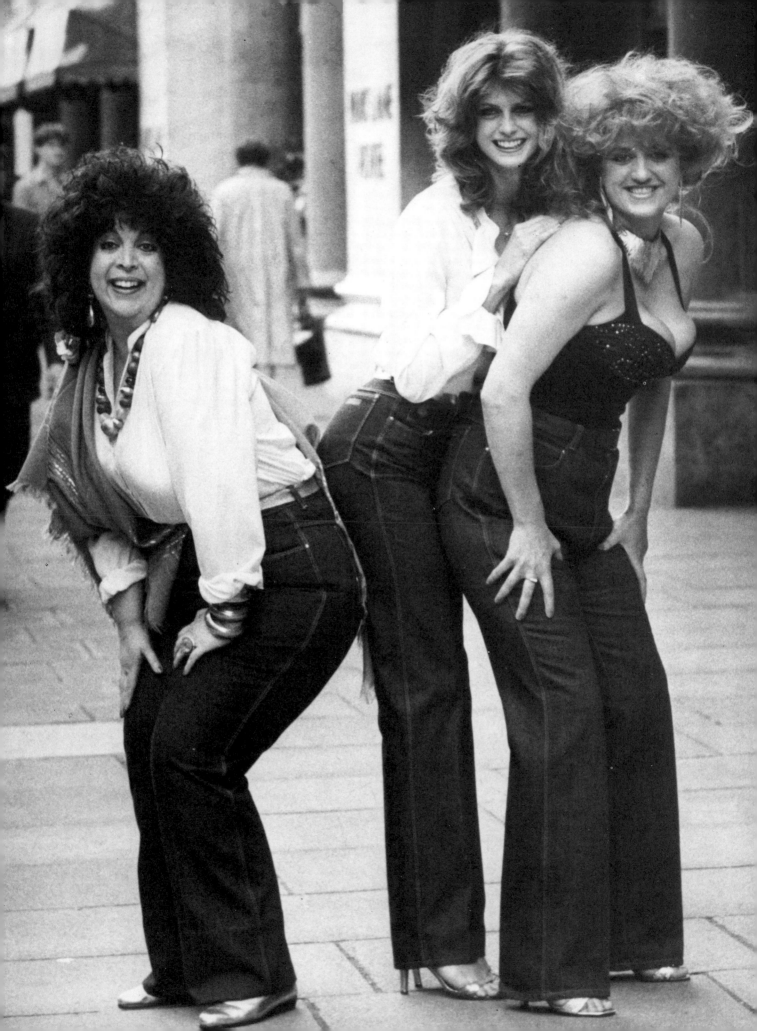

them up with a silk shirt, high heels and gorgeous jewellery, or down, with an old T-shirt and running shoes. People even wear them to the office these days. Every year we read that jeans are out, that denim is dead, and then some new style, some new way of treating the fabric, like stone-washing, comes into the shops and sales zoom. I don't think denim will ever be out, it's too useful and too comfortable. Its devotees, and that includes most people, simply won't let it die. You can now buy jeans especially cut for women in very large sizes.

Throughout my life until quite recently my weight always fluctuated so wildly that I never had the chance to wear anything until it was worn out. The first time that happened was with my much-loved jeans from Macy's. They simply fell apart, but first they went through that wonderful, soft, comfortable stage that jeans reach when they are old and have been washed hundreds of times. An old pair of jeans and a black turtle-neck sweater are still my idea of heaven – my own 'personal classics'.

Classics and designer clothes

Personal classics are those things that you keep year after year. The longer you have them the better they feel and the more you love them. Whatever new things I buy I find that every winter I go back to a favourite sweater, a perfect skirt. The brown flared brushed cotton skirt *(facing p. 168)* is what I wear when I don't know what to wear! I bought it about five years ago at Jungle Jap. It was £25. I remember the price because I thought it was a lot and I didn't buy the same skirt in black which they also had in my size. I could kill myself now that I didn't. This skirt is a perfect example of a garment that was made for a size 12 but would fit almost anyone. It has an elastic waistband and is cut so beautifully that it looks good on everyone who tries it. I've worn it with shirts and waistcoats, with my black turtle-neck sweater, and under another skirt or dress as a petticoat. I've made a calico pattern from it and copied it. When it falls apart I'll copy it again.

Separates can be incredibly versatile, but because it's easier for outsize manufacturers to turn out endless arrays of shapeless tent dresses, it can be difficult to find good separates if you're big. Most manufacturers have not yet cottoned on to the fact that we want the same kind of clothes as slimmer women have; and most outsize sweaters and shirts feature that extra bit of detailing, the stripe on the sleeve, the puffy short sleeve on a blouse, that makes them tacky. I know I keep mentioning men's clothes, but here again it makes sense to look in the men's department for simple cotton shirts and good-quality classic sweaters. Also keep an eye out for skirts with elastic waistbands. You can always make your own skirts or trousers or culottes, the kind of things that you simply cannot find in your size. Separates can look just as stunning and dressy as a dress. You can wear your blouse or sweater tucked in, or leave it out and belted as we've done in the picture of Denise on p. 124. One of my favourite summer outfits is a cream or white skirt, with a big T-shirt loosely belted over it. Here again, the accessories you choose can add your personal mark. Check out Denise's sexy little ankle boots with her tweed jacket and skirt to see what I mean.

The tweed jacket that Denise is wearing in this pic is a size 16 from a standard size mail-order catalogue. This proves two things – one, don't be afraid to try on

Modelling jeans at the launch of Gloria Vanderbilt in London, 1981, with Francis Shingler (centre) and Eve Ferret

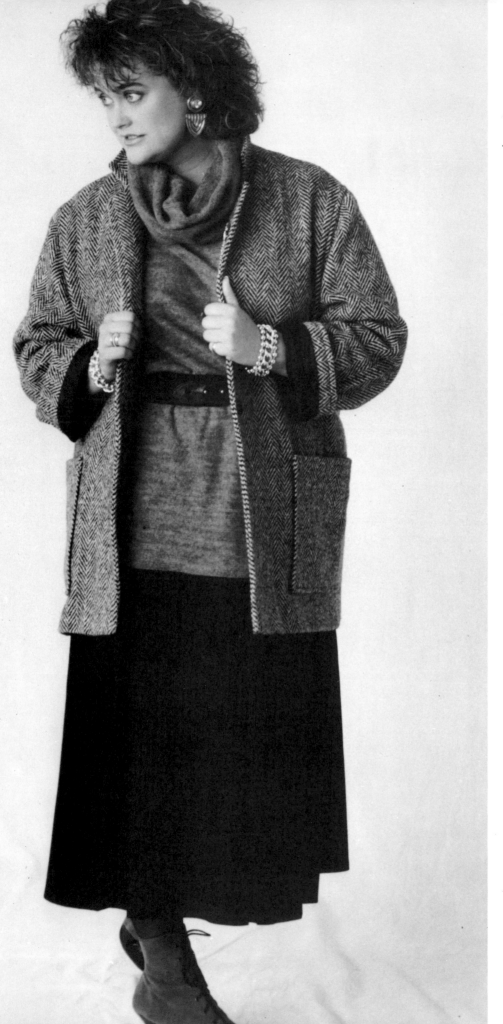

Left: Denise Smith gives this tailored black skirt and tweed jacket from a mail-order catalogue her own special sparkle with strong jewellery and sexy ankle boots

Right: Mandy Crane wears her favourite skin-tight jodhpurs with a jacket in bold checks from her own company, Gorilla Farm

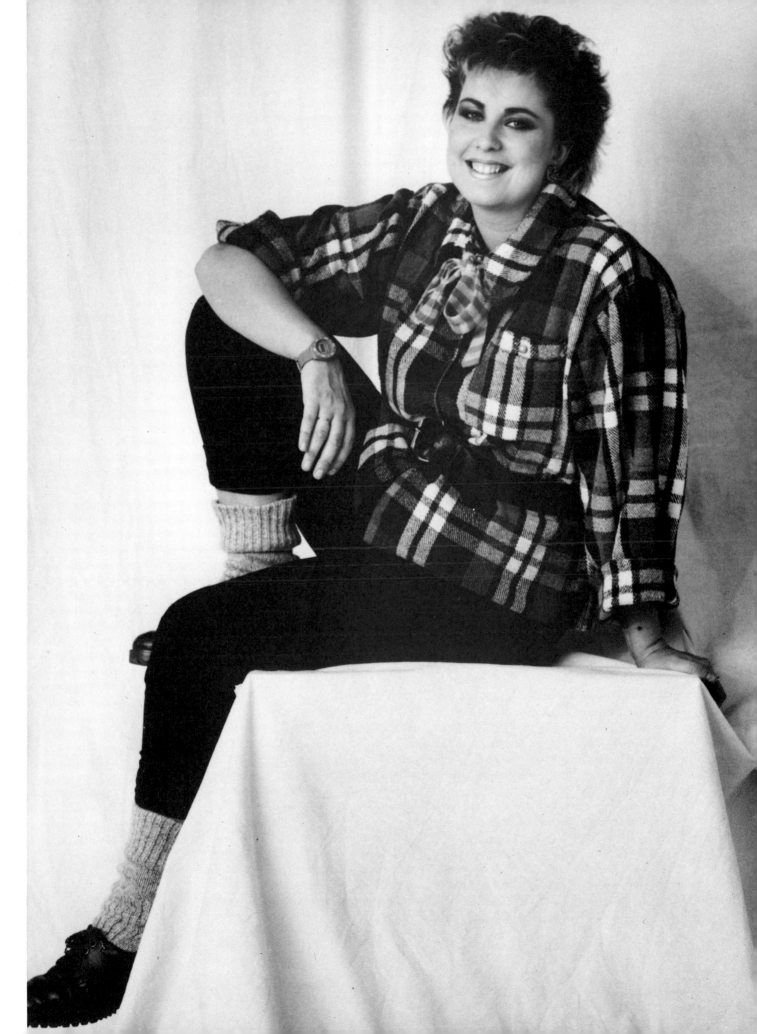

something that's smaller than your usual size. A size 16 is supposed to be for a 40 in/102 cm hip. Denise's hip measurement is 50/127 – so, so much for the size label. The other point to be made here is that mail order can be a great way to shop if you don't live near a large shopping centre, or just hate to go shopping. If, at first, a particular catalogue seems dreadful, and I'm afraid many outsize ones do, persevere and look through all the pages. Hidden away among the antiquated polyester floral smocks and iron-clad tailored suits, you can sometimes find some nice 'sportswear', a good pair of jeans, a corduroy skirt, a good-looking tracksuit. And, of course, anything you order can always be returned if it doesn't fit or you don't like it.

Elizabeth Osborne in one of my own 'personal classics', a Dorothée Bis wool smock dress c. 1976

T he Dorothée Bis black and brown check smock that Ozzie is wearing *(opposite)* is another of my favourites, and demonstrates that a smock dress needn't look baggy and shapeless. Black tights and flat black shoes complete the classic French schoolgirl look. They are also supremely comfortable. I've been wearing them since they became fashionable during my own mid-teens, when to dress like a beatnik and hang out in Greenwich Village cafés was all the rage.

All the other women featured in the book had special things that they'd had 'for ever' and that they loved to wear. By updating your shoes, your hair, your jewellery, you can make that favourite dress or sweater feel new each season.

❝ Until fairly recently my very favourite skirt was a French Connection print, a patchworky sort of thing, that I thought was the best thing in the history of clothes. It flowed, it drifted, it moved when I moved, and everyone said I looked like a three-piece suite in it. They were probably right in so far as the pattern went, but I thought it was just the bee's knees, and if it wasn't falling apart I would be wearing it now. ❞

Denise Smith

❝ I like very narrow skirts to just below the knee and a big top. The simpler the clothes are the better they look. No paisleys and absolutely no crimplenes. I usually wear flats. I walk very quickly so I'm always falling over in high heels. Last time I wore high heels I was doing a video in Los Angeles and they brought me a pair of these gold mules from Fredericks of Hollywood that had six-inch heels. Well, your leg muscles change when you don't wear heels and I needed a crane to hoist me up into them. I was so uncomfortable. It was quite funny because at first I couldn't walk in them at all, it was like having odd feet. ❞

Helen Terry

❝ I don't go for the special-occasion garment. The occasion's special enough without feeling uncomfortable because you're wearing something new. I would much rather wear something that I know I look good in and that I like and feel comfortable in. ❞

Claire Rayner

❝ I have the most incredible thing that I got a couple of years ago. It's a huge cape which is all glittery. It's green with pink stars, like a magician's cloak. I use it as my dressing-gown. I love getting home in the evening and getting into, not my jim-jams, but my cloak, the way an old-fashioned bloke would get home and put on his smoking jacket. It's wonderful. ❞

Vicki Pepys

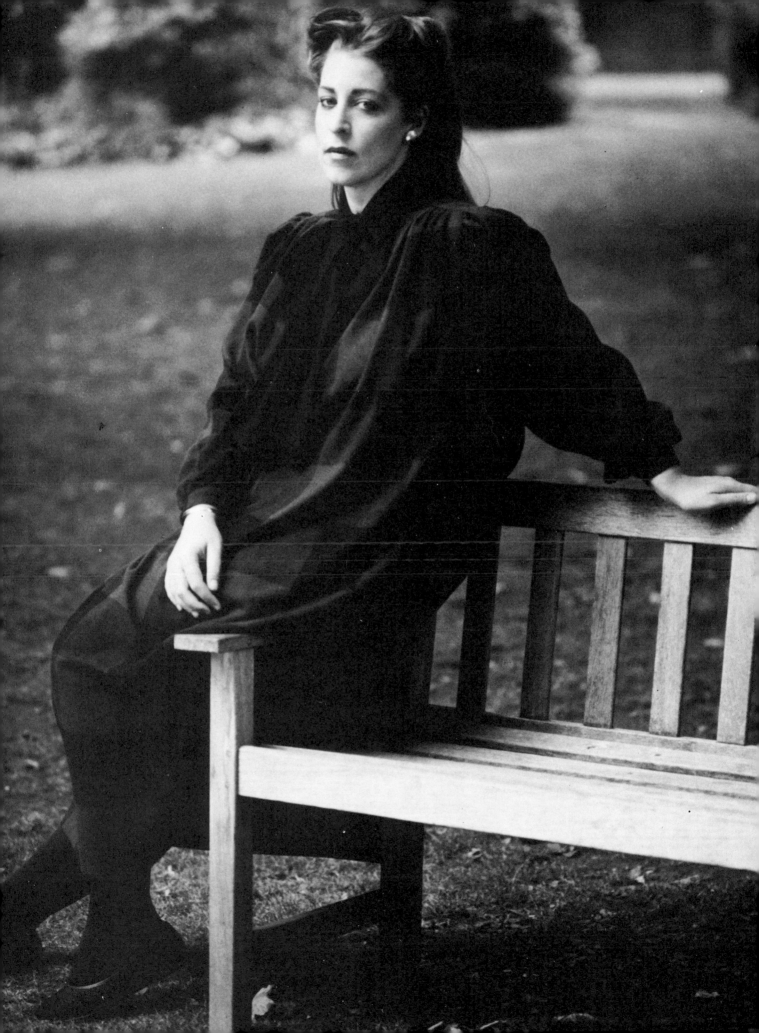

I look back at some of the 'expensive' things that I've bought over the years and they turn out to be the cheapest, simply because I've worn them so much. I then turn to my closet, which I must confess still has its share of hardly ever worn 'bargains', and it's pretty clear which things were the best value.

With that thought in mind let's turn to some more designer clothes. Good clothes, expensive clothes, are usually cut more generously than cheap ones, which tend to be skimpy. Wait for the sales and then go to the better boutiques and buy the best you can afford. You can be pleasantly surprised at what you will find to fit you. Most of the clothes in this section are several years old, some more, and they are still going strong.

The one exception is the pair of Japanese dresses that we photographed on Angela and Ozzie *(p. 130)*. The recent rise of the Japanese designers is a godsend to big women. Though a lot of the new clothes are *enormous*, they couldn't be more different from the badly cut shapeless tents that have always been pushed our way. The big, loose, flowing shapes are a return to more classical times when the drape and movement of the fabric was everything. Their ideas are filtering down to the cheaper end of the market and there has never been a better time for finding large, well-cut, interesting clothes.

One thing to remember when trying on these new bigger clothes is that if the dress or top was cut to be big on a size 12, it should also be big on you. I know that it is easier said than done, and that sometimes just to find something that goes over your head is all that you can hope for. But when big styles are 'in', and they are from time to time, try to choose things that still look big on you. There's nothing that looks worse or makes you feel more uncomfortable than something that is tight under the arms or pulling across the back.

If the big baggy look is just too much for you, you can always belt it as we've done with Ozzie's dress in our 'Japanese' picture. Incidentally, this kind of dress looks just as terrific over trousers.

We've given this outfit a medieval flavour with the flat leather sandals and loosely wrapped 'turban' made from a piece of old Japanese fabric held together with safety pins.

A good-quality coat can last you for years and is definitely one of those things that is worth splashing out on. I've already discussed my trusty trenchcoat that is now in its sixth year and still going strong. In the coat picture *(pp. 136-7)* Carole is wearing a luxurious grey flannel wraparound coat that is definitely a classic; that will, as they say, go on for ever and never date. In spite of the fact that Carole is a size 24 this coat is a size 14, as is the belted, large-shouldered, wool melton coat that Mandy is wearing. Very often good designers cut their clothes generously and you can fit into a smaller size than you would think.

The 'leopard'-lined jacket was specially made three years ago by designer Michiko Koshino, but you can get the same effect with a man's bomber jacket, either new or second-hand.

A perfect example of personal classics are the clothes that Kate Franklin chose to wear for her photographs. They are both by designer Bill Gibb and they've been in Kate's wardrobe for years. The intricately patterned knit poncho worn with the frilly white shirt and western style calf-high boots *(facing p.129)* is Kate's favourite outfit, and has been since she bought the poncho about ten years ago.

Breaking all the rules! Vicki Pepys wears horizontally striped T-shirt with army-surplus shorts. Janis Townes in shocking-pink bibbed shorts, size 12, and loose white T-shirt (one of the few garments I've ever seen where one size did really fit all!)

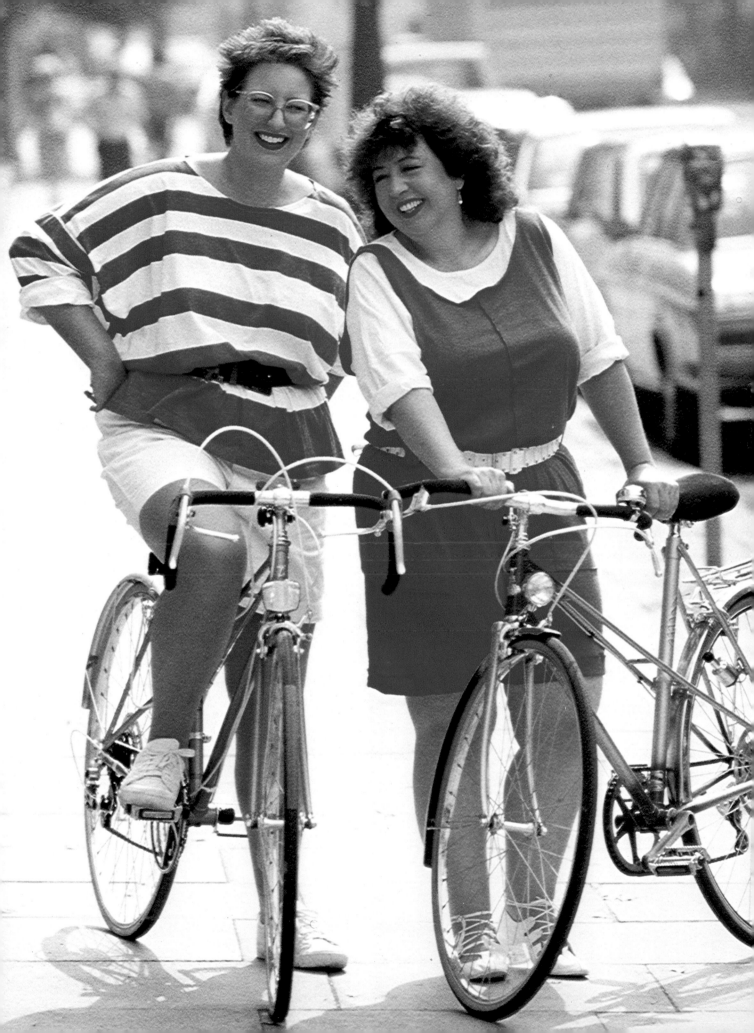

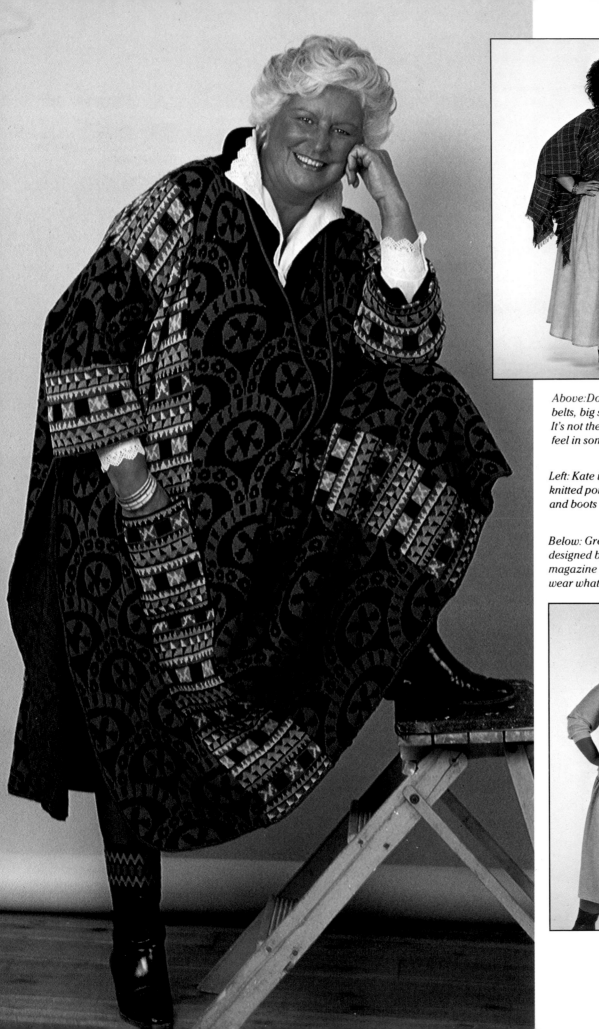

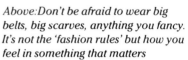

Above:Don't be afraid to wear big belts, big scarves, anything you fancy. It's not the 'fashion rules' but how you feel in something that matters

Left: Kate in her favourite outfit – knitted poncho, frilly white shirt and boots

Below: Grey sweatshirt top and skirt designed by me for Woman's Realm *magazine in 1983. 'Why shouldn't we wear what everybody else wears!'*

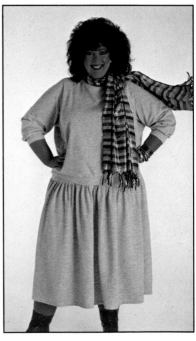

The magnificent evening dress *(facing p. 144)* in which, I think, she looks like a Grecian goddess, she bought in 1977. The pastels and creams, which emphasize her lovely silver hair, are just the kind of colours that big women too often shy away from. Dark colours may make you look marginally slimmer, but what we're talking about in this book is not looking slimmer, but looking better. When choosing clothes look for colours that make you feel good, that suit you, that emphasize the colour of your hair, your eyes. The right colour can make your face come alive, your skin look fresh and clear. If you feel you need more help with choosing colours, there are some excellent books on the market that can help. Don't be afraid to buy one or borrow it from the library. After all, you have just as much right to look terrific, to look your best, as anybody else, and wearing the right colours really makes you feel good.

The only brand-new thing in this designer section is Sue Formston's enormous black/grey/brown sweater by Joseph Tricot. I had been to Sue's house and had my usual rummage through her closets to choose what she would wear for her pictures. We had it all worked out and then on the day of the shoot, she walked into the photographer's studio wearing this sensational outfit *(p.134)*. All my plans went out the window. I knew I had to have a picture of her in this. It all worked so well, this gorgeous chunky sweater, the geometric scarf (that came, incidentally, from a different shop) and her own culottes that had been made for her by a friend. What I like particularly about this sweater-scarf combination is the mix of different patterns, the enormous squares of the sweater, picked up and accentuated by the tiny squares and stripes of the scarf. It provides an object lesson in the perfect mixing of patterns.

Accessories

Jewellery and other 'accessories' are something that all fashion writers talk about constantly. There's a good reason for that. You really can alter the look of a whole outfit just by changing the accessories. The way you use them can be the beginning of discovering how you like to look. They also provide a cheap way of trying out something new. You may love red but may not yet be ready to splash out on a red dress or sweater. A bright red scarf is a good way of trying it out in a small dose.

I am crazy about scarves, big ones. I like to take a large, square shawl, fold it into a triangle and loosely wrap it twice around my neck tying it in the front. I love wearing different patterns in complementary colours. I wear lots of browns and rusts and I'm always on the lookout for scarves in these colours. If you find a scarf you like but it's too small, you can always buy two of them and sew them together. Scarves make great belts, especially over summery, floaty clothes. Try folding a large scarf into a long rectangle and hanging it over one shoulder. Then tuck the ends under your belt for a stunning Russian Dr Zhivago look.

I first got into head-wrapping after a particularly disastrous haircut several years ago. I went around for months with my head covered up waiting for my hair to grow. That's when I became a headwrap pro. Once again, the trick here is to think big. One scarf looks flimsy and dull, two is better, but three, well, that's fabulous. You can wrap the first one tight and build on top of that. I like to twist another scarf and wrap it over the first around the hairline. You can see an

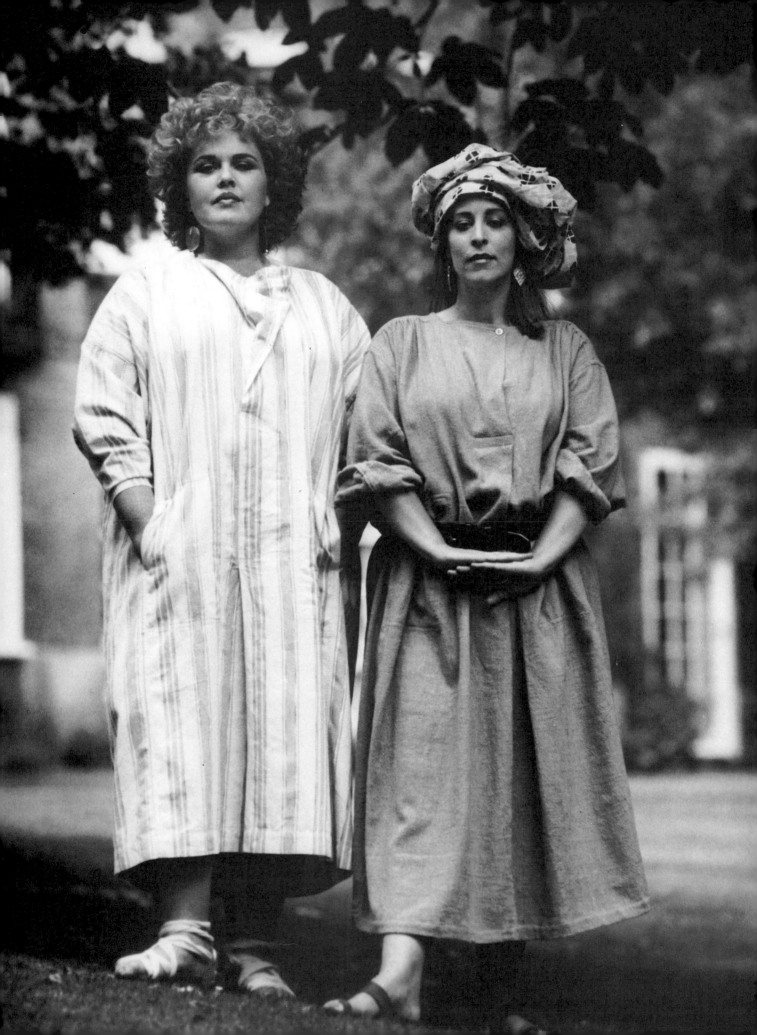

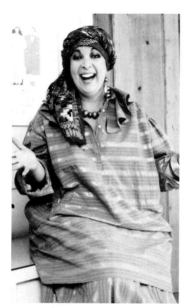

Above: A loose smock top can look great over a matching skirt, especially in a wonderful fabric like this with its horizontal gold stripes

Opposite: Recently, the Japanese designers have spearheaded the return to loose, flowing shapes. Angela Troak wears her cotton stripes free and flowing. Elizabeth Osborne loosely rolls her sleeves, lets her belt hang low and adds a strip of fabric softly wrapped into a turban for a medieval effect. Both these dresses are size 12

Below: Liz Birru in an exotic head-wrapping which is simply a large strip of fabric folded and knotted like an enormous hair ribbon

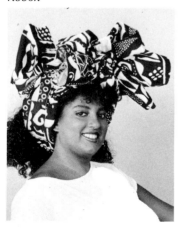

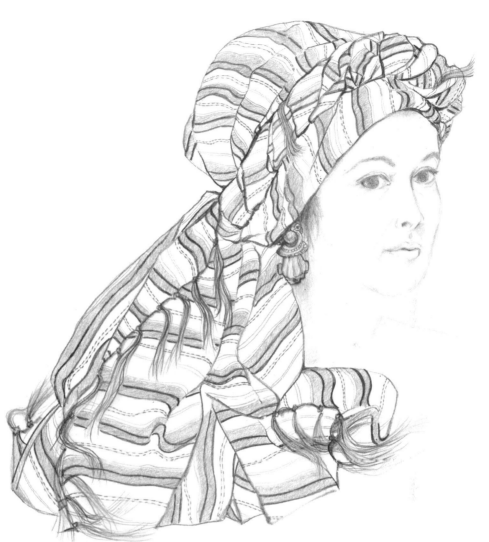

example of this double wrapping in the picture of the gold striped outfit *(above left)*. I then wound a small gold lamé scarf into the first twist and let the fringed ends hang down over my ear.

You can use a scarf to look elegant or bizarre. It can add the final finishing touch to a stunning dress or lift a simple T-shirt and shorts out of the doldrums. Any piece of fabric that you like can make a scarf. The black and white 'head-dress' that Elizabeth is wearing *(left)* is just a big square of fabric wrapped around and knotted. Here's one area where being brave and experimenting really pays off. As Louis B. Mayer said in Hollywood, 'Do it right. Do it big. Give it class!'

Some of my favourite scarves have been real cheapies that I've bought at various Woolworths, or their equivalent, on my holidays. Italian and French chain stores are particularly good for scarves. They have great patterns and colours and are surprisingly reasonable. Also look out for beach wraps known as kangas or pareos. They are big and wonderful for wrapping all of you, from your head to your whole body.

The one thing that I no longer buy cheap (with the exception of my beloved espadrilles) is shoes. I used to be a shoe freak. I bought lots of shoes, always

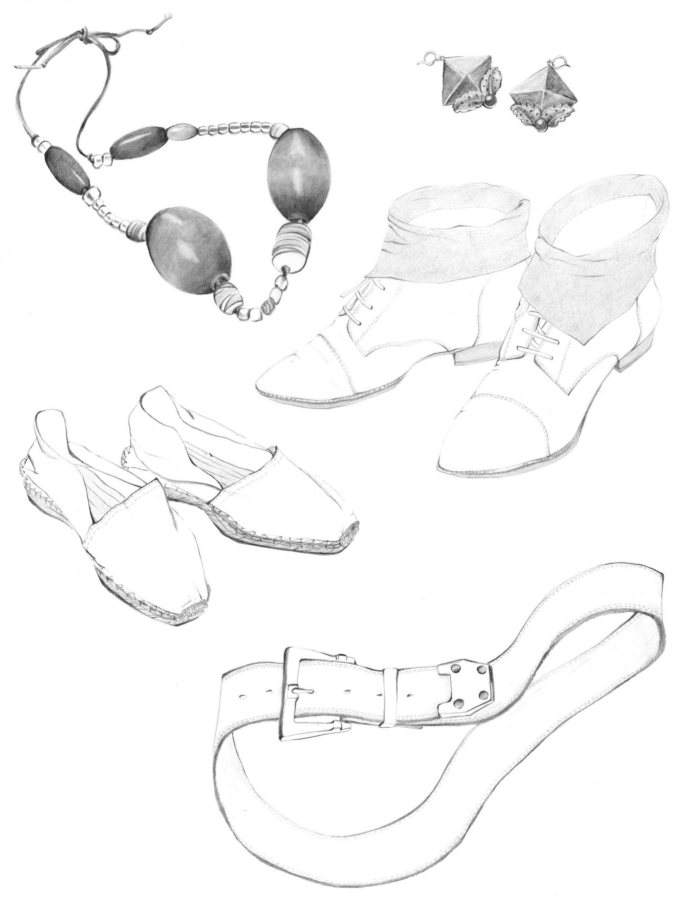

cheap. They never fitted me right and they always hurt. I found myself wearing sneakers and running shoes all the time because they felt so good. I then bought my first pair of really good boots in a sale two years ago. They were beautiful, they were Italian, and I never even dreamt that they would be comfortable as well. They were. I can walk further in them than in my sneakers. And they always make whatever I'm wearing look elegant. Since then I vowed to buy only good shoes, even if that meant buying fewer pairs. After all, my feet have a lot to carry around, I might as well treat them well.

Belts and jewellery are other investments that pay off. I love to wear belts and I think that there's hardly anyone, no matter how big, that doesn't look good in the right belt. As I always say, 'your waist is there, you just have to look for it!' Once again, big is better, when it comes to belts. I always steer clear of skinny little numbers, I don't think they really add a thing, and self-belts, belts made of the same fabric as the dress, are something else I've never gone for. My favourite belts are men's belts or big fabric cummerbunds that you can wrap around twice and tie in the front. In these pages you will see two belts over and over again. One is a man's belt that I nicked from my father when I was seventeen. The other is a heavy black belt that I bought at Biba when I first moved to London in 1969. It cost £1, which at the time wasn't cheap. It still looks good and could have been designed yesterday.

Jewellery is another area where you can play around and try things out. What I've discovered is that when I get the right bracelet or the right pair of earrings, I wear them over and over again. I prefer big jewellery on myself and on other big women. It's a question of proportion. I once asked designer Monica Chong (who is tiny herself) what she thought big women could and couldn't wear. She answered that we could wear anything as long as the proportion was right. I think this applies especially to jewellery. There's so much wonderful costume jewellery around these days, much of it big and bold, that putting together a few favourite pieces shouldn't be a problem for anyone. Don't worry about wearing the same things over and over. Designer Wendy Dagworthy, one of the most stunning women that I know, always wears an armful of bangles that run practically up to her elbow. She changes her earrings, sometimes adds a necklace, but those bangles remain. They are perfect and have become very much of a personal hallmark.

When you're choosing jewellery, try things on. I know that it can be rather intimidating. Some snazzy jewellery shops seem to expect you to buy expensive things without even touching them first, much less trying them on. But be brave and insist that they remove things from the cases and let you try. After all you're there to (possibly) spend money and there's no way you should if you don't know what something's going to look like. This applies especially with earrings which come in so many different shapes and sizes. Try *both* earrings on to make sure that they suit the shape of your face before buying.

Beware of matching sets of big jewellery, earrings that match the necklace, necklace that matches the bracelets. Too much matching stuff is boring – 'symmetry is the antithesis of style'. True style comes from the unexpected touch, the one perfect thing that makes an outfit, like the diamanté crocodile wending its way up Sue Formston's scarf in the picture on p. 134, or the leopard print scarf that Carole is wearing with her red suit *(facing p. 112)*.

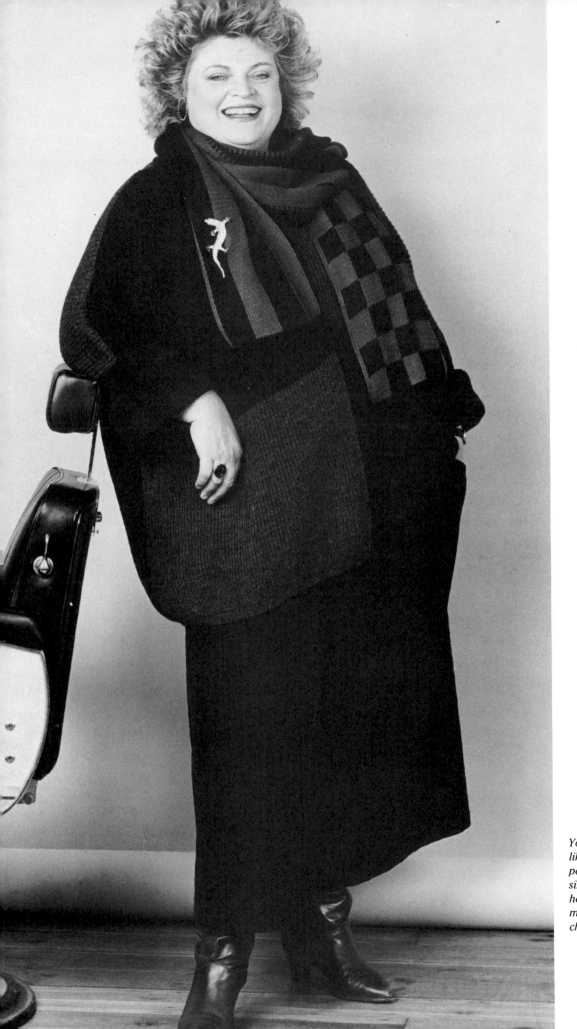

You can find marvellous things like this enormous geometrically patterned sweater in standard-size shops. Sue Formston wears it here with shiny boots and home-made culottes for a look that's chic and stunning in any size

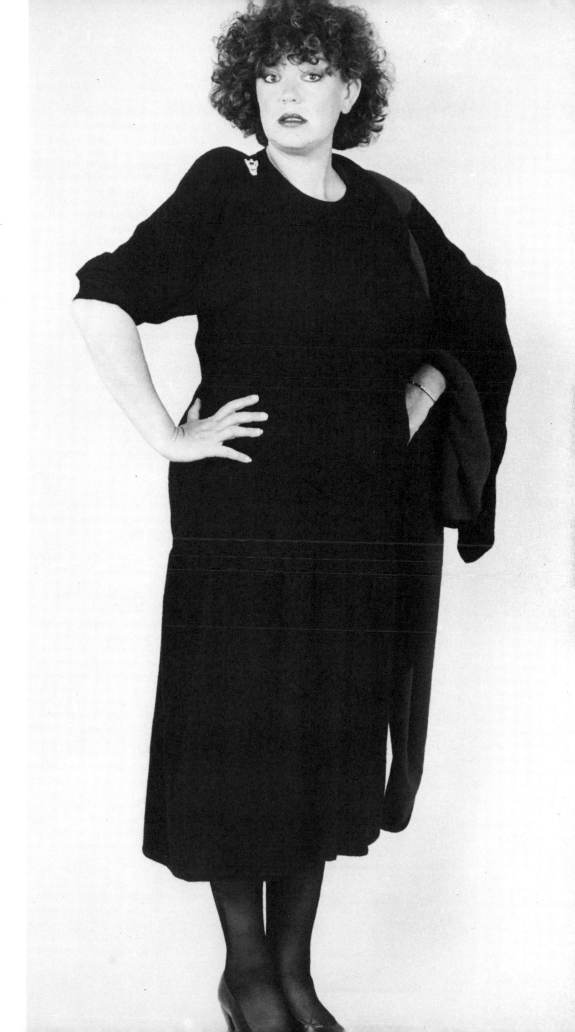

Wearing black doesn't have to mean you're hiding. Meredith Etherington-Smith's black cashmere two-piece and large shawl is sexy and dramatic

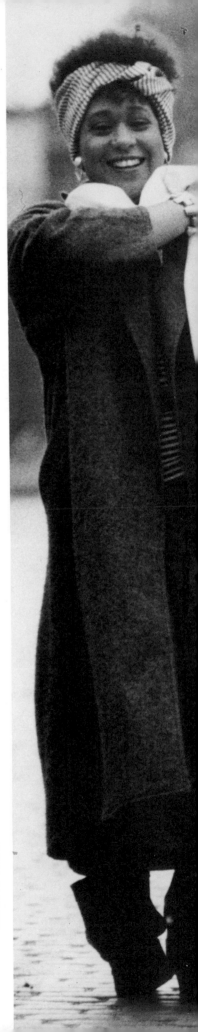

Once again, you don't have to spend a small fortune to look sensational. I buy fewer accessories now than I used to. I think that once again it's about confidence. When you know what you like, when you trust your own taste, you can buy that one really good pair of shoes, the perfect leather shoulder bag, the more expensive bit of jewellery, because you know that you'll love them and get a lot of wear out of them. For the past year, almost every time I've gotten dressed up, I've worn the same pair of silver-coloured earrings made out of dozens of tiny ball bearings. They cost £20 which I thought was a lot at the time, but I've worn them so many times that their cost now seems negligible.

> **❛ First of all, pick a colour that suits you, and buy or make an outfit in that favourite colour, something quite plain. Then accessorize it in as interesting a way as possible. Add bangles, things on the shoulders, maybe a scarf or a cardigan, then perhaps patterned tights and interesting shoes (even shoes that clash with the colour of your dress) so when people look at you they think, 'What an interesting person, *and* there's a lot of her, so she must be *very* interesting! I must go and talk to her!' ❜**
>
> *Vicki Pepys*

Outsize shops

I thought long and hard about what outsize shops to include in this book. Should I have a list of sources at the back of the book, and include all the shops, all the mail-order catalogues, all the possibilities? I was in the midst of accumulating a list when I had a phone call from a friend. 'Where', she asked me, 'can I take a friend, who has never been to London, to buy some clothes? She is very big and she has great taste and only wants to buy really terrific things.'

I realized then that when faced with the reality of someone without a lot of time to waste running around, there weren't many places that I could advise her to go. If she had all the time in the world she could have gone to the obvious outsize chains and the outsize departments of the London department stores, in the hope of finding that one good-looking thing that does occasionally slip on to their rails. But this woman was a tourist here without the time or the inclination to go on an endless pilgrimage.

It made me realize anew how bleak the situation is, even in a large, cosmopolitan city like London. Of course there are exceptions and it's always worth having a look at each new outsize shop that opens. Even within one shop there can be a tremendous variety of merchandise, some dreadful, some much better. But the general feeling among the women I interviewed is that they only go into an outsize shop 'under duress' – if they need something they cannot get anywhere else, like underwear, trousers, or bathing suits.

> **❛ Outsize clothes really are dreadful. They are the dregs of fashion in terms of style, colour and fabric. It's because it's assumed that the people who wear those beastly things are decrepit and totally ignorant and they never go out of the house. ❜**
>
> *Joanne Brogden*

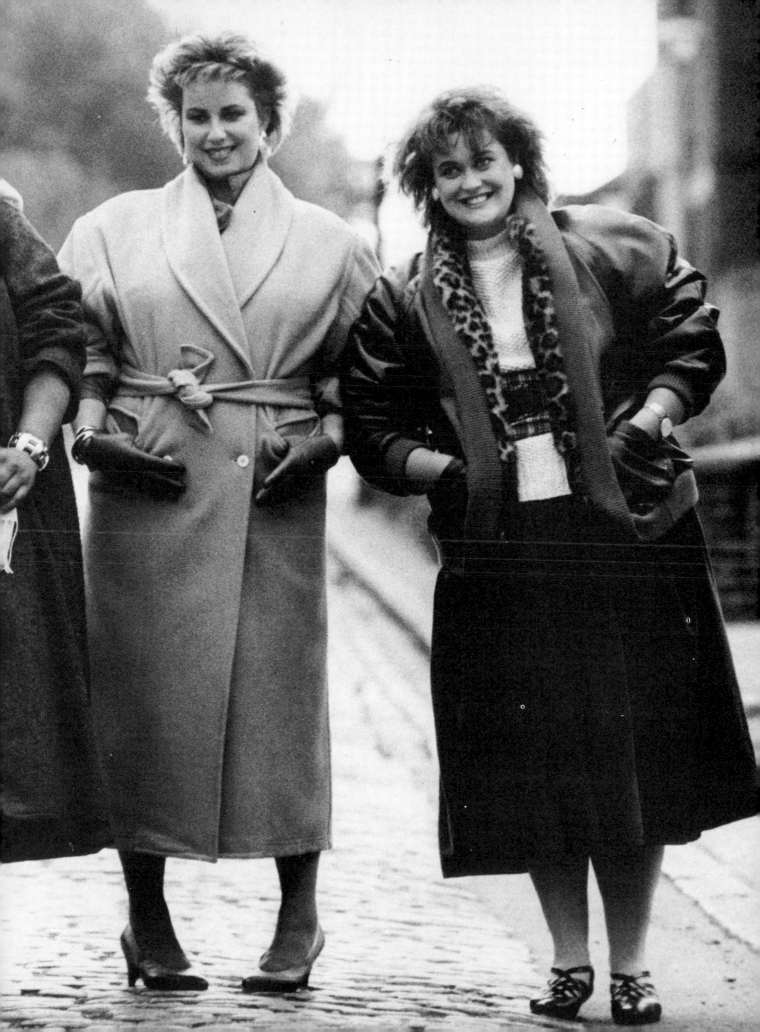

> ⁶ If you look at the fashion landscape, it stops short with a great crevasse between the size 14s and the rest of the countryside, which is uncharted territory. People simply do not think about it. They don't put it into their plans. Large ladies are deeply underprivileged. It just isn't fair, and it's stupid, old-fashioned thinking, because women have got larger over the last hundred years but the minds in the fashion business haven't. It's not a lack of clientele; there are certainly the customers out there. It's a lack of brave spirits actually prepared to say, 'Right, I'm going to open a shop for large ladies.' ⁹
>
> *Meredith Etherington-Smith*
>
> ⁶ I hate the material, I hate the cut, they're never long enough and they're always ghastly. Twice I've been in an outsize shop and both times I got stopped by people asking where I got what I was wearing. Much to the displeasure of the assistants I answered, 'Well, I never buy anything here!' ⁹   *Sue Formston*

Previous page: Two coats and a jacket that prove you don't have to settle for the powder-blue tent of your local outsize shop. From the left: Carole Burton, Mandy Crane and Denise Smith

There seems to be some indication that people are slowly waking up to the vast potential of the outsize market and new companies, mail-order and retail, do spring up all the time. Unfortunately, they also disappear. I think this may be for two reasons. The first is that the kind of clothes that they are doing simply do not fill our needs. The second is that sometimes we don't even know that they exist. A woman came to one of the first meetings that I had to plan this book. I had never met her before. She came in the most wonderful red sweatshirt with a big cowl neckline. It was really big and loose and well-cut. 'Where on earth did you get that?' I asked. 'Diana Clothes,' she answered. I had never heard of them, nor had any of the other seven women who were seated around my kitchen table that night.

By the time that I called the office of Diana Clothes the next week they were out of business. The reason given to me by the sad owner was cash-flow problems. It seemed to me that cash-flow problems were inevitable if no one knows you are there. We must put more pressure on fashion editors and let them know that we want to know what's available in our size. Only if new companies are given publicity can we find out that they exist and lend them our support.

The few outsize garments that I have included are here because they are fabulous, in any size; they are not just the best of a bad lot. The mere fact that such things do exist makes it even more annoying that there aren't more of them.

Carole fell so much in love with the red suit that I photographed her in *(facing p. 112)*, that she just had to buy it. The same goes for Denise's white boiler suit in the photograph on p. 141.

The brown satin dress that Angela is wearing *(facing p. 144)* is studded with large bronze sequins and is exactly the type of sophisticated, luxurious evening dress that is usually so hard to find in our size.

The grey-and-white striped cotton dress that Elizabeth is wearing as she lounges on the garden steps with Vicki *(opposite)* is cool and floaty. It's wonderful to wear loose over a bathing suit or white cotton trousers, but here we've belted it and added a grey linen waistcoat to give it a sharper, more tailored, city look.

With a little imagination you can sometimes find uses for a garment that the designer may never have intended. The ruffled summer party dress that Kathy is

Stripes, whether vertical or horizontal, look cool and crisp on a hot summer day. Elizabeth's tent dress from an outsize shop is belted and 'waistcoated' for a tailored effect (left). Vicki (right) drapes her Betty Jackson drop-waisted peach and white stripes with her favourite 'cheap coral'

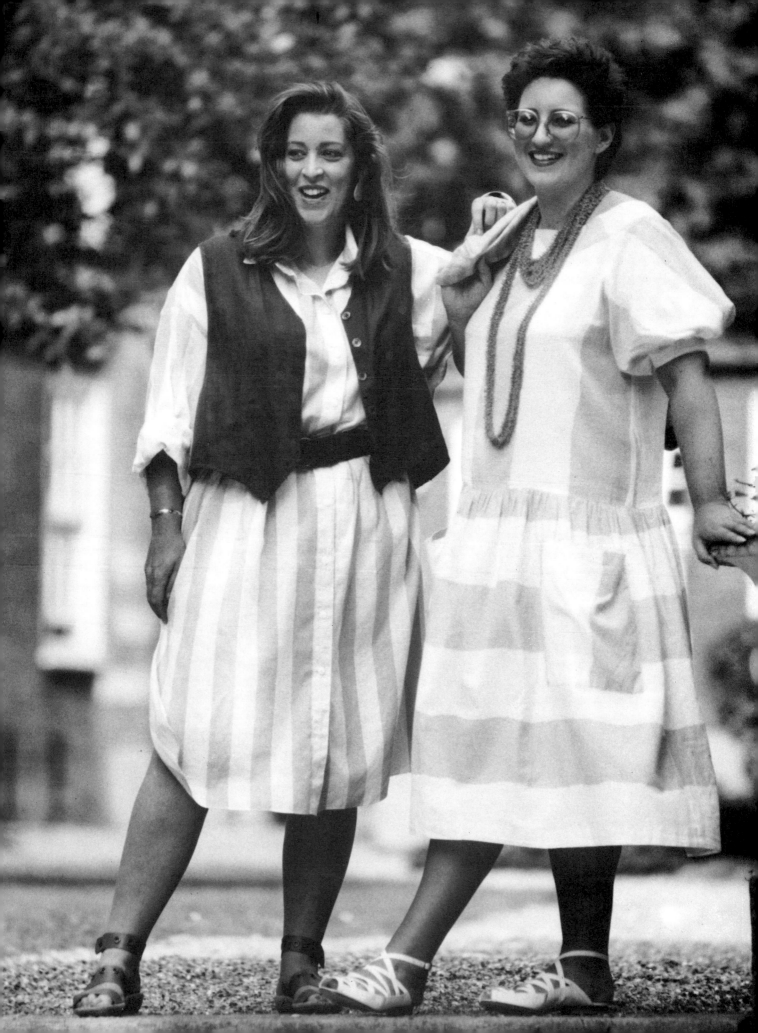

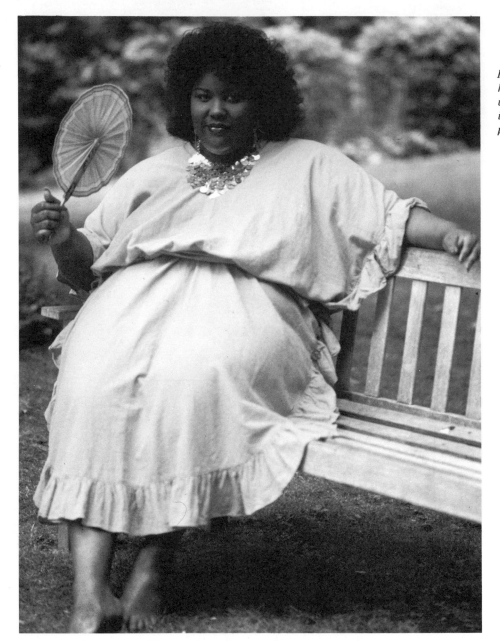

wearing *(above)* is really a rather shapeless cotton housecoat from an outsize shop, in a stunning shade of bright turquoise. By belting it, blousing it up over the belt and adding some exotic brass jewellery, we've turned it into something much sexier.

Shopping

If you are not satisfied by the latest offerings of your local shop featuring 'fashions for the fuller figure' then what? The answer is to go to any shop selling 'normal' clothes. I know it can be difficult, even humiliating, to confront the stares of saleswomen who obviously think you're out of your mind even to walk through the doors, but that is something we must overcome. Sometimes it can be easier to go shopping with a friend. You can give each other moral support and encouragement, and having an ally along can give you the confidence to try things on that you might never have dreamed of.

> **❛ You've got to be prepared to pay a bit more. People who are a size 10 can find cheap things that are reduced. Well, you just don't get that in big sizes. Anything half-way good goes straight away – that's if it's there in the first place. ❜**
> *Denise Smith*

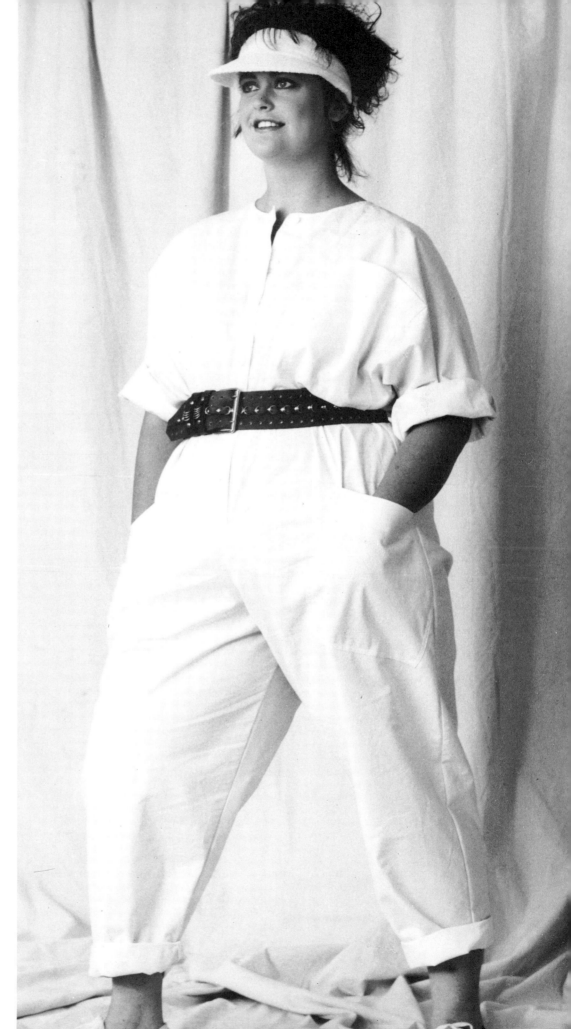

Don't listen to anyone who tells you there are things you mustn't wear if you're large. Denise's hips measure 50 in/127 cm, yet you'd have to go a long way to find someone who'd look as good in this white boiler suit as she does

Overleaf: Liz Birru wears her own cotton jersey drawstring-waisted dress from a standard-size shop. Proof that it pays to try things on no matter what the size label says.

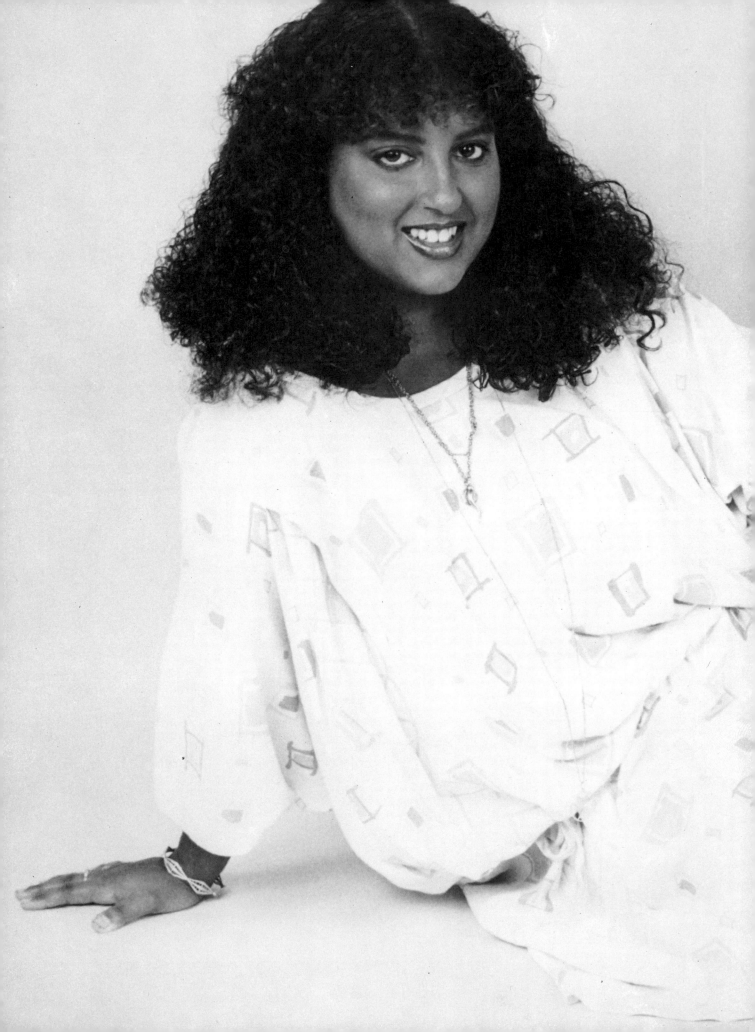

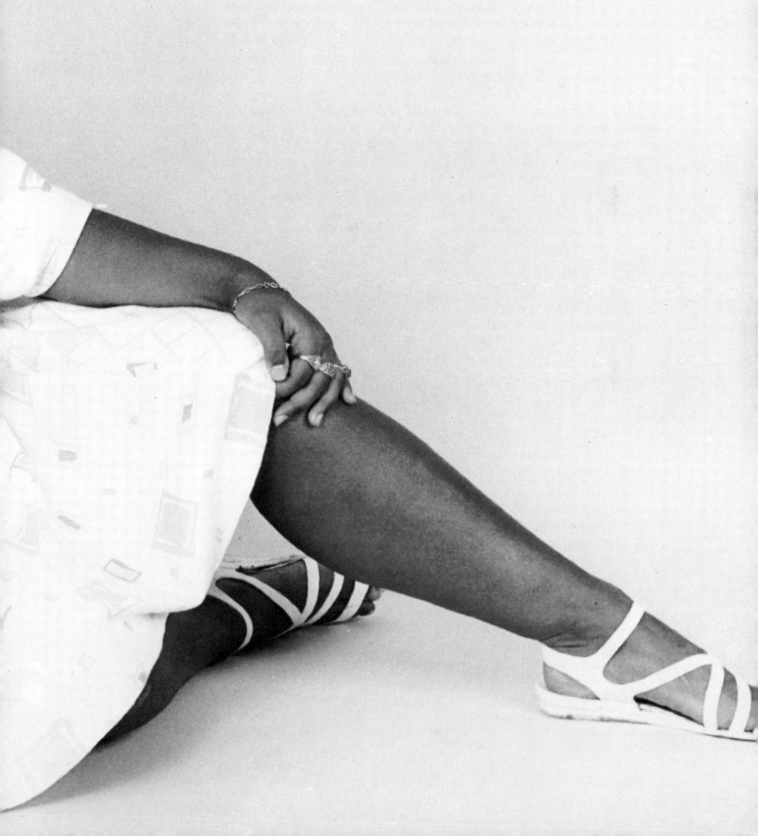

❧ You have to look in places where you wouldn't normally look. Don't ask, 'Have you got it in my size?' because they'll always say no. Then you'll look yourself and find a size 12 dress which measures 60 inches round the bust, but they haven't told you about that.

I don't like trying things on in shops, I prefer to take things home and try them there. So I always take a tape measure with me when I'm shopping. I can then measure the hips and the bust of whatever it is that I like and then I take a chance. I always make sure it's something I could exchange or have a credit note for. ❧
Sue Formston

❧ I never go out looking for a particular something. But I'm always on the lookout for something that's 'me'. If I see it I get it there and then. I think you have to have a special little purse where you put your bits of money, so that you always have some cash available, because if you see something, you've got to grab it; you may never see it again. ❧
Janis Townes

❧ It is most important *not* to go looking for a particular size. If you shop around there are loads of manufacturers, mainly continental, where size doesn't enter into it. I sold an Italian dress that was a size 14 recently to a woman who is a size 22. She looked gorgeous and walked out of the shop six feet above the ground. Don't apologize for yourself when you are shopping. Don't say to the saleswoman, 'I'm sorry but I don't suppose you have anything in a size 20.' Why should we apologize for ourselves? Be positive when you shop. And don't be afraid to try on, and don't listen when they say they only go up to a size whatever, just go and look for yourself. Be determined! ❧
Angela Troak

I feel that most of you reading this book could probably write this section yourselves. As big women we are all used to having to look for that one dress that's cut just a bit bigger. We check armholes, the width across the bust, the hips, the length. I've reached the point at the age of thirty-eight, where I can really tell, just by holding something up, if it will span my hips, my own danger point. What I can't tell, however hard I look at something on the hanger, is how it will look on me. Sue Formston says she never tries things on in the shop, but just makes sure she can bring it back if it's not right. This is a solution if you absolutely cannot bear to try things on while you shop, but I would suggest that if you can, you should summon up your courage and try. On one of the first TV programmes I ever did about finding clothes for big women, one of my 'models' said she'd always wanted jeans but had never been able to find them. I came into the studio for our dress rehearsal with four or five different pairs for her to try. The first three pairs were too big. 'I thought you told me you couldn't find jeans,' I asked her. 'Well, I never really tried them on before,' she admitted.

It's essential that you do try things on whenever possible. Don't just think of yourself as a 'big' woman and therefore assume that anything that's big enough to go around you is OK. We all have different shapes. We get big in different ways, and a certain style may fit both you and me, but look great on you, awful on me. There is just as much variety in what suits us and what doesn't as there is for slimmer women.

Opposite above: Angela Troak's brown satin evening dress peppered with sequins – big can be sleek, elegant, sophisticated

Opposite below: Kate Franklin ethereal in softly falling pastel chiffon

Opposite right: Jan Murphy – men's pyjamas and dressing-gown, dressed up with heels and sprinklings of diamanté jewellery make great party wear

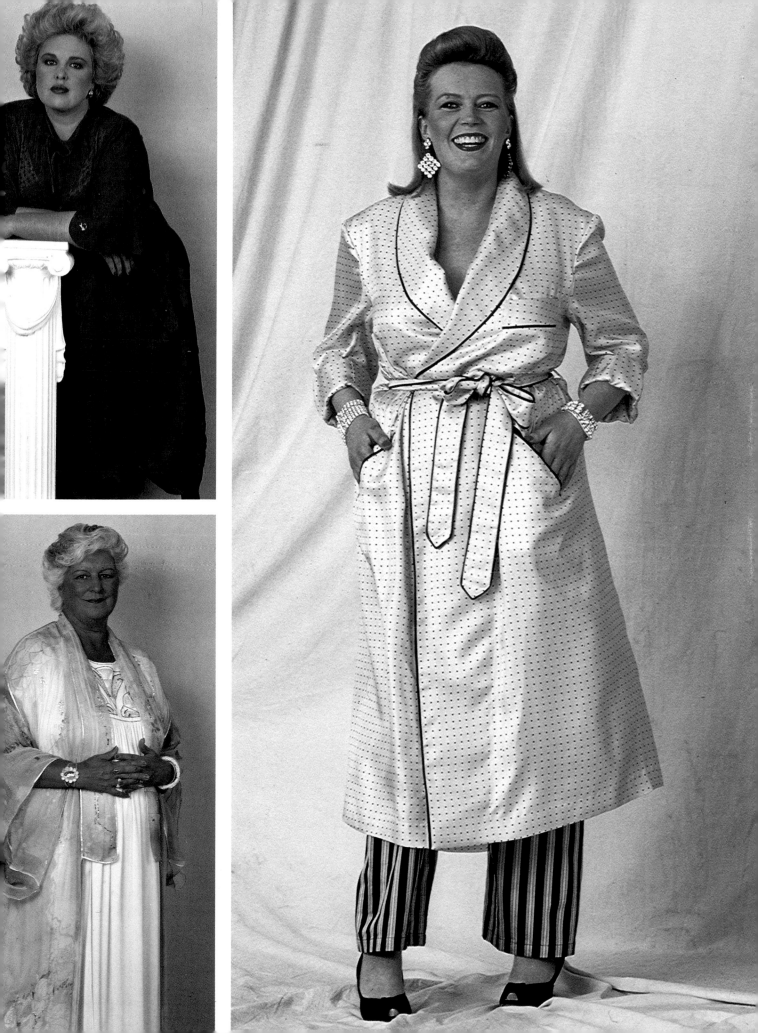

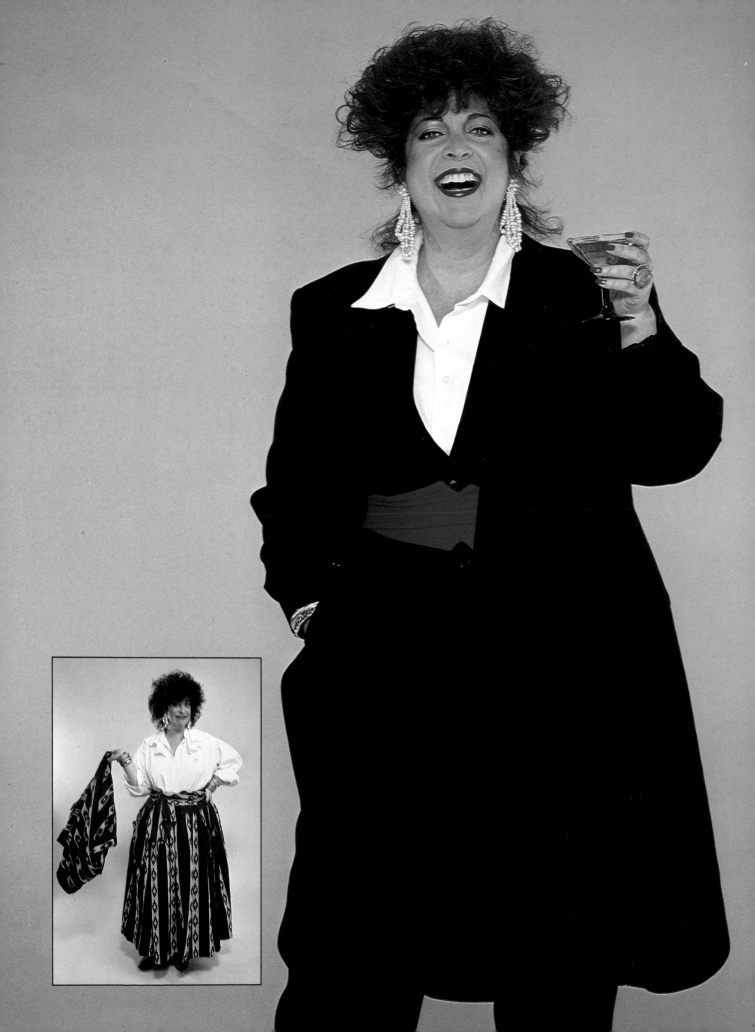

Angela Troak came to my flat in London for her try-on session. She brought so many beautiful things with her that I just had to try them. One of them was a long black linen dress cut like a man's nightshirt. 'I hate that on me,' she said, 'I think it looks dreadful!' I tried it on – I loved it. 'You can have it' she offered. I then looked through my own closet and came out with a dress that I had had for two years and never worn. It was beautiful but it made me look busty and matronly. Angela tried it on. It was sensational. Many people would look at us and think we are the same size. We may be, but we are certainly not built the same way; Angela's smaller bust and wider shoulders gave this dress a completely different shape, and she and it looked terrific. The moral of this story is always try things on first. Don't be afraid to try something on that's unlike anything you've had before. You may be pleasantly surprised.

A last word about size labels – if you go around thinking 'I'm a 22 and I'm never going to try anything on that's smaller', you'll severely limit your choice. The pink shorts that Janis is wearing as she prepares to conquer the city streets on her bicycle *(facing p. 128)* are actually a size 12. It's just as silly to be put off buying something because the label says it's bigger than you're used to. So what if it's a 26. All that matters is that it fits you, is comfortable, and that you like it. After years of buying my clothes too small, it's such a relief to actually have them fit me properly. Now when I'm buying things, trousers and jeans in particular, if I'm between sizes I always opt for the bigger. Then I don't have the constant worry about things shrinking in the wash and I'm more comfortable to boot.

> ❝ For me wearing nice clothes is incredibly important. It says who I am. One of the best things people can say to me is, 'You always look nice.' I don't think they realize it's because I'm very careful about the things I wear. I would never wear anything that's too tight. I think that's a mistake a lot of big women make, wearing things too small. It makes them look twice as big when they wear something that doesn't fit them. I wish women would have the confidence to say, 'OK, I'm a size 26, and I'm going to wear this, *and* it's going to look good.' ❞
>
> *Carole Burton*

Problem-solving

There are certain problems that have come up again and again in these interviews; the difficulty of finding good underwear was one. Decent bathing suits that don't make us look like an armoured tank are another.

Second-hand man's tailcoat and trousers worn with glitzy earrings and bright red cummerbund – the man's tuxedo I'd always longed for

Inset: A winner for summer evenings – long Ikat patterned skirt made even more glamorous by its matching scarf – an easy-to-copy idea for home dressmakers.

> ❝ I have a problem with knickers/underpants. I don't want unattractive knickers, but I'm stuck with them. One day they'll realize that you can be fifty inches around the hips and have pretty knickers, but not yet. ❞   *Denise Smith*
>
> ❝ One thing they never get right is proportion. Things are wider but not longer. Tights go around my hips but don't reach my crotch. All these things just take a bit of sense to work out. ❞   *Elizabeth Osborne*

> ❛ It's very hard to find good trousers for large ladies, so pregnancy trousers are the ones I usually buy. They're very easy over the stomach and then they go in nice and close over the legs.
>
> I do buy larger-size bathing suits, but I take out those hard-pointed little pads. You just cut those out and you're well away. ❜   *Kate Franklin*

As I hope you have realized by now, I don't believe in rules where clothes are concerned. What you like and feel good in is what you should wear. There is only one garment that I feel strongly enough about to actually lay down a rule. That is the bra. I have seen so many big women ruin a perfectly wonderful dress or sweater by wearing a bra underneath that is too small. I know it's virtually impossible to find gorgeous bras in big sizes, but this is one area where I feel that compromise *is* necessary. I long ago gave up looking for pretty bras, and decided to opt instead for ones that fit. They do tend to look rather surgical and colour choice is usually limited to black and white, sometimes beige if you're lucky, but at least they fit and eliminate the awful 'four-tit' syndrome. You know the kind of thing I mean – two breasts in the bra and two above it. I think it's better to wear no bra at all than to look like this. If you want to wear sexy underwear for private moments in the bedroom, then by all means do, but always have at least one good, well-fitting, albeit ugly bra to wear under clothes that cling. You'll be amazed at the difference it makes.

Another purely physical problem that I've had to deal with through the years is 'thigh-rub'. This is the sore, sometimes agonizing, condition that results when two heavy thighs rub up against each other with each step. It is for me a seasonal condition, brought about by hot summer days and the absence of tights. It was even more terrible during the days when we all wore stockings and the top of my thighs bulged out over the tight stocking tops. But then, I wore a garment called Chafe-eze, a kind of strip of silky fabric that covered the area between the tops of your stockings and the bottom of your underpants. The widespread adoption of tights saw the sad demise of Chafe-eze. Thigh-rub is a rather embarrassing problem and one that I thought only applied to big women. Then, several years ago, on a very hot day, I happened to be taking a train trip with a thin friend. We were sitting in a rather secluded section of the railway carriage, when she withdrew a small container of Johnson's baby powder from her handbag. She glanced furtively around the car, hiked up her skirt and, sprinkling her inner thighs liberally, sighed with relief. 'What are you doing?' I whispered in amazement. 'Thigh-rub,' she answered, 'I always get it in this weather.'

Realizing that this thin friend also suffered from what I had hitherto considered to be one of the awful humiliations of being fat was strangely liberating. I set out to tackle it, and not allow myself to suffer any more of its discomfort. The things that cause it the worst are tights that don't fit properly and bare thighs in hot weather. Always make sure that your tights are long enough so that the seams which connect the legs and the gusset don't hang down between your thighs and rub. As far as bare thighs are concerned, I try to avoid them, especially if I've got a lot of walking to do and it's hot. In the summer I am most comfortable in light white cotton trousers which I wear under practically everything, T-shirts for lazing around in, belted Victorian nighties for parties, and big, loose dresses like the one Ozzie is wearing on p. 127, or even under the Wendy Dagworthy outfit on p. 90.

Thigh-rub can be at its most annoying at the beach. In the water it's fine, and when I've had a chance to dry it's fine. It's that awful period when you're damp and salty and sandy that causes the trouble. This used to be particularly bad when I had to walk home to my parents' house, which is only a couple of minutes from the beach. But that two-block walk in the scorching summer heat could be agony. Then, last summer I found the solution. I began to wear my white cotton trousers over my bathing suit and under whatever beachcoat, shirt or caftan I have on. For those of you who are used to changing into your swimming clothes at the beach, this may not sound very earth-shattering. For me, however, it was an important landmark in my struggle to come to terms with my size. The reason was simple. On Fire Island everybody goes directly from their house to the beach wearing only their bathing suits. For me to appear on the beach wearing my trousers and actually disrobe there was rather unorthodox, and set me apart, in my own mind, from everyone else. But I was, at last, comfortable. No more thigh-rub, no more chafing, just cool airy cotton where once there was pain.

This is a pretty good general principle to follow; look for comfort above all else, and to hell with what anyone else thinks. Feeling good and being mobile in your clothes are the most important things.

> ❛ The place where you think you'll be at your most uncomfortable is on the beach, with everybody else topless and thin. It *can* be a bit embarrassing sitting up and playing cards for hours on end with everything you've got bulging out, but nobody's really looking. They're all wondering, 'Who's going to win this card game?' They are not thinking, 'Oh, look how fat Vicki is.'
>
> I felt fine on the beach this year. I actually went topless…when I was lying down! And I love the water, I always feel so graceful and wonderful. Luckily I'm quite a strong swimmer, so rather than sit on the beach all the time, I learned to do a bit of synchronized swimming.
>
> There are always those days when you think 'I'm so fat, I can't go out', but nobody's looking at you, they couldn't care less really. Mostly it's a thing that's in your mind. As long as you don't go up and punch them on the nose, they're not going to take a blind bit of notice of you. ❜   *Vicki Pepys*

Thigh-rub is not the only problem I've had with my legs. Many big women with heavy thighs have calves that taper gracefully to end in ankles as slim and delicately formed as those of any slim woman. Not me. My problem doesn't stop at my thighs but continues on down the full length of my legs to take in my knees, my calves and my ankles. Even when I was skinny, the legs were not.

Most women dread walking by a construction site. I never worried that the catcalls and whistles would taunt me because I was *fat*, but only because I had such enormous legs. As a teenager I used to come home from school every day on the Fifth Avenue bus. I can remember getting off the bus one afternoon, I must have been around fifteen, and as I crossed Fifth Avenue on 88th Street a delivery boy who was be-bopping his way down the street with a carton of groceries looked up and saw me coming. He stopped dead in his tracks and yelped at the top of his lungs, 'Whooo…look at those fat legs, mama!' I was absolutely crushed. I walked the rest of the way home in a red daze of embarrassment. I still can't cross that corner in front of the Guggenheim Museum at 88th Street and Fifth Avenue without seeing that boy and hearing his remark.

When I was a teenager I even went to a new diet doctor who specialized in getting the weight off a particular 'problem area'. He sat me on his examining table in a flimsy little white robe, looked hard at my legs, and said yes, he could see the problem, but there was nothing he could do for me until I dieted some more, and got my weight to well below the 'average' for my height. Only then would he be able to start a course of injections directly into my legs that would 'melt the fat away'. I never did manage to get as thin as he wanted me to be, but his promise and the hope he held out to me sustained me for a long time. It kept me going just to know that when I did get thin enough this man could then, as if by magic, inject away my legs.

Remembering this incident now emphasizes how much my own views have changed in the last twenty years. There has been a lot of TV coverage lately about new methods of sucking fat out of the body. These documentaries inevitably feature the latest miracle surgeon who can overnight reduce the size of a woman's behind, or her thighs, by one barbaric method or another. It's not so different from what the doctor in New York promised me so long ago, but now when I see the terrible things that are done to women's bodies in the name of thinness and in the pursuit of beauty it makes me furious.

I was living in Italy in the early sixties when tall leather boots for women first became fashionable. Until then I had always worn either big floppy rubber wellingtons, or fur-lined storm boots, both of which slid on over shoes and were therefore wide at the top. I had, therefore, in spite of my big calves, never encountered the problem of boot buying that was to become such a nuisance in later years. I've already mentioned that I used to be somewhat of a shoe freak, and living in Italy was the perfect place to indulge that passion. I was eighteen years old and had spent the summer studying Italian in the small city of Perugia. One of the great pleasures of my time there was the shoes. They were beautiful and they were incredibly cheap by New York standards. Throughout the summer months my friend Mila and I paid regular visits to all the local shoe shops, whose window displays and merchandise changed constantly. But now it was autumn and a new phenomenon appeared in the display cases – boots that were shoes as well. They were tall and they were skinny and every shop had them. Mila couldn't wait to try them on.

We sat in the shop and waited to be served. When the young Italian salesgirl came over to help us we all three went outside into the cold and looked through the frosty glass at the lighted display. Mila pointed to a particularly spectacular pair of black boots. Back inside the shop a large box was produced, and from it Mila carefully removed the most beautiful boots I've ever seen. They were black glove leather with a long zip up the side and a little cuff of black fur around the top. Mila slipped her foot into one of them and zipped it right up; it came to just underneath her knee. The salesgirl looked at me and asked, 'Anything for you, *signorina*?' I didn't dare say that I wanted to try the same boots on, because I knew and she knew that they wouldn't fit. We went outside again and looked in

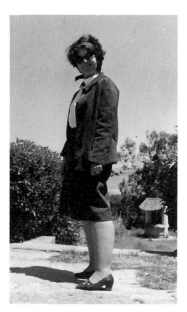

Looking back at this picture of myself at age eighteen, when I was living in Italy, my legs don't seem all that fat! But I couldn't find any high boots to fit me

the window and I pointed at a very pretty pair of ankle boots, black suede with two tiny buttons on each side.

I bought my boots and Mila bought her boots, and I felt terrible. I somehow knew that Mila's boots were just the beginning. I could tell that this was a fashion that was here to stay, it wasn't just a flash in the pan. I could also tell that these new tall boots were never going to fit me. We went through that winter hobbling around on the cobblestones, me in my short black suede, Mila in her tall black fur trimmed leather.

Several years later, when I was back home in New York, I was reading the *New York Times* one day when I saw a small line drawing of a pair of boots. Even in the drawing you could tell that these boots were big. Over the drawing were the enticing words 'all types of boots with extra wide tops'.

I dragged my mother with me for moral support and we headed down to West 35th Street. There it was, Treemark Shoes. We stopped to look in the windows before venturing inside; across the back were boots of every shape and description, tall boots and short boots, suede and leather and patent. And the same way that I had known immediately that Mila's boots would never fit me, I now knew, standing in the rain on West 35th Street, that these boots would.

So we went in. It was like arriving at some rather surreal cocktail party. The place was full of enormous women, surrounded by piles of cardboard shoe boxes. They were being served by sweating, shirt-sleeved New York salesmen, who maintained a constant line in joky chat.

Now there are no shoe salesmen in the world like those in New York. They have no pretence of being fancy or chic or smart. They know what they want to sell you and if you know what's good for you, you buy it!

My own salesman asked me my size; then, without even waiting to hear what I wanted, disappeared, screaming back over his shoulder 'I've got just the thing for you.' He reappeared a couple of minutes later with a huge stack of boxes. He plonked them down on the floor in front of me, sat himself down on a little stool, and proceeded to do battle with my calves. Together, between the two of us, we huffed and puffed and stretched and pulled and tugged and eased and cajoled until one pair of boots were made to, I wouldn't exactly say slide, more like crawl, up my leg. The trick at Treemark was that a lot of their boots were elasticized so that they would fit almost anyone. Now my own legs are particularly big and, although I do have several pairs of boots from Treemark that I've worn quite happily through the years in total comfort, I must confess that I have just as many pairs of those elasticized numbers that I've never worn. I've never been able to. These were the ones that took half an hour to get into in the shop, with the salesman, his fingers turning blue from the effort, insisting, 'Don't worry, they'll stretch, they'll stretch.' Well, they didn't stretch because for those boots to stretch I would actually have had to be wearing them, and, once out of the shop and alone in my bedroom, without the added muscle power of the man from Treemark, try as I might I was never again able to get them past my ankles.

There were quite a few years where the only boots I could buy were very heavy sheepskin-lined practical things with zippers up the front over the instep. However, thank God, over the last couple of years ankle boots have become fashionable again and even I, albeit with a bit of searching, can now find a reasonable selection of boots wide enough and short enough to do the trick.

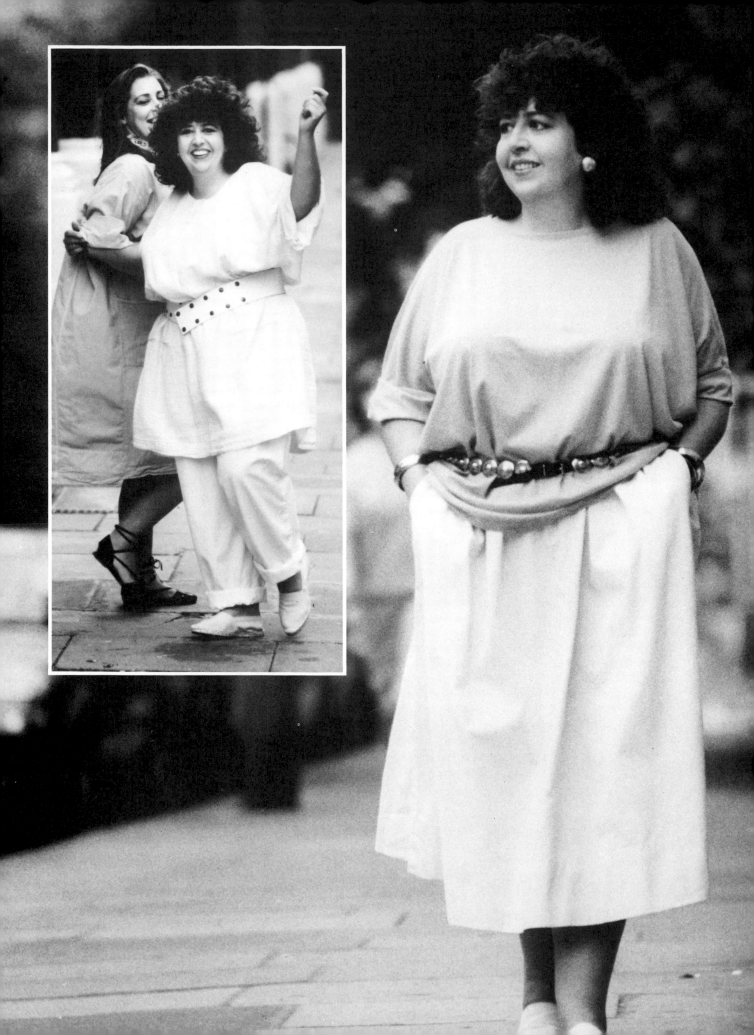

10

MAKE IT OR GET IT MADE

> 6 I haven't the time, the patience or the inclination to make my own clothes. I want the thrill of going out and shopping like everybody else. In desperation I have made things, but I'm a great bodger. I once made a pair of jeans. My mother and I had a running joke – we said I could make denim legs on suspenders because I always wore long shirts over them so it didn't matter what the top looked like! 9
>
> *Elizabeth Osborne*

Making your own clothes is one of those complex issues that angers many big women. 'Why', they protest, 'should we have to make things? It's degrading to have to sew our own things just because we are unable to find what we want in the shops.'

It's a sentiment I've shared. Why indeed? On the other hand, I've also derived a lot of pleasure from making myself something from start to finish.

Making your own can be one way of getting exactly what you want. Janis Townes wears simple white home-made skirt that's seen many summers – a change of T-shirt, jewellery, and shoes brings it up to date year after year

Inset: This well-cut tunic can be worn as a dress or as a top over trousers or a bathing suit. It's infinitely versatile and there's a pattern for it on pp. 155-7

> 6 I suppose the really difficult time for me must have been in my teens – fifteen, sixteen. The clothes in most shops only went up to a size 14 and I was finding it difficult to buy things. I desperately wanted to wear the same as everyone else. I could just squeeze into a size 16, which I did. Then when I looked back at the pictures, I thought, 'How awful I looked in those clothes that didn't really fit me.' After that I thought, 'No, I'm never ever going to do that again. I'm never going to wear anything that doesn't fit me well!' My sister bought a sewing machine and taught me how to use it and I started making my own things. Soon I had more clothes than anybody else and they were much nicer. I took off from there and never looked back.
>
> I taught myself to make patterns. At first I copied what my friends were wearing, very simple things, but I've gotten quite good now and if I see something I like in a magazine, I can just make up a pattern for it and make it. The only thing I don't make is coats. 9
>
> *Carole Burton*

> ❝ I do have one or two very basic patterns that I bought, one for a shirt, another for trousers, but after you've been making things for a while you know how to cut things out. I can probably make myself a pair of trousers, without a pattern, in about an hour from the beginning to the very end. I must confess that I ruined many a piece of fabric on the way to where I am now, but now, if I want to go out tonight, and I've got nothing to wear, I just sit down and make myself whatever I want. ❞
>
> *Carole Burton*

I also started dressmaking when I was a teenager. Early on I tackled a very intricate *Vogue* designer pattern for a Chanel suit. It was gorgeous, with a twelve-gore skirt and a silk-lined jacket with a matching silk blouse. I slaved over that suit for a week, working late into the nights, and barely able to drag myself out of bed in the mornings to go to school. It was absolutely beautiful. It didn't exactly suit the lifestyle of a sixteen-year-old schoolgirl, but I used to take it out and just look at it, at my handiwork, for years afterwards.

A Chanel suit is one extreme; you can utilize your sewing skills in simpler ways.

> ❝ Don't be put off buying something because it looks too small. It's fairly easy to do some simple alterations. Learn to look at how things are made and to look for extra material in the seams. Sometimes there is an incredible amount of fabric crammed into seams that can be let out. You can make the tiniest pair of pleated trousers fit by simply removing the waistband, releasing the pleats and adding a new waistband. As long as you wear a top *over* them, no one's going to know. If you get a dress that you really like, you can actually wear it till it almost falls apart and then make a pattern out of it. I did that with a favourite dress from last summer that started life as a black dress with big flashes of colour on it; I then chopped it up and it became three dresses, in different African prints, and a jacket. ❞
>
> *Vicki Pepys*

There are certain mainstays of my own wardrobe that I simply cannot find in the shops and if I had not made them I would have had to go without. I long ago gave up the complexities of designer patterns and I now stick to very simple basic shapes. The white skirt that Janis is wearing on p. 150 is an old standby of mine. It couldn't be simpler, just two rectangles gathered on to a waistband with pockets in the side seams.

I did actually copy and make a rather complicated pattern for my favourite Kenzo brown-striped skirt. I then made it up in several different fabrics. One of these is the plaid that you see facing p. 168.

The American designer Sharon Minetta made the matching plaid shirt. That's my own antique lace collar, which I added. I've had this particular outfit for about five years now. Plaid is one of those classics. You can wear it staid and traditional in the British way, a plaid kilt with a white blouse and velvet waistcoat or jacket. Or you can jazz it up as the Italians do and mix different coloured plaids together, layering one on top of the other.

If you enjoy sewing, then making yourself clothes can give you a lot of satisfaction. If you truly hate it, don't have the time, or simply can't be bothered, then it can be a life-saver to find a friend who enjoys it and will make things for you. If you can afford a dressmaker, that can be another good solution. I say this not because I think it's right or just that we should *have* to make clothes but simply because sometimes making a particular garment is the only way we'll ever get it! It's a question of what is practical. And after years of compromising with the limited choice of things that are available, it can be tremendous fun choosing fabrics that you really do like and making them or getting them made into styles that suit you perfectly.

> ❛ I'm very interested in fabrics and what can be done with them. I have a wonderful dressmaker. Alice doesn't need patterns. If I see a design I like, I draw it for Alice and she does the rest. I always try to take advantage of what's around. We went to Spain recently and I had two leather suits made, with full-length skirts and jackets, one with a waistcoat. Spain is full of shops that tailor to measure, so I just picked one that looked nice. In Singapore, my husband Des had an evening suit made, so I had a couple of jackets made too, one in black-on-black figured fabric and one in green. They're gorgeous. 'It doesn't matter what size it is,' I said. 'Who cares about the size, you just make it my size.' ❜
>
> *Claire Rayner*
>
> ❛ Someone was making something for me not so long ago, which was a lovely luxury, and I said, 'Look, the one mistake people always make when they make me clothes is they don't believe the measurements when they get them in front of them.' He was a really old-fashioned pattern cutter, very sweet, and he said, 'Well, I don't know, it looks pretty horrendous on paper.' I said, 'Of course, but don't make the mistake of cutting it small because you think you've gone wrong with the measuring tape. If in doubt cut it larger!' ❜ *Meredith Etherington-Smith*

Just for fun, I've included three pattens in this section for three of my favourite and most useful garments, ones that I would be lost without.

The first pattern is for an enormous top/dress. This is a fairly recent addition to my wardrobe, but now that I've got it I don't know how I ever lived without it. It has a rather special place in my heart. I was working in France – it was the first time I'd actually been abroad to film – and the only free time I had was the morning before I was due to fly back to London. I got up early and scurried around the broiling streets of Juan-les-Pins, picking up a basketload of French goodies to bring home. I was on the way back to the hotel, struggling under the weight of my Brie, when I passed a tiny, makeshift clothing stall in the street. With that practised eye that all big women have, I spotted this large faded blue cotton 'thing' hanging amidst all the tiny numbers on the rail. I pounced. 'How much?' I inquired. It was dirt cheap. I tried it on behind a curtained partition. 'I'll take it,' I beamed. 'We have it in other colours,' the young salesgirl told me enticingly, and pulled out a white one, a yellow one, a black one.

I searched my now depleted wallet. 'Do you take credit cards?' She pursed her lips and clucked her tongue in the French manner, as she returned the garments to the rails. Of course not, I thought, where do I think I am, Bloomingdales?

'Hang on to them, I'll be right back!' – and I headed for the nearest bank where I changed every remaining penny of travellers' cheques that I had with me. Let's hope the BBC pays for the taxi to the airport, if not I'm sunk.

And I bought that top in every colour they had, and if they'd had more I would have bought them too. I have, literally, lived in them all this summer and know that I will all next summer too. I may even wear the darker coloured ones in the winter with a turtle-neck sweater underneath. Janis and Ozzie are wearing them on p. 150. As you can see, you can either wear this as a dress or as an overtop. You can belt it or leave it loose, and it is really big. So often the big loose tops made for smaller women lose their style on us. Even though we can get into them, they're not as big as they are supposed to be, they cling around the bum or under the arms. This one, believe me, is big and fits every woman you see in this book.

The ones I bought in France are made in cotton, but I think you could make it up in almost any fabric. It would be great in light corduroy, or wool, and sensational in lightweight denim.

The trousers I've already talked about in Chapter 7, but here they are again. I've been making them for five years now; when they wear out, I just make some more. I make them up in heavy cotton drill that gets lovely and soft when it's washed. I always have a couple of white pairs for the summer, when I live in them. I wear them with T-shirts or sweaters, or dress them up with longer tops and even dresses like the beige Japanese dress that Ozzie is wearing on p. 130 which I belt or leave loose. You can leave them long as in the pattern, and roll up the cuffs as I do, or if that's not your style, you can cut them off and hem them to whatever length you like. They are sublimely comfortable any way you care to wear them *(between pp. 88 and 89)*.

The third pattern in this section is a knitting pattern from knitwear designer Jennifer Kiernan. This sweater is one of the first things I bought when I started campaigning for better clothes. It was actually meant to be a dress, but on me it made the perfect sweater over jeans. It's the sweater I was photographed in for my first fashion session for *Fashion Weekly (p. 105)*. I've worn it many times over the years for TV shows and photographs, and women always write wanting to know where they can get it. Jenny doesn't make it any more herself but she has made a pattern for it especially for this book.

In addition to the bright green one in the photograph *(facing p. 168)*, Jenny also made it in a classic cocoa colour with various shades of rust and brown for the yoke, a pastel peach with contrasting shades of raspberry and purple for the yoke, and a bright crisp white, with clear jewel colours around the yoke. The white one looks particularly alpine and would make a great sweater to take with you on a winter holiday.

Remember that making something for yourself doesn't have to be a sign of defeat. The perfect skirt, the culottes, the pair of trousers that actually do fit, can be a cheap and useful way of making life easier.

One-size top

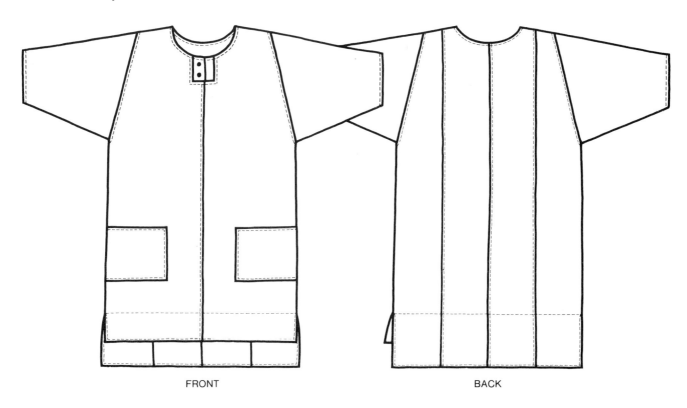

FRONT   BACK

MATERIALS:

3½yd/3.2m of 45in/114cm wide fabric. Two ⅝in/1.5cm buttons; matching thread; graph or tracing paper.

Fabric suggestions: cotton gaberdine, poplin, seersucker, Viyella, lightweight wools

MAKING PATTERN

Following layout diagram overleaf, copy the pattern and all markings full size on to graph or tracing paper. Cut out the paper pattern and pin on to the fabric following the layout in diagram.

TO MAKE UP

Seam allowances of ⅝in/1.5cm are included in the pattern unless otherwise stated in the instructions. Unless stated otherwise, press all seams to one side and topstitch ¼in/6mm away from seam.

1. Matching pieces marked A, stitch the two fronts together at the centre front.

2. At corners marked B on the front opening, snip the corners in ¼in/6mm. *(See diagram 1.)*

3. Fold the front facings in half where marked on pattern. Place one on top of the other so that one folded edge is ¼in/6mm from the raw edge of the other. *(See diagram 2.)* Stitch together at lower edge.

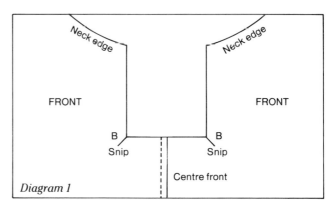

Diagram 1

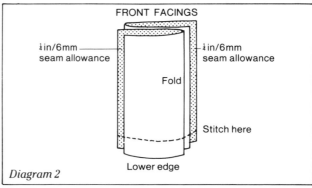

FRONT FACINGS

¼in/6mm seam allowance   ¼in/6mm seam allowance

Fold

Stitch here

Lower edge

Diagram 2

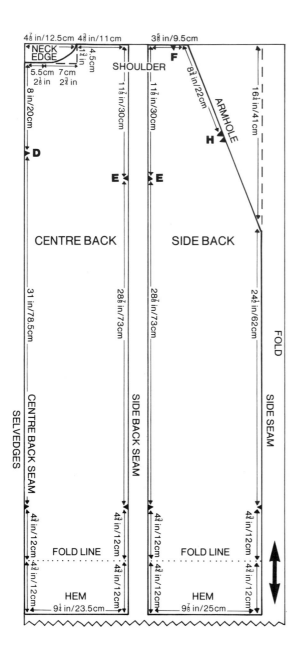

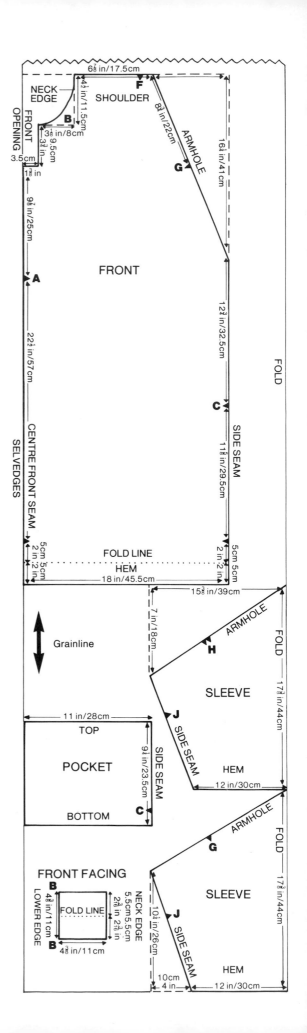

Pattern and layout for one-size top

4. Matching corners B on the front opening with corners B on the front facings, stitch together taking a ¼in/6mm seam allowance. *(See diagram 3.)*

5. Turn facing upwards. Sew each facing to side edges of front opening from neck edge to corner B ¼in/6mm from the edge *(see diagram 4)*, taking care to stitch through the front and both raw edges of one front facing, but not the folded edge of the other.

6. Press seam away from neck and topstitch on the right side.

7. Press under ½in/1cm twice along top edge of pocket. Stitch close to edge. Press ⅝in/1.5cm around remaining edges of pocket. Place pockets on front side, edges matching C at side seams. The lower edge of pocket should measure 14in/35cm up from hem edge. Stitch pocket in place close to the edges.

8. Matching back pieces marked D, stitch centre-back seam together.

9. Matching pieces marked E, stitch side backs to back panel.

10. Matching pieces marked F, stitch front to back at shoulder seams.

11. Turn under ¼in/6mm twice around neck edge and the top of facings, stitch down in place.

12. Press 4¾in/12cm to wrong side at back hem. Turn raw edge under ¼in/6mm and stitch in place.

13. Stitch sleeve to armhole, matching Gs and Hs and easing the top of the sleeve into the armhole.

14. Press 2in/5cm to wrong side along front hem edge, turn under ¼in/6mm on raw edge of hem and stitch down close to edge. Topstitch ¼in/6mm from lower hem edge.

15. Matching pieces marked J, join the front to the back starting from the sleeve and going down the side seam to the hem, stopping 2in/5cm away from front edge. Press seam open.

16. Topstitch around side opening ¼in/6mm from edge, catching seam allowance down. *(See diagram 5.)*

17. Press under ½in/1cm twice at sleeve edge and stitch in place.

FINISHING

On right side of front facing, machine two ⅝in/1.5cm buttonholes ¾in/2cm apart, beginning the first buttonhole ½in/1cm away from top and side edges. Sew the buttons to the left facing in line with the buttonholes.

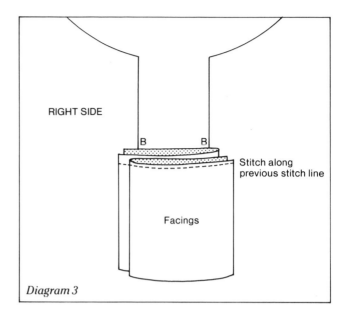

Diagram 3

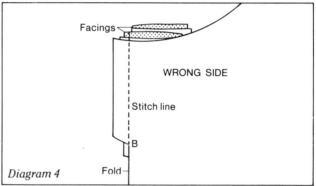

Diagram 4

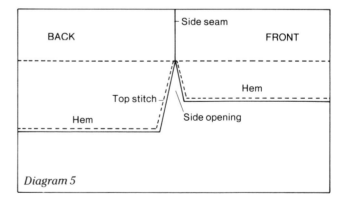

Diagram 5

Trousers

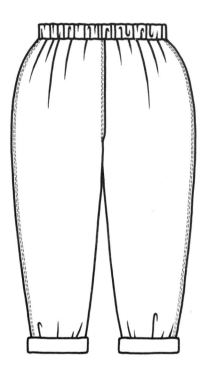

MATERIALS:

60in/150cm wide *or* 36in/92cm wide fabric *(see table below)*; ¾in/2cm wide elastic cut according to waist measurement plus 1¼in/3cm; matching thread; graph or tracing paper.

Fabric suggestions: cotton gaberdine, tracksuiting, wool flannel.

Size chart

	16	18	20	22	24	26	28	30
Waist	30in	32in	34in	36in	38in	40in	42in	44in
	76cm	81cm	86cm	91cm	96cm	101cm	106cm	111cm
Hips	40in	42in	44in	46in	48in	50in	52in	54in
	102cm	107cm	112cm	117cm	122cm	127cm	132cm	137cm
Fabric required								
60in	2yd	2¼yd	2½yd	2¾yd	2¾yd	3yd	3yd	3¼yd
150cm	1.85m	2.1m	2.3m	2.5m	2.75m	2.75m	3m	3m
36in	2¾yd	3yd	3¼yd	3½yd	3¾yd	3¾yd	4yd	4yd
92cm	2.5m	2.75m	3m	3.25m	3.5m	3.5m	3.7m	3.7m

MAKING PATTERN

Following layout diagram 1, copy the pattern and all the markings full size on to the graph or tracing paper. Cut out the paper pattern and pin on to 60in/150cm wide fabric as shown on cutting layout diagram. To cut out the 36in/92cm wide fabric, fold the fabric length in half lengthwise and pin the trouser leg pattern pieces side by side on the fabric, with the pockets below.

GRADING PATTERN TO REQUIRED SIZE

Measurements given in the diagram are for size 22. For smaller sizes reduce the pattern as follows. For each size down, take away ½in/12mm from each side seam at the waist and hip, graduating to nothing at the hem edge and take away 1in/2.5cm from the waistband edge to shorten the crotch length. Shorten the leg length (if necessary) by 1¼in/3cm at hem edge. For the larger sizes add on the measurements given above.

TO MAKE UP

⅝in/1.5cm seam allowances have been included unless otherwise stated in the instructions. All the seams are sewn with right sides together, the edges neatened and pressed open unless otherwise indicated.

1. Stitch front to back, matching As, leaving open between A and B. Snip into the seam allowance close to end of stitching at these notches.

2. On the front only, topstitch close to and ¼in/6mm from side seams between these notches making sure the seam allowance is not stitched down. *(See diagram 2.)*

3. Stitch pocket pieces, matching Bs, to side front and side back. Stitch the pocket pieces together and press towards the trouser front.

4. Topstitch the rest of the side seams, matching stitching to the topstitching on the pocket openings.

5. Stitch fronts together, matching Cs. Press the seam towards the right-hand side and topstitch close to and ¼in/6mm from seam.

6. Stitch back pieces together, matching Ds. Press the seam to the left-hand side and topstitch close to and ¼in/6mm from seam.

7. Stitch the front inside legs to back inside legs matching Es and the centre-front and centre-back seams.

8. Press 1¼in/3cm to wrong side at waistband edge and turn under ¼in/6mm along raw edge. Stitch close to this edge leaving an opening at the centre back to thread the elastic through.

9. Turn under 1¼in/3cm at hem edge and turn under ¼in/6mm along the raw edge. Stitch in place close to this edge.

10. Cut the elastic to the required length plus 1¼in/3cm. Thread the elastic through the waistband. Overlap the ends of the elastic by ⅝in/1.5cm and stitch together.

FINISHING

Sew the gap left at the centre back of waistband. Roll up the trouser hem to the length desired.

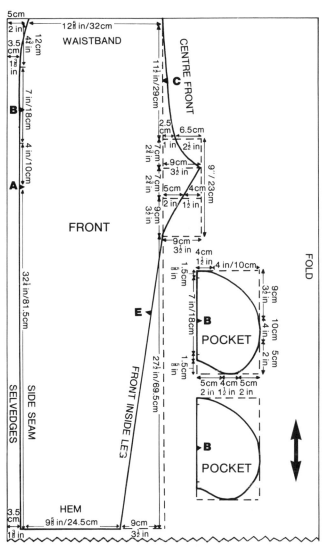

Diagram 1: Pattern and layout for trousers

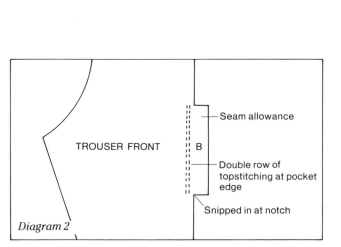

Diagram 2

NB *Measurements on the trouser pattern are for size 22 (American size 20) and should be adjusted to a larger or smaller size as necessary following the instructions given in the pattern under 'Grading pattern to required size'*

Dot-dash sweater (Jennifer Kiernan)

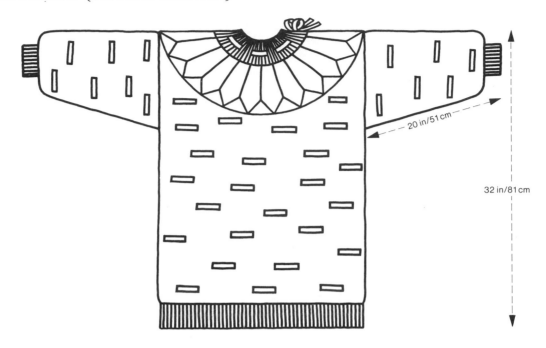

Yarn: 26 25g-balls mohair; 11 odd balls of coloured double knitting wool for dashes and yoke.

Needles: 4½mm (UK 7/US 6) for rib; 6mm (UK4/US 9) for body; 5mm (UK 6/US 7) for yoke.

Size: Large.

Tension: Knit 13 sts and 18 rows to 4in/10cm.

Measurements: Centre front to yoke = 26in/66cm; yoke depth = 6in/15cm; armhole depth = 12in/30.5cm; sleeve seam = 20in/51cm; underarm = 64in/162cm.

Abbreviations: k = knit, p = purl, st = stitch, tog = together, inc = increase, st st = stocking stitch.

BACK AND FRONT *(both alike)*
With 4½mm needles and base colour, cast on 80 sts and work 21 rows in k 1, p 1 rib.
Next row: In rib, inc once in first st then every 4th st across remainder of row to last stitch, inc in this (101 sts).

Change to 6mm needles.

Now work remainder of body in moss stitch (k 1, p 1). Place a total of 24 dashes over the body piece at random. Work straight for 22½in/57cm or to desired length.

Dashes: Always worked with two threads of yarn and in garter stitch, 6 st wide by two rows deep.
Always start a dash with the right side of work facing, and leave a 2in/5cm strand of wool to tie off.

Shape yoke: Still working in moss stitch, work 46 sts. Turn, leaving the remaining 55 sts on a spare needle. Work back to armhole edge.
Next row: Moss st 42 sts. Turn – slip 1, work back to edge.
Next row: Moss st 38 sts. Turn – slip 1, work back to edge.
Next row: Moss st 34 sts. Turn – slip 1, work back to edge.
Next row: Moss st 30 sts. Turn – slip 1, work back to edge.
Continue decreasing in this way until 18 sts remain. (Place one more dash in this area).

Then continue decreasing, but working 2 sts less each row (as follows):
Next row: Moss st 16 sts. Turn – slip 1, work back to edge.
Next row: Moss st 14 sts. Turn – slip 1, work back to edge.
Continue decreasing in this way until 2 sts remain.

Transfer all these 46 sts on to a spare needle, plus 9 sts from the centre of the work. Rejoin yarn at the last remaining 46 sts and work across row.
Next row: Moss st (from side edge to centre) 42 sts. Turn – slip 1, work back to edge.
Next row: Moss st 38 sts. Turn – slip 1, work back to edge.

Repeat the shaping as for opposite side.

Now place all 101 sts on same needle, making sure the right side of the work is facing forward, and commence yoke.

Yoke: Proceed in stocking stitch.
Cast on 5 sts at the beginning of row, knit across these, k 101 sts of body on to the same needle, cast on 5 more sts. These go over the shoulders. (111 sts.)

Next row: P.

Next row: Introduce colours for yoke, all in single thickness
yarn.

K 1 colour, *k 9 base, k 1 colour*, repeat * – *
across row.

Row 2: P 2 colour, *p 7 base, p 3 colour*, repeat * – * to
the last 9 sts, p 7 base, p 2 colour.

Row 3: K 3 colour, *k 5 base, k 5 colour*, repeat * – * to
the last 8 sts, k 5 base, k 3 colour.

Row 4: P 4 colour, *p 3 base, p 7 colour*, repeat * – * to
the last 7 sts, p 3 base, p 4 colour.

Row 5: K 5 colour, *k 1 base, k 9 colour*, repeat * – * to
the last6 sts, k 1 base, k 5 colour.

Break off base colour and proceed in colours.

Row 6: P across row in colours:
p 6, *p 10 colour* – repeat * – * to last 5 sts, p 5.

Row 7: K 5, *k 2 tog, k 8* – repeat * – * to the last 6 sts, k 6.

Row 8: P across row in colours.

Change to 5mm needles, and continue to work in colour as
follows:

Row 9: K across row.

Row 10: P across row.

Row 11: K 5, *k 2 tog, k 7*, repeat * – * across row to last 6
sts, k 6.
Work 3 rows st st.

Row 15: K 2 tog, k 3, *k 2 tog, k 6*, repeat * – * across row
to last 6 sts, k 4, k 2 tog.
Work 3 rows st st.

Row 19: K 2 tog, k 2, *k 2 tog, k 5*, repeat * – * across row
to last 5 sts, k 3, k 2 tog.
Work 3 rows st st.

Row 23: K 2 tog, k 1, *k 2 tog, k 4*, repeat * – * across row
to last 4 sts, k 2, k 2 tog.
Work 3 rows st st.

Row 27: K 2, *k 2 tog, k 3*, repeat * – * across row to last 3
sts, k 1, k 2 tog.
Work 3 rows st st (44 sts).

Change to base colour and k 1, p 1 rib for neck. Work 4 rows
in rib.

Make eyelets: K 1, *cast off 2 sts, work 4 sts,* repeat * – * to
last st, p 1.

Next row: Cast on 2 sts over each hole.
Work 2 rows in rib.
Cast off in rib *loosely.*

SLEEVES *(both alike)*

With 4½ mm needles and base colour, cast on 34 sts and
work 22 rows k 1, p 1 rib.

Change to 6mm needles.

Inc 1 st in every st across next row (68 sts).
Work in moss stitch, increasing 1 st at each end of every 6th
row until 86 sts are on needles.
Place 12 dashes over each sleeve.
Work until sleeve measures 20in/51cm including rib (or to
desired length). Cast off loosely.

TO MAKE UP

Slip stitch the shoulder seams and neck edging.
Slip stitch sleeve head to body – it should come down
12in/30cm each side of shoulder seam.
Slip stitch the side seams and sleeve seams.
Tie off all dashes ends, leaving 2in/5cm inside.
Very carefully steam press seams and yoke.

MAKE NECK-TIE: Take 12 strands of wool 48in/122cm
long. Plait in groups of 4. Tie knot at each end, leaving
1in/2.5cm loose. Thread through eyelets in neck rib and tie
in bow at front, back or side according to preference.

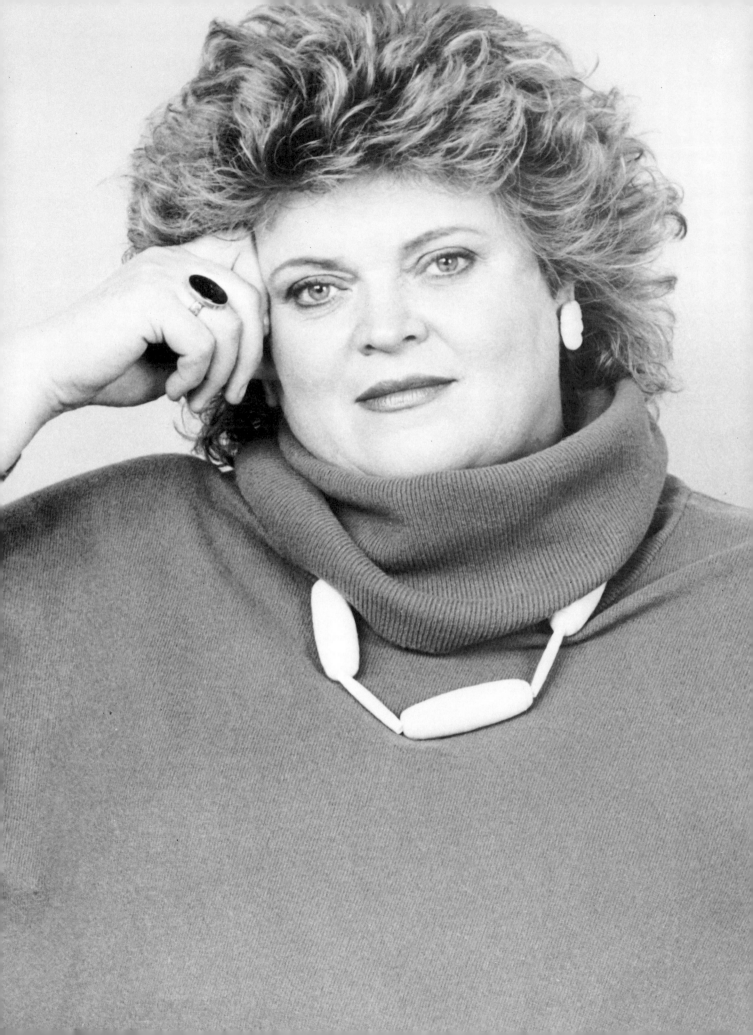

11

PAMPERING

I thought long and hard about whether or not to include a section about make-up in this book. So much has been written about women's unhealthy dependency on it. We all know women who are ashamed to leave the house without first 'putting their face on'. I've even met women who are embarrassed to let their *husbands* see them without make-up. At the opposite end of the spectrum are those women who feel it is an essential aspect of women's liberation to dispense with make-up altogether.

My own attitudes fall somewhere between these two extremes. I consider myself a liberated woman – and I wear make-up. I don't feel the 'need' to wear it. I wear it, when I wear it, because it gives *me* pleasure to do so. For me, wearing make-up falls into that general category that I'll call pampering. Into this category go those things that I do for myself, when I have the time, when I'm in the mood, and when I want to give myself a lift.

A classic sweater dress like this can be something you keep for ever. Sue Formston bought this one in 1977 and it's still going strong

---

6 Skinny women pamper themselves so why on earth shouldn't big women? Because they feel that they aren't allowed to, they aren't allowed to be glamorous, and it's rubbish. One thing I've never done but I'd love to do is have a facial. It sounds like such a good idea, you go in feeling like an old dog, shut your eyes, and twenty minutes later there you are. 9
Helen Terry

6 The chiropodist is something that I love. I don't go as often as I'd like to but I'd go every month if I got it together and could afford it. The chiropodist just makes you feel so wonderful. I find feet particularly ugly and it makes you feel nice to have them pampered and cared for – you just walk so much lighter. 9
Jan Murphy

6 In the bath I use a loofah. They're marvellous, they get your circulation going. I use one on my face as well. I get one of the long ones, cut it up into hand-size pieces and when it's very soft I use it on my face once or twice a week.

Whatever my favourite perfume of the moment is, I have the bath oil, the moisturizer, the whole works, and I love to have a gorgeous long lovely bath and oil myself and go to bed feeling like a dream. 9
Angela Troak

Too often big women don't pamper themselves. We feel that we are not entitled to those physical pleasures that slim women take for granted. Our bodies are not worthy of this loving attention. For years I never looked at any part of myself below the neck. I didn't want even to see that part of me, so consciously to spend time caring for it was out of the question. But once I stopped trying to alter my body, once I stopped punishing it, I found that I began to enjoy physically pampering myself. When you accept that your body is indeed you, then you can treat it like the treasured possession it is.

There are so many simple ways that you can pamper yourself. Using body lotion all over, conditioning your hair, putting aromatic oils in the bath, soaking in a tub filled with bubble bath, all pleasurable tactile pursuits that involve you with giving pleasure to your body and therefore to yourself.

When I die and go to heaven I personally hope that what I find there is one big jacuzzi. I've only ever been in one three times, and the first time I was so embarrassed about exposing my naked body to the other bathers that I almost broke my neck trying to get into the water unobserved. Once in, however, I never wanted to get out – it was bliss.

Water is obviously my thing. I love showers and the only improvement we've made to our ancient flat is to have a shower installed. We have a special massage shower head that was easy to install; it pounds away at those stiff muscles that I get at the back of my shoulders until I feel like I could float right up through the ceiling.

Having a sauna is another highly sybaritic experience that you may wish to indulge in. I've met some fascinating women in saunas. Their lack of shame about displaying their variously shaped bodies did a lot to help me to accept my own nakedness.

Obviously having a sauna or a jacuzzi are not the kind of things that most of us do every day. There are however two things that I do do every day that are an important part of caring for myself. The first is to drink a great deal of water. I always tend to retain a lot of fluid, especially just before my period. I find that by drinking about eight glasses of water a day my fluid-retention problem has diminished considerably. All that water keeps the kidneys in good working order. It has also made a tremendous difference to my skin. It's much smoother and softer than it used to be and I'm certainly not getting any younger!

The second thing I do is to care for my skin in the simplest possible way. I wash with soap and water and then I moisturize with Equalia. Ever since I hit puberty I had the same flaky dry patch of skin on my chin. No matter how much moisturizer I slapped on it always came back after several hours. One day I happened to borrow a friend's Equalia. It was like magic. The dry patch disappeared, never to return. The moral of this story is: always try out different products until you find the one that suits you.

Hair

As for my hair, I like it big, like me! I keep it cut rather ragged and spiky and I dry it in such a way as to get maximum volume out of it. I either scrunch-dry it with a strong setting foam, with my head hanging upside down, or I let it dry naturally and then set it on heated rollers. (I've had the same set since I was seventeen.)

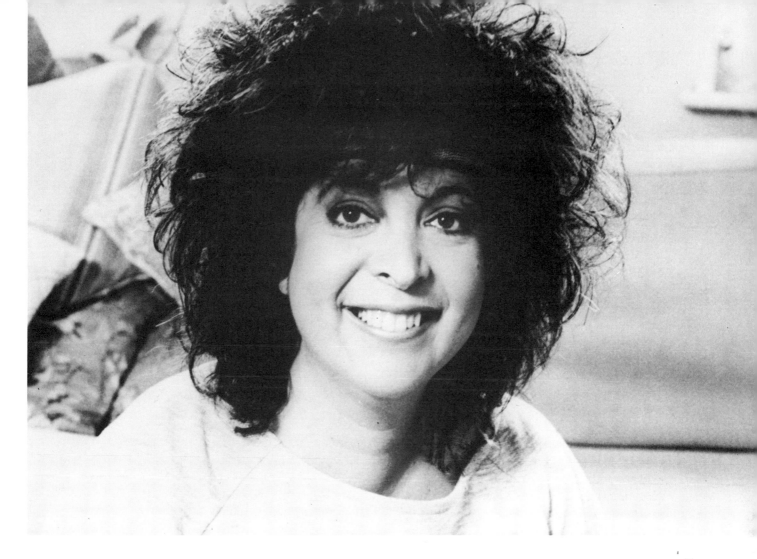

Here my layered hair was 'scrunched' dry with setting mousse and then lightly backcombed

After setting it I brush it out and then back-comb it to give it the fullness I like. This is how we did the hair for the ball-gown picture *(facing p. 89)*. With a slightly different comb-out we got the more traditional Sloane Ranger look *(between pp. 88 and 89)*

Now that my hair is longer I quite often wear it as you see it in the red tracksuit picture *(facing p. 96)*. This couldn't be easier, just bend over, brush all the hair to the top of your head and secure it with a covered elastic pony-tail band. It's the messiness of this look that gives it its appeal. Just let the bits hang down as they will, don't try to neaten it up too much or you'll spoil the effect. This topknot is the perfect easy base for different head-wrappings that you may want to try.

> ❛ For years I had long hair cut in a way which covered the sides of my face, because I thought that my cheeks were so big that I had to hide them. Of course by hiding a part of my face I was also hiding the things that give people an indication of the kind of person you are, your smile, your expression, etc. I finally decided that I was going to have my hair cut. It was at the same time that I decided that I wasn't going to diet any more. It totally changed the way I look and people said 'My God, you look so much better, you look completely different.' Although my head might have looked a bit like a pea on a drum, I had more of a face all of a sudden, more to play with, more to put make-up on, more to smile with and more to laugh with. ❜
> *Mandy Crane*

We did our own head-wrapping over the rather elaborate French roll for our 'Dress for Success' picture *(facing p. 97)*. This was the only style that was completely new to me, and although it was a smaller, more compact style than I ordinarily wear, I loved it. The hair was back-combed, which is essential if you have a shaggy cut like mine, before it was swept up and back into the French twist. The fringe was then tonged for lift. For the more natural looks my hair was simply left to dry and then smoothed over with a brush and hot hairdryer.

Make-up

As far as make-up is concerned I very rarely use it at all during the day. I certainly don't feel the need to put my face on before I leave the house. This is quite a change from my early twenties when I wouldn't go out without a full face of make-up, right down to false eyelashes. These days, when I've got to look 'done up' in a hurry, I usually go for a quick flick of lipstick and dark glasses and put a bit of translucent powder on my nose.

I do, of course, wear make-up when I'm working. Having my make-up done professionally taught me one very important thing – don't be afraid to experiment. It's very easy to get stuck in a make-up rut. Since I was fifteen I'd been using the same brown eyeshadow and eyeliner that toned in with my eye colour. Then a movie make-up artist suggested I try purples and lavenders. These colours, which contrast with, and therefore emphasize, the brown of my eyes, make them appear darker and more dramatic. Another good dark colour, and not as hard as black, is navy blue, especially if you like an Italian movie-star look!

For Chapter 7, in which I appear in so many different styles of clothes, we re-did my make-up for each shot. In some, like the tracksuit and the trenchcoat, it looks like I'm hardly wearing any make-up at all. The fact is, I was wearing tons. It takes a long time to get that flawless-complexion look, let me tell you. It don't always come naturally! In other shots, the Arabian Nights for example, Paula Owen, our make-up artist, really piled on the eyes. Believe it or not, this is more the sort of thing I'm likely to do myself than is the natural look. It's at night, for going out to dinner or for parties, that I really go to town – eye make-up, blusher, lipstick, the works.

When I do my own make-up, I very rarely use foundation. I find that it's the one thing that tends to make me look overly made up. But I do use a loose translucent face powder which I apply with one of my favourite luxuries, an enormous

---

❛ When I started having make-up artists when I was with Culture Club, that's when I started feeling a lot better about it all. I thought 'God, you can do this with a bit of paint.' When I do my own make-up I usually just wear foundation, sunglasses and lipstick because I can't be bothered to do my eyes. The Grace Jones school of make-up. I do play around a lot with my make-up when I'm on stage, and with my hair. I do all sorts of things with it. I've even had it done with silver aluminium powder that turns it steely grey. I've been growing the front bit for a couple of years now, I'm going to grow it till it's right down to my knees. The rest I have cut every four weeks or so. ❜   *Helen Terry*

fluffy make-up brush. I put a bit of powder into the lid of the powder box, dip my brush into that, and then tap the brush on the edge of the lid to shake off any excess powder. Otherwise you can end up looking like you've dipped your face in the flour bin.

I use a blusher that is as close as possible to the rosy colour that my cheeks get when I've been out in the fresh air or exercising. I apply it directly to that part of my cheek that goes rosy on its own. I find it disconcerting to see women with pinky rosy cheeks and a large slab of orangy blusher an inch below that. My way may not be how the make-up pundits advise you to do it, but I think it looks most natural.

I've always enjoyed making up my eyes. Being quite dark I can get away with quite a lot of eye make-up before I start to look tacky. Mimi Kimmins, make-up artist *par excellence* at Thames Television, taught me a wonderful way of applying eyeliner without getting that hard edge that can look so harsh. Using water-soluble cake eyeliner in brownish-black I apply a line of well-diluted eyeliner above the upper lashes and let it dry for several seconds. Meanwhile I rinse out my eyeliner brush and then, with the clean brush dipped in water, I re-moisten the upper edge of the dried line and spread it upwards over the lid. It's basically just a method of blending the liner upwards to soften and smudge the effect. After this has dried I put on my eyeshadow.

I find it impossible to use kohl or liner on the edge above the lower lashes – my eyes are rather sensitive, they run and the liner disappears down my cheeks – so I apply a bit of powder eyeshadow under the lower lashes from the middle of the eye to the outside corner. I always blend this and all eyeshadow well with a Q-tip. You should never see an edge where the make-up stops and you begin.

Something that I never thought would find its way into my exceedingly messy make-up bag is an eyelash curler, but I have recently discovered its magic. It's not the actual curling process that I find appealing, it's the fact that it lifts the lashes up and away so that they don't hang down over your eyes. This has the effect of making your eyes appear larger and, most important, wide awake – invaluable for those days when that is exactly how you don't feel. Use the curler first, then apply your mascara. Don't do it the other way around or your lashes will stick to the curler and may pull out. Ouch!

When I was a teenager I overdid the eyebrow tweezing bit. I think it was mainly as a protest against my father who was appalled when he first caught me at it. Would that I had listened to him then. I tweezed so much that I discouraged the growth and my brows are now rather sparse. I fill them in with a brownish-black eyeshadow powder which I think gives a much softer look than pencil. I have a very fine sharp-angled little brush that allows you to apply and blend at the same time.

I'm a great fan of good make-up brushes. They are a worthwhile investment that can last you for ages. Often the brushes that come packed together with blusher, shader or powder are too small and stiff. You can get a more natural, subtle effect with a larger, softer brush. Cheaper brushes also tend to lose their hairs all over your face as cheap paintbrushes do when you're painting your walls. Good brushes can make the process of applying your make-up a lot of fun – like working on a great painting or work of art which is, after all, what your face is, isn't it?

> ❛ I love bright lipstick. I've got some really horrible plastic coral beads, they only cost 90p, and I've never stopped wearing them. They're a bright, bright orange, and I wear them with lipstick the same colour. ❜ *Vicki Pepys*

An invaluable part of a brush collection is a lipstick brush. Lipstick applied with a brush looks much lighter and lasts longer. If you're interested in it really staying put, apply one coat with your brush, then blot with a tissue, and apply a second coat.

Be careful with lip-liner pencils. If you do use one, make sure to blend the line in very thoroughly with your lipstick. I've seen many a good make-up job ruined by a mask-like dark line around the lips. I find that I get just as sharp and neat an edge with my lipstick brush.

For touch-ups during the day I use natural Corn Silk pressed powder. It's colourless and ideal for blotting up excess oil and removing shine.

After I've applied powder and/or blusher, I slightly darken my beauty spot. I use a light or medium-brown eyebrow pencil just to bring it back to the colour it was before the other make-up obscured it.

Between pp. 168-9 you will find colour drawings with guidelines indicating how various make-up looks in our photos were created. Paula Owen, who did all these make-ups, offers the following general tips for applying make-up:

- Your make-up should always give definition to your features, never over-power them.
- Use as little foundation as possible to get the maximum effect. Try applying it with a damp sponge for a smooth finish.
- Use a minimum amount of powder for a natural look.
- Always blend very well for a natural soft look. (What appealed to me most about Paula's eye make-up was that no matter how dramatic the look, no matter how heavy the make-up, it never looked hard or harsh. To achieve this soft look Paula blends, and blends, and blends!)
- She suggests conditioning dry lips with Blistex or Blistese. She also uses it under and even over lipstick to keep lips moist.

Paula's *don'ts* include:

- Don't use too much blusher. It looks phony and unnatural.
- Don't use colours that overwhelm your natural colouring.
- Don't use too much mascara. Nothing looks worse than lashes clotted together with black sludge.

> ❛ I'm fanatical about taking my make-up off no matter what time I go to bed. I think that's important. I use a cleanser, then soap and water, then a toner. And I use Vaseline to remove my eye make-up. It's wonderful for your lashes. ❜
> *Angela Troak*

Above left: My favourite skirt of all time and the subject of many home-made copies

Above right: I made the skirt, Sharon Minetta made the blouse, and together they add up to a classic plaid 'dress' in cool washable cotton that fits perfectly

Below: Jennifer Kiernan's sensational sweater, here made up in vibrant green. You can make it yourself – see pp. 160-1

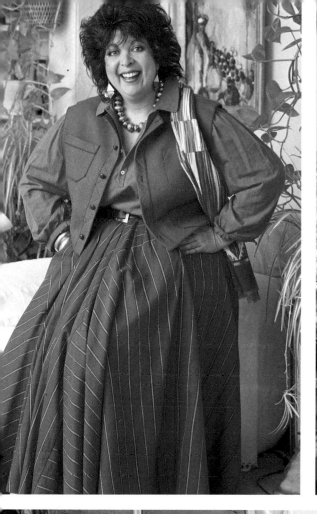
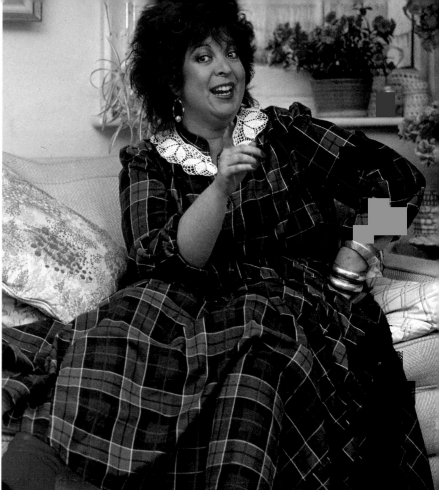
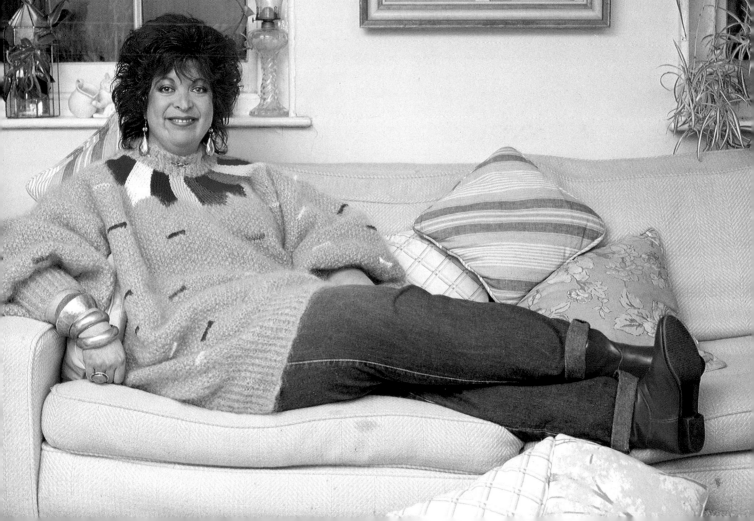

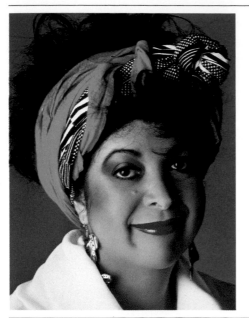

Nancy Roberts

brownish-black brow powder

yellow-gold down centre

orange-red powder shadow on outer and inner corners and up to brow!

Soft purple powder under eyes — close to lashes. Black mascara.

Soft red blush.

Brightest orange lip-liner + lipstick.

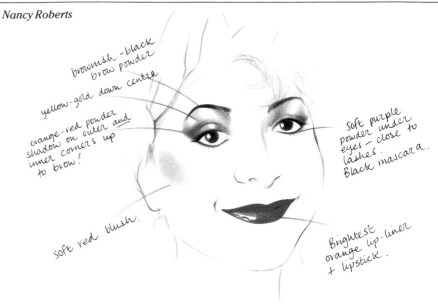

Jan Murphy

Soft yellow amber — all over lid up to brow

light brown brow powder

navy powder used as eyeliner next to lashes above and below Black mascara.

Soft red blush

Hollywood red — liner and lipstick!

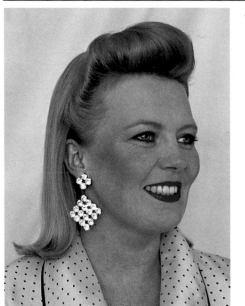

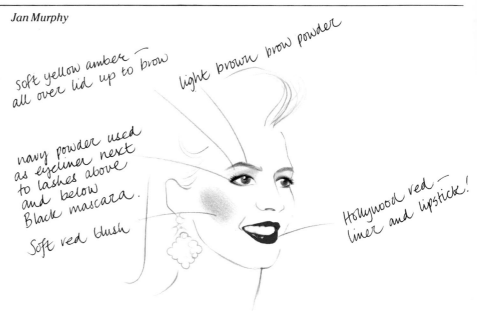

Meredith Etherington-Smith

touch of fuschia — extending outwards

lavender-grey — all over lid and up to brow.

light brown powder on brows

deep purple in socket and outer top lid brown pencil on eyeline + dark brown kohl inside

black mascara.

fuschia lip liner and lipstick.

pale fuschia blush

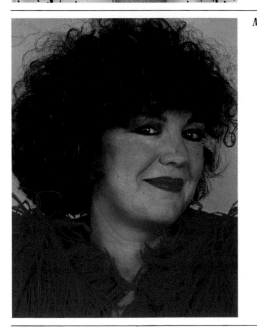

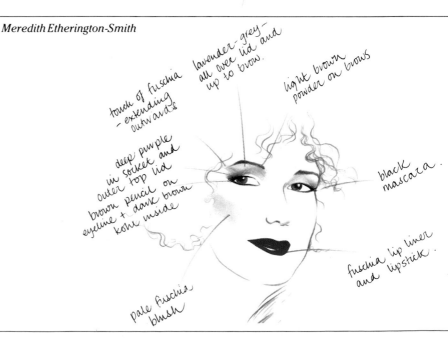

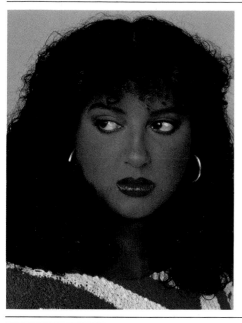

Liz Birru

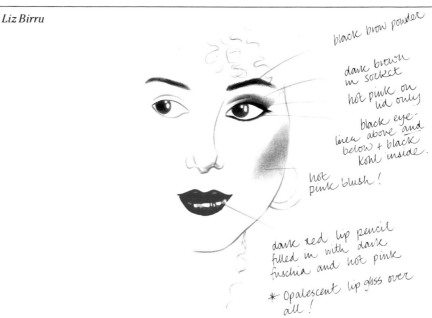

black brow powder

dark brown in socket

hot pink on lid only

black eye-liner above and below + black kohl inside.

hot pink blush!

dark red lip pencil filled in with dark fuschia and hot pink

* Opalescent lip gloss over all!

Mandy Crane

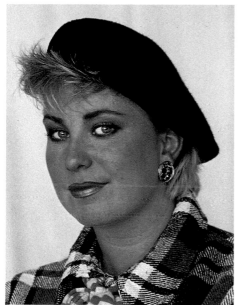

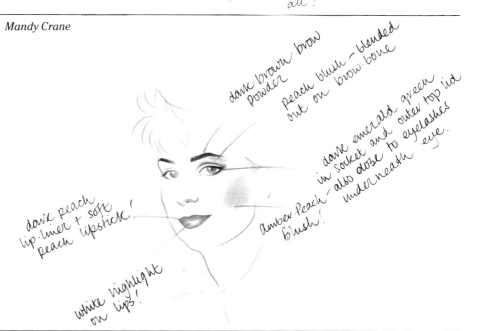

dark brown brow powder

peach blush - blended out on brow-bone

dark emerald green in socket and outer top lid - also close to eyelashes underneath eye.

Amber Peach blush!

dark peach lip-liner + soft peach lipstick!

white highlight on lips!

Angela Troak

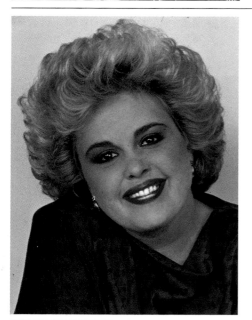

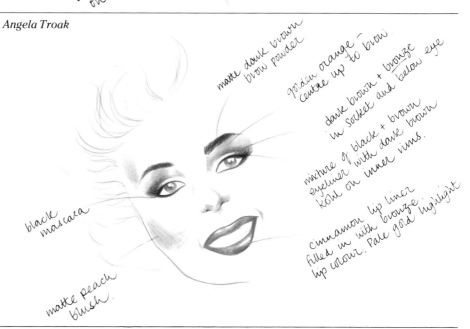

matte dark brown brow powder

golden orange - centre up to brow

dark brown + bronze in socket and below eye

mixture of black + brown eyeliner with dark brown kohl on inner rims.

cinnamon lip liner filled in with bronze lip colour. Pale gold highlight

black mascara

matte peach blush.

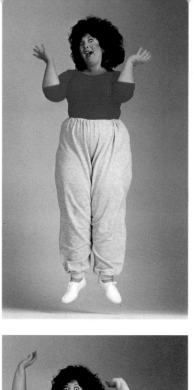
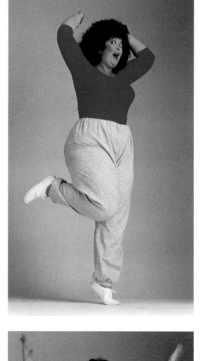
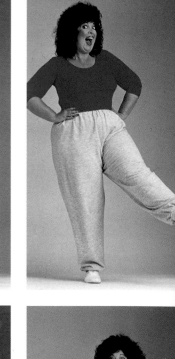
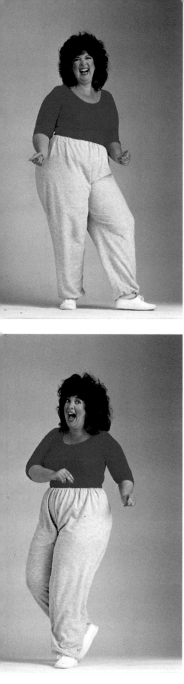
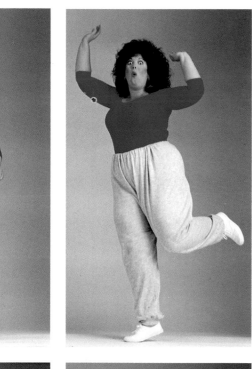
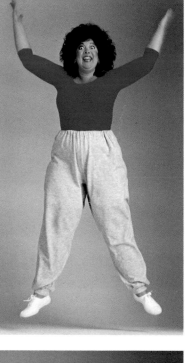
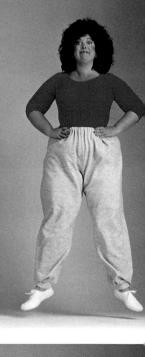
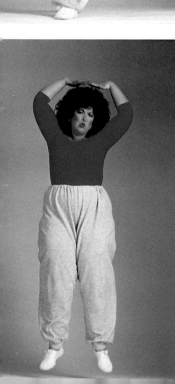
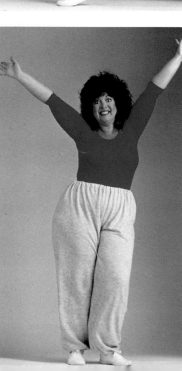
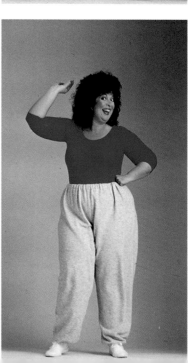
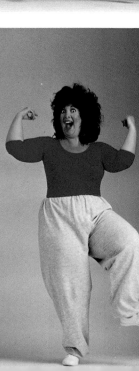

12

HEALTH

When I was seven and in my second year at the Hoffman School, a new toy arrived in the playground. I stood at the window with my classmates and watched as four workmen uncrated an enormous concrete turtle. We could hardly wait till recess to get out and take a closer look.

That turtle became the most popular thing in the playground for the next two weeks at least. It stood five feet tall, a prehistoric dinosaur in our midst, and all round its shell small niches had been let into the moulded concrete to serve as footholds.

The bell would ring signalling playtime and children would grab their coats and race down the steps and along the path to the turtle, excited and eager to get there first and be assured of their turn. Everyone from the tiniest nursery-school kids to the big shots in the sixth grade stood in line, laughing and shoving and waiting to clamber up its sides and perch on top for their moment of glory.

Everyone that is, but me. I would purposefully head off in the opposite direction, wandering towards the swings, or out to the edge of the softball field, where, studiously and with the utmost concentration, I would gather armfuls of the spring flowers that grew there in abundance. Then, seated in the high grass, and, always watching my schoolmates and the turtle out of the corner of my eye, I would feign total involvement in the intricate task of turning the daisies into chains.

I wanted to climb that turtle more than anything in the world, but I was afraid. Afraid that I wouldn't be able to, afraid that my feet would slip out of the niches and I would fall, but most of all afraid that I would look silly. Silly and clumsy and ridiculous and fat.

I waited for my own try at climbing the turtle until many months after it had first been delivered. My schoolmates had long ago lost interest and moved on to something else and now only the occasional climber could be found there. On this particular day there was a ball game going on in the field and the turtle was deserted. I slowly pushed the toe of my shoe into the lowest foothold. I could feel my heart beating in my ears, as I pulled myself off of the ground. I held on for dear life as my foot found its next hold, and as I climbed up and up, I kept a lookout for a stray ballplayer, a teacher, anyone who might see me and begin to laugh. I made it unobserved to the top. I threw one leg over the round concrete

'Moving in ways I never thought possible'

shell and sat there trying to catch my breath. The cold rough stone pressed against the insides of my thighs. The palms of my hands were red and marked with the texture of the concrete, and there was a tear at the waist of my cotton dress. But I had made it. I sat there for just one moment, feeling terrific and proud and full of accomplishment, before I glanced around and saw a group of my classmates heading in from the ball field, straight in my direction. I still had time, if I hurried, to get down before they saw me and, throwing caution to the winds, I slid quickly down the opposite side of the turtle, missing most of the footholds along the way and arriving on the hard ground with a thud and a long red scratch down my right knee.

That about sums up how I've always felt about exercise and sports. I know climbing a concrete turtle isn't exactly a sport, but it sure was fun. Fun, that is, for the other children who climbed it every time they felt like it, and with every climb built up confidence in their own physical capabilities. I was always so frightened, so embarrassed, so terrified of being laughed at because I was fat, that I never did anything physical unless I had to.

My childhood and adolescent memories are riddled with recollections of avoiding sports: faking sickness to get out of going to day camp; having one sore throat after another to avoid skinny dipping at sleepaway camp; finding an excuse to leave the beach in a hurry the moment my girlfriends decided to join in with the boys' volleyball game. How could they?

One of the things that I did try, that I was forced to try, and that stands out in sharp relief even against the general background of physical humiliation that I faced as a fat child, was rope climbing. We never knew in advance when it would be included in our schedule. We'd troop through the big double doors of the high school gym, a cluster of giggling girls in bright green gymsuits, and I'd stop dead in my tracks at the sight of the long rope dangling from the rafters like a hangman's noose. Because of course my hands and arms couldn't possibly pull up the rest of me. Their strength was totally out of proportion to the weight they were asked to hoist. And yet I was made to try. No teacher ever said, well, look at Nancy's arms and look at Nancy's body. Unless Nancy is Superman there is no way Nancy can lift that body up on those arms.

Why do teachers persist in inflicting these cruelties on fat children? Is it to punish them for being fat? Do they really believe that humiliating the child is the means towards making her curb her appetite?

The habitual excuse offered is that these impossible challenges build character. Nonsense! I refuse to accept that to set a child up for failure is an aid to her development as a human being. All it does is leave her with inhibitions and the awful fear of making a fool of herself.

> ❛ Gym class was hell. I couldn't do handstands and jump over horses because I was too big, but the teacher used to say 'There's no such word as can't.' I used to get notes from my mother saying I was ill when we had a gym day. It made me so miserable. People are cruel because they think that when you're fat you're greedy and undisciplined, and they want to punish you for that. They won't consider that there may be other reasons why you are big. ❜ *Jan Murphy*

I now know that many of my contemporaries, no matter what their size, felt self-conscious and insecure about their bodies. They hated enforced participation in sports just as much as I did, but there was one major difference. In the same way that I never saw a fat person portrayed as attractive, able and confident, so I never saw a fat person successfully participating in any kind of physical activity.

The sporting personalities that I saw on television and in the newspapers were all thin. I had no role model to copy, so I assumed that I just wouldn't be any good at these things. I didn't realize till much later that I really had no idea if I was good at them or not, because I was always so embarrassed that I never even tried.

Nevertheless, there were two physical activities that I did enjoy. First there was swimming. I learned early how to ride the Atlantic waves on Fire Island. To be buffeted about by them, to dive headlong through the clear hard water just before they broke, was one of my great thrills. I knew no fear in that water. I stayed in for hours on end and only after repeated cries from my mother who stood watching from the shore would I emerge, lips blue, fingers and toes white and shrivelled.

And then there was dancing. From the age of nine when, dressed in black velvet and white cotton gloves, I first learned the intricacies of the rumba and the foxtrot from the music teacher at the Hoffman School, to my teens, when my boyfriend Jeffrey and I could knock the socks off all the other lindy dancers in our class, dancing was a passion.

Dance classes

One of the most rewarding moments of the past five years for me came shortly after the transmission of my 'Large as Life' television series. I was shopping in my local supermarket when a slim, smartly dressed woman came up to me. 'I just want to thank you', she said, 'for what you've done for my daughter. She's twelve years old, and very unhappy about her weight. You see we're all slim in our family, me and her two sisters. We've just moved to London from the country and she's been terrified about starting at a new school. But watching your programmes has made her feel so much better about herself, I had to tell you.' I looked beyond the woman to where her daughter stood. She had dark hair and was dressed in a long brown raincoat that covered her completely from head to toe. We smiled at each other across the supermarket aisle, and I knew her so well. I saw myself standing there, shy and self-conscious and filled with the pain of being fat at twelve. We spoke for a few moments, then, too shy to continue, she withdrew her hand from mine with an almost inaudible 'goodbye'. I watched her walk away down the aisle with her slim mother. Just before they disappeared into the crowd of shoppers, the girl looked back over her shoulder at me and a broad grin spread over her face. She waved and was gone.

In one of the programmes in that 'Large as Life' series I had discussed the question of exercise for big women. I hadn't done any dancing or any swimming for years when, in the spring of 1982, I found myself bitten by the exercise bug. I thought to myself, OK kid, you may be fat, but there's no reason for you to be unfit. The first thing I did was to join a local swimming pool. It wasn't the Atlantic rollers, but it was pretty good for central London. Next I decided to do some exercises. I started off alone in my apartment with a simple set of gentle stretches. I felt better, more flexible and limber. But, being naturally gregarious, as well as rather undisciplined by nature, I soon got bored exercising alone.

I looked into the possibility of going to an exercise or dance class. There were certainly enough of them around. The newspapers and women's magazines were full of stories about the latest exercise phenomenon. These same articles stressed how large amounts of weight could be lost and body shapes altered by rigid adherence to the new fitness regimes.

This wasn't at all what I had in mind. I really couldn't see myself attending a class where I might find myself surrounded by women who were there simply because they were hoping to lose weight.

It was at about this time that I heard about a group of women in Canada who were trying to help each other through the problems of being 'overweight'. They met weekly to discuss their problems and also did a regular exercise class.

What a wonderful idea. A class where all the women would be like me. Where I would feel comfortable and unashamed about my size. Surely there must be such a thing in London. I looked through all of the papers listing 'fitness' classes but the only ones that seemed to be geared towards bigger women were also geared towards losing weight. So I decided to start a class of my own. A class where big women could come without fear of being reprimanded about their size. Where they could come and start to discover that moving could actually be enjoyable, where they could begin to feel happier and more self-confident with their bodies, and where they could, above all, have a good time.

Knowing nothing whatsoever about how to begin, I called for assistance upon my good friend, dance teacher and choreographer, Michael Manning and together, using his skills and my body we devised our 'Big, Beautiful and Fit' dance classes.

I was terrified of doing anything dangerous, anything that could possibly hurt women, who, like myself, might not have done any exercise at all for many years. We planned each exercise carefully and then went to see an orthopaedic surgeon to check out our programme. He gave us a piece of advice that was at odds with much of the current fitness dogma, but which was to become the cornerstone of our class. He told us always to remember that pain was the body's way of warning of possible injury, and that if an exercise or a movement was causing pain it should be stopped immediately.

After some alterations, he approved the set of exercises that we were planning as the lead-up to the dance section of the class. These exercises were all based on gentle stretches. There were to be no hurried movements, no jerks or bounces, and certainly no 'going for the burn'. We watched out particularly for bad backs, and weak knees, and emphasized the importance of each woman working at her own pace. At the end of this chapter you will find instructions for some of the exercises that we do.

As I said earlier, I've always loved to dance, and so dance-centred the classes would be – everything from disco routines à la *Saturday Night Fever*, to flamenco and a simple ballet practice barre. We aimed to make the classes dance-centred, enjoyment-centred, and absolutely nothing to do with losing weight.

The first night of class arrived and with it twenty women, all eager, all nervous, and all different sizes. This was one of the surprises of the classes. Many of the women who came that night and who still come are far from fat. They come because they don't feel comfortable in the competitive atmosphere that exists in most exercise classes. They, like me, resent having their bodies criticized, resent being extolled by some rock-hard perfectly formed dancer to 'pull in that sagging tum', 'tighten up those flabby thighs'.

For many of the women who came, it was their first experience of any kind of movement class. They came wearing every imaginable type of garment, track-suits, baggy trousers, loose dresses; one or two brave souls came in leotards even then.

It was a pleasure to see those women who had been the most self-conscious, the most covered up, gradually start to peel off the layers of clothes, the layers of inhibitions. Michael was a perfect teacher. He was enthusiastic and encouraging and fun. And he treated us like normal people, putting the emphasis on our movements and not on our size.

Still frightened of hurting someone, I insisted that he go very slowly, I criti-cized him severely for anything that I felt might be too difficult. About two months after class had started I asked the women for their reactions. They only had one criticism – it was too easy, they wanted more!

My favourite description of the classes came from Lynette, one of those who came to that very first night. She described them as a step into normality for large people, the first door that, once opened, gave her the power to open many others.

Exactly a year after that first dance class, Janis Townes and Elizabeth Osborne, two of the women who had come on that very first night, started teaching a class themselves.

❛ The first night of dance class I walked in and saw all the other big women, it was the most wonderful experience. Even looking in the mirror, which I thought was going to freak me out, didn't. You just see your image and you check to see if you're doing the exercise properly, you're not thinking 'Oh God, that sticks out there', because everybody looks the same. I say the same, but that's not true, in fact I didn't realize how many shapes there were, or how many different sizes of women thought they were big. It really ranged from what looked to me to be skinny to women who were really big.

Although I love dancing I would never have thought of doing a class. I suppose that was the last frontier. You think you've got to look like Margot Fonteyn before you can even walk into a dance class where you just know that everybody is concerned about their image and wearing those glamorous leotards.

It's made a big difference to my life. It's another reason to hold your head up. When people say, 'What do you do Saturday mornings?' and I say, 'I teach a dance class', they don't know what to say. Their whole idea of you has to change. You're not saying, 'Well I'm sitting at home eating two pounds of chocolates all on my own, because no one will take me out.' You're out there doing things, for goodness sake. And they certainly can't tell you you're not fit, because you're often fitter than they are, you run up those stairs and run for the bus, and put your legs in places they could only dream about!

Janis Townes

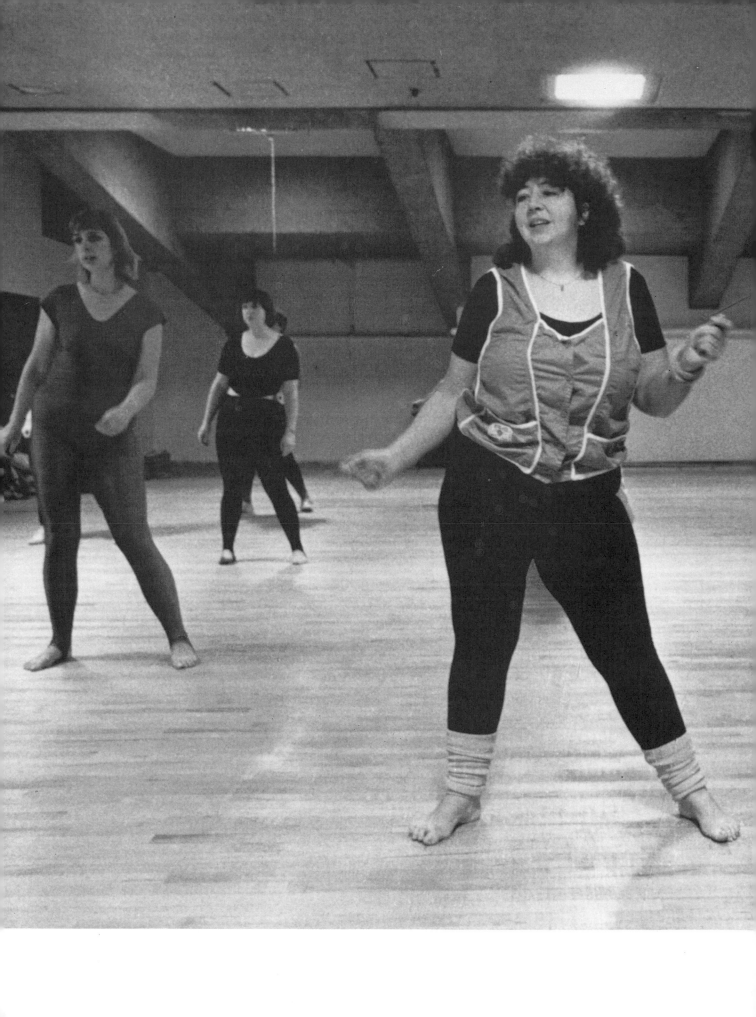

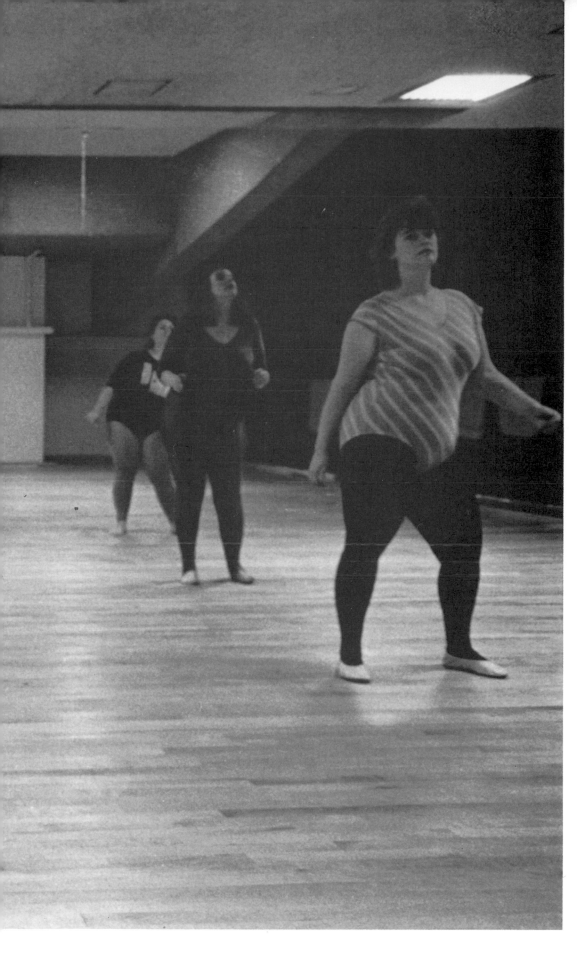

'One, two – step, kick!'
Janis in charge

❛ It's not just a dance class, we feed ourselves spiritually. Women come, feel at home, have a laugh, and eventually they feel totally unselfconscious about their size and their shape. There's lots of big women who are good dancers, but they don't do it because they feel too inhibited about their size. But here we're doing complicated dance routines and there's a real buzz going around the room. The moving and the dancing become almost a sensual pleasure, and fat women aren't used to being sensual. Or if they are, they hide it very carefully. The only time they may get this same sort of pleasure is if they're very secure with one man they've known for a long time and the lights are out. For big women to take joy in their bodies in the way that I think many slim women take for granted is a lovely thing to see.

The class has affected whole areas of these women's lives. Some of them who have been married for a long time felt that they were failing in their roles as wives because they didn't look right. But they don't apologize for the way they are any more. They've gained a lot of confidence. On Saturdays we have the use of the pool and one woman who is fifty-eight learned to swim for the first time. She went on holiday and spent the whole time in the water after having sat by the side for thirty years covered up from her chin to her knees.

As far as teaching the class is concerned, I hope I'm doing it when I'm sixty-five, because I just love it. ❜

Janis Townes

❛ Doing the dance class does actually make me feel high, the physical release. I hadn't moved for such a long time. I'd swum when I was younger and I'd played tennis, but for a long time I'd avoided any kind of exercise like the plague. Not because I didn't enjoy it, but because I couldn't get the right clothes to do it in and be comfortable in...I'd be playing tennis in a dress, and I was convinced everyone was laughing at me.

Coming to class, being with a group of other women who knew exactly how I felt, who had all been there, made it possible for me to become active again, to say to myself, 'Yes, you can do it!'

A few weeks after class had started I took the kids that I teach out for the day. Now there are attitudes and ways of behaving that you develop that just grow over the years, and it would never ever have occurred to me to join in a rounders game with the children. I would have been the one cooking the hot-dogs. But I just thought that day – 'I would like to play rounders.' When I was at school myself I was never any good at it. I tried to get 'struck out' as soon as possible so I wouldn't have to play. But on this day I stood there in front of the kids that had been making comments about my size ever since I'd been teaching them, and I whacked this ball and scored a rounder, and the kids thought it was just great, 'Miss has scored a rounder.' No one laughed at me. It was a moment of awakening. ❜

Elizabeth Osborne

The classes have taught me something very important. Health is more than just being thin. It is assumed that big people are unfit. If this is true, if we are unfit, then surely it is because we have been too ashamed, too self-conscious, to participate in the kind of activities that promote fitness. If you are afraid to go cycling, afraid to go swimming, afraid that you will become the object of ridicule if you do these things, then obviously you are not going to be as fit as someone who does.

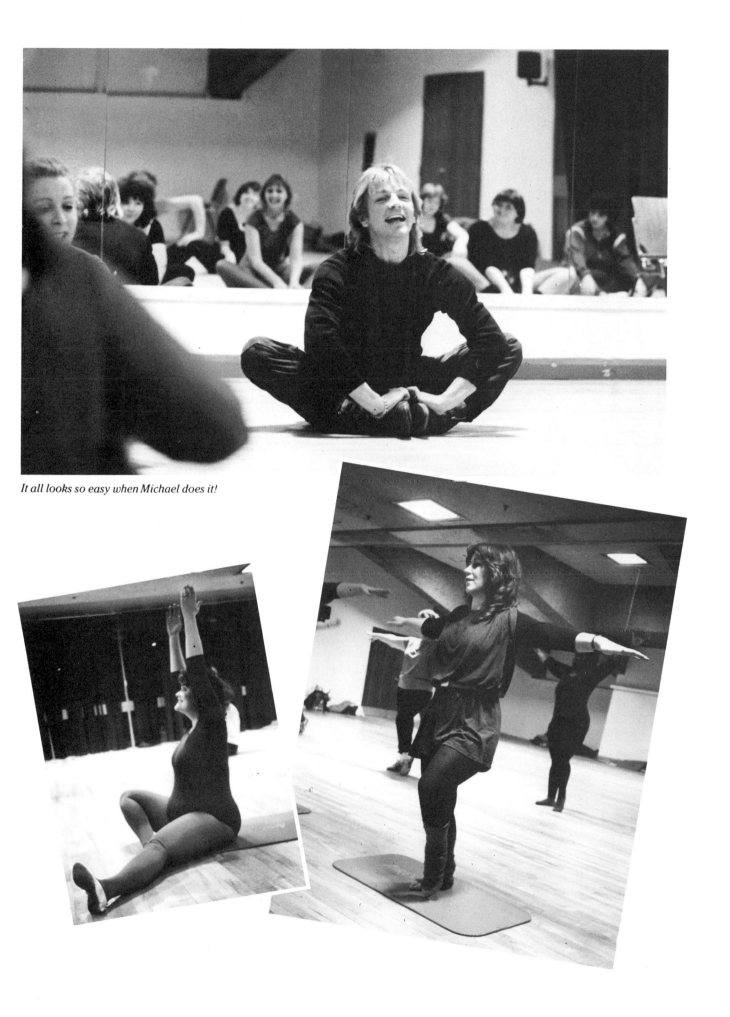

It all looks so easy when Michael does it!

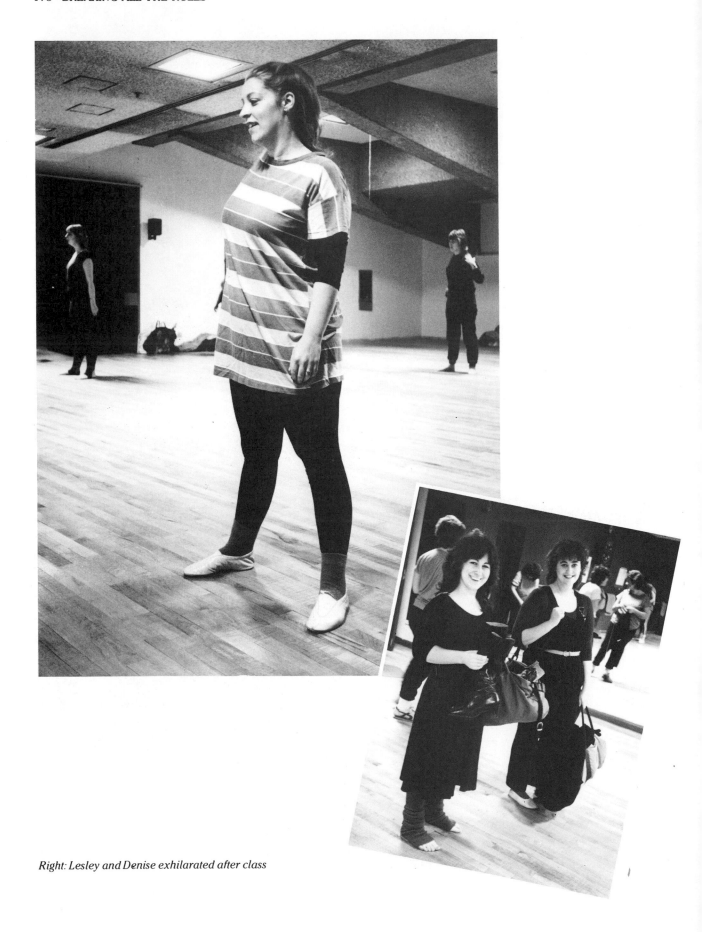

Right: Lesley and Denise exhilarated after class

On the other hand, those women in this book who do take part regularly in some form of exercise feel good, healthy and strong. Their size hasn't stopped them and it needn't stop you. If there is something that you've always wanted to do, get out there and do it.

If you'd like to start your own class try to do it at a local health centre where there are other facilities to enjoy. Our own classes are held at the London Central YMCA, where we also use the swimming pool and the sauna. Being with other women in a non-competitive situation can often give you the courage to participate in those things that you may have been too embarrassed to try before. It can be easier to put on a bathing suit and go swimming or strip for the sauna if you are not alone.

Enormous strength can be derived just from meeting and talking with other women who share the same feelings about their bodies. For many of us the time spent together over coffee after class is as valuable as the time spent exercising on the mat.

Finding other women for your class needn't be a problem. Local newpapers and radio stations can usually be persuaded to run an article or give a mention. They usually get interested if you make it clear to them that you are planning to start a movement class for big women that has nothing to do with losing weight! You can always take out an inexpensive classified ad in the local paper if you find that idea less daunting than seeking 'free' publicity.

The right choice of teacher is vitally important. You must find someone who enjoys *dance*, not just exercise, who appreciates the purpose of the class, and who can help you to feel relaxed about 'bodywork'. The personality of your teacher is the key to the success of your class. You should leave your class

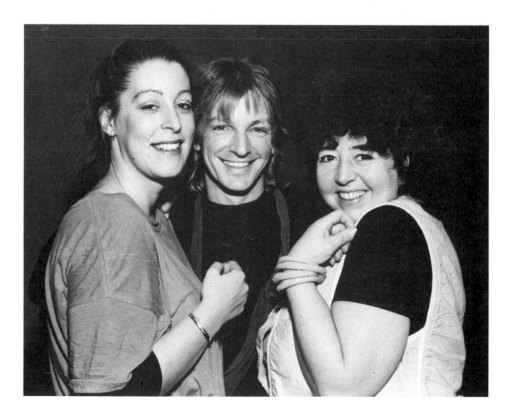

Dance class teachers: Elizabeth Osborne, Michael Manning and Janis Townes

feeling not only that you've had a good workout, but that you've had a wonderful time. The teacher's personality (or lack of it) sets the tone for the atmosphere within the class, so make sure you get someone you *like*. Advertise (put a card up, or leave one at the administration office) at local dance studios or health centres, and then interview potential candidates until you find someone you think is right.

If after your classes have started you sense a note of what I call fat discrimination (remarks about you losing weight, or criticism of your ability that relates to your size, etc.) creeping into your teacher's tone, or he or she begins to ask you to do things that you all feel may be dangerous and that hurt, you must feel free to discuss this with him or her. Remember that these are *your* classes, and that you will have had a lot more experience of moving a big body around than they will. Sometimes certain movements that seem perfectly easy to someone slim can be difficult for us, simply because of our added bulk. Don't be afraid to point this out to your teacher. Eventually you may, like Janis and Elizabeth, choose to teach a class yourself. There is absolutely no reason why you should not. As long as you make yourself aware of what particular exercises might put a strain on certain parts of the body and either avoid them or warn members of your class with problems in these specific areas to avoid them. You should also, of course, love to dance, be excited about conveying that enjoyment to the women in your class, *and* be good at making up new dance routines. It is wonderful to see a big woman teaching a dance class. It's something that really does break all the rules.

In the last couple of years I've discovered that I also love walking. The more I can walk, the better I feel. I go to the park, wear my running shoes and do a steady 20–30 minutes fast walking. I may not be running like the joggers that pass me, but I know that I am doing what feels right for my body. Walking, like running, swimming, and cycling, is an aerobic exercise. When done at the proper pace and for the correct amount of time, all of these exercises increase the strength and capacity of your lungs and of your heart. They also make you feel energized and capable of anything. When I'm doing one of my 'serious' walks in the park, and not just strolling around the neighbourhood, I always check my pulse rate to make sure that I am keeping it at the optimum exercise rate for my age and size as suggested by any number of books on aerobic exercise.

Another aerobic exercise that is very popular with many of the women I've spoken with is swimming. Not only is it enjoyable, it is an ideal exercise for bigger women. Our body size gives us added buoyancy and the water supports us so that injuries are very unlikely.

Every woman who talked to me about her own exercise routine stressed one point – the sense of achievement she felt. It's the sense of breaking out of the mould. Just as dressing beautifully breaks down the 'fat and ugly' stereotype, so getting out there and doing something energetic starts to dispel the 'fat and lazy' image.

> ❛ **I swim three times a week. I do fourteen lengths at 8 o'clock in the morning. It's great, really fun and I feel very healthy. ❜**
> *Kate Franklin*

> ❛ At school I was very athletic, I played netball, I sprinted, and did discus and the shot. That's when I started gaining weight – all muscle. I thoroughly enjoyed athletics and although I was getting bigger, there was never any pressure put on me to slim. I was very fit and could outrun everybody. Friends would say, 'Oh you can't run', because I was supposedly too big to be a sprinter, but then we'd race and I'd beat them all. ❜
>
> *Carole Burton*
>
> ❛ I ride whenever I can. Horses are big animals and they're very strong so size is no excuse for not having a go at it. ❜
>
> *Mandy Crane*
>
> ❛ I do at least six dancing lessons a week and I work out at home every Sunday. I'm always going to a lesson and coming out sweating. People think it's because I'm about to have a heart attack, they're thinking 'quick, get the stretcher', but it's because I've worked. ❜
>
> *Liz Birru*
>
> ❛ I couldn't stand organized games at school, it's so very boring. As soon as there are rules I'm not interested. But I swam a lot, and I still do. We walk every morning and I've got my little stationary exercise bike. Most evenings I do about three miles on that, while I'm watching television.
>
> There are all kinds of health. All I know is that I feel fine and that I'm as healthy as I know how to be. ❜
>
> *Claire Rayner*

My own exercise routine is rather erratic. I don't let it become a fetish. Like 'fetish eating', I steer clear of 'fetish exercising'. I go through periods when I am very keen and others when I'm more relaxed. I've reached the point where I don't need to exercise to feel good about myself any more than I need to diet.

I think it's important to see things like exercising, like dressing up, or putting on full make-up, as things that you choose to do because they make you feel good and give you pleasure. When any of these things becomes an obsession, a crutch, that's when they spell trouble. When you can't go to the supermarket without getting all dolled up, when you can't leave the house without 'putting your face on', and when you feel worthless because you've not done your exercises, then you've got a problem.

Doctors' attitudes

Going to the doctor can be torture if you're big. Many doctors blame absolutely everything from an earache to an ingrowing toenail on the fact that you're overweight. One woman told me that if she walked into her doctor's office carrying her head under her arm, he'd tell her that it had fallen off because she was too fat. I've had the feeling from many doctors that I'm not entitled to their care or their sympathy as long as I'm fat. After all, their reasoning seems to go, why should they take care of me if I won't take care of myself.

Since that day five years ago when I first read that 95 per cent of women put back all the weight they lose on diets, dieting recidivism figures have been widely publicized. Any number of newspaper articles and television programmes make reference to these figures and yet this doesn't seem to stop most doctors making their patients feel like failures if they don't manage to maintain a weight loss. This never ceases to amaze me. It's as if all the latest research, all the latest findings, make no impact whatever on what was taught many years ago in medical school.

The horror stories concerning diet doctors and medically sanctioned methods of losing weight are heartbreaking. Many women have attended specialists to be given diet pills and massive injections, sometimes containing ingredients as bizarre as horse urine. One woman told me of a doctor in Harley Street who was so popular and so busy that, to save time, he administered his own brand of miracle injection straight through her tights. I've known women who've gone to hypnotherapists to curb their compulsive eating behaviour, who've had staples put in their earlobes to curb their appetites. They've had operations to remove excess fat around the buttocks and thighs. They've had intestinal bypass operations to reduce the amount of food that the body can digest, and they've had parts of their stomachs partitioned off with staples to reduce their capacity for food.

I once did a TV programme with three women who had had their jaws wired together so that they could only take in liquids. One of these women had had her wires removed several months earlier and had promptly regained all the weight she had lost, and more. This sad fact seemed to make no difference to the two women who were still 'wired up . They were determined to go on with this barbaric practice, visiting the dentist once a month to have the wires loosened so that they could clean their teeth, and always keeping a pair of wire clippers handy in case they needed to be sick.

On the same programme with me was a particularly slim nutritionist who did admit that actually *maintaining* the weight loss could be a problem. At her own clinic they were at the moment trying out a new method that seemed to be working very satisfactorily. After the required weight loss had been achieved and the jaw wires removed, a plastic cord, that could only be removed with special shears, was fastened around the 'patient's' waist. This cord had a bit of slack in it, to allow for a weight gain of approximately three to four pounds. If a patient put on more than three or four pounds then the cord became tight and uncomfortable, cutting into the waist. It was at this point, naturally, that the patient knew it was time to return to her diet.

The woman who sat next to me on that afternoon programme telling this story to me and to the three women who had had their jaws wired, didn't seem bizarre in any way. And yet she thought it was perfectly sane that this almost medieval form of restriction should be used on women who were bigger than she was.

There exists an attitude that says that fat people are no more than research animals, guinea pigs on which to try out the latest diet fantasy. One large woman told me of a particularly gruesome three-week stay in hospital. The doctors were supposedly trying to locate a medical reason for her extreme overweight. During this time she had to obtain all of her food from a vending machine, she had four blood tests a day, was plunged into a tank of water and then put into an iron casket. These were presumably some sort of tests, but although she remained in hospital for three weeks, no one ever explained to her the reason or purpose for any of them.

❝ My doctor is the only person who ever puts any pressure on me. He says, 'You're now thirty-nine, when you're fifty you'll have rheumatoid arthritis.' He's not really got a leg to stand on, I have my cholesterol checked from time to time, and my blood pressure is as low as anything. I'm actually frightfully healthy, very energetic. ❞

Meredith Etherington-Smith

❝ I don't go to doctors. I haven't been to one in a long time. When I was quite young my mother took me to a doctor because she knew that I was miserable about my weight and the school had put pressure on her to take me. I remember this doctor himself was rather overweight. He asked me to touch my toes which I couldn't do and still can't do and the shame was dreadful, I felt so impotent. He was looking at me and I was only about nine years old – fat and vulnerable. He was very aggressive, it was as if he wanted me to be thin the next day. I felt he was asking me to do the impossible because I knew I wasn't any more greedy than my friends who were thin, so how could I lose that weight? I've avoided doctors ever since...I don't know why he wanted me to touch my toes really. I think he just wanted to show me and my mother that I was fat. But he didn't have to do that because we both knew. ❞

Jan Murphy

❝ I go to a female doctor now who's never mentioned weight. I even went to a dietician to get a special diet because I'm allergic to milk, and I thought she'd get me on those scales, because they love scales, don't they? You can't walk into a doctor's office without ending up on a pair of scales, but she said to me 'Now, we want a diet that *maintains* your weight, don't we?' I was amazed. ❞

Janis Townes

Thankfully all doctors are not insensitive to our needs, and we can do a lot through our own behaviour and attitudes to better our lot. Doctors are, after all, people. Some of them we get along with, some we don't. It can be difficult to change doctors but sometimes it's worth it. If you feel that your doctor isn't paying proper attention to other aspects of your health because he's blaming everything on your weight, then tell him. If he still doesn't give you the care you think you deserve, then change doctors.

I've found that it's all a question of being assertive. I don't think doctors are accustomed to fat people talking back to them. Several years ago I was in an automobile accident. I suffered whiplash and pains in my back for some time after. I naturally went to a doctor right after the accident. Several months later I was still suffering back pain and I went to see a specialist. He looked at me sceptically as I described the pain, and I just knew from the look on his face what was coming. 'Listen,' I said, 'I know what you're thinking, and it's no good telling me to go on a diet because I won't. I spent too much of my life miserable as a compulsive eater and I've no intention of going back to that now!'

He was, to put it mildly, stunned. So was I, at my effrontery, but I also felt good. He looked at me for a moment, and then smiled resignedly. 'Well,' he said, 'I guess we'd better treat the Nancy Roberts we've got here and now, and not the one we could have.' It was that easy. I think I was lucky; I get the feeling I was dealing with one of the more enlightened members of his profession, but it worked.

Sally, a young mother on one of my programmes, spoke of the doctor who told her that if she didn't lose weight she'd be dead in five years. She was carrying her second child at the time and was understandably distressed by this information. She's since moved to another town and changed doctors. With some trepidation she went to her first appointment. Her new doctor surprised her by telling her that she was obviously meant to be a 'big girl' and she should work at coming to terms with that fact. He then expressed the far from common sentiment that it was important for her to be happy and relaxed the way she was.

Happy and relaxed – two states that don't come easily to those of us who consider ourselves fat. The amount of tension and anxiety associated with being fat in our society is incalculable. The psychological pressures felt by those of us who live our lives as 'bigger' women are impossible to describe to people who don't share our problem.

In an age when we accept that our state of mind has tremendous influence over our physical health, it's time we examined the correlation between being fat and the stress-related illnesses normally associated with obesity from a new perspective.

Recent studies, explored by Kim Chernin in her excellent book, *Womansize – The Tyranny of Slenderness*, suggest that it may not always be the physical fact of being fat that leads to the 'obesity-related illnesses' so common in our culture, but that these illnesses may in fact be brought on by the tension and anxieties of being stigmatized because of our size. No other physical characteristic except skin colour is so stigmatized in our society. Those of us who have suffered the pain and humiliation of being treated as outcasts in a society that hates fat, who are under constant pressure to diet, to conform to a size that may not be natural for our own bodies, are certainly more susceptible to stress and therefore to the stress-related illnesses than are people who lead their lives free of these pressures.

My own recipe for a healthy life these days has a lot more to do with what I'm doing than with what I'm eating. But just because I don't diet any more, it doesn't mean that I'm not conscious of what I eat. I'm as aware as the next woman of the latest nutritional findings, and I try to cut down on foods that I know are bad, not just for me, but for everyone. But this has nothing to do with losing weight, just creating a healthier body. I've cut down on sugar, on salt, on fats. I try to eat more fibre. Every time I cut myself a slice of wholemeal bread or throw a baking potato in the oven, I think of those years of going without, those years when these same things were tantamount to poison, and how unhappy I was then, and it seems crazy that something so utterly unimportant should have made me so miserable.

I've come a long way since those days in the playground at the Hoffman School, since those feelings of fear, of shame, of not being able to take part. I've realized that being healthy doesn't mean spending one's life thinking about food and one's appearance. It means, instead, exploring one's potential, enjoying one's family and friends, and seeking out and taking pleasure in all the marvellous things that life has to offer. It means having the courage to climb the turtle.

> ❛ **Life's for living, in the end. There are so many marvellous things to see and do and be part of, that it's nonsense to be fanatical about dieting.** ❜
>
> *Joanne Brogden*

> ❛ **The main way that people can help themselves is to stop putting things off. People say, 'When I've lost weight then I'll do so and so.' Well that can go on for years, then suddenly you wake up one morning and think, my God, what happened to all that time!'** ❜
>
> *Mandy Crane*

Exercises

The following is a list of some of the exercises that we do in our classes. They can form the basis of your own class, or you may prefer to do them on your own at home, or with a couple of friends. Many of them you will recognize. They have been around for ages. Some I can remember from my own dreaded days in high school gym class. Others were given to me by my doctor when I was suffering from neck and back complaints after the car crash that I've already mentioned; these are movements which are well known to exercise teachers and physiotherapists the world over.

Although the exercises are ones that I've known for years, what is new is my attitude towards doing them. I no longer see them as something that I am forced to do by some outside influence, but as something that I do for myself. They make me feel supple, strong and full of energy. If you should decide to give them a try, I hope they do the same for you. When I do them alone I like to put on background music. It should be slow and soothing, nothing with a steady beat that you might be encouraged to keep up with. The point of these exercises is to do them at your own speed, not at the tempo of a fast dance record.

You should always check with your doctor before starting any exercise programme. It is important not to overdo things at first. Depending on your level of fitness (I had done *nothing* for years when I started) you may begin by doing the exercises only twice a week, building up to three or four times a week. You may enjoy doing them so much that you want to do them every day. It's entirely up to you.

These exercises are designed to stretch and strengthen all parts of the body gently. You should never bounce, jerk or yank as you do them, but always move gradually and slowly into the stretch. If you always move as if you were moving through quicksand, then you will avoid injury. If something does hurt – *stop*! Pain is a warning and should be treated as such! It is natural to feel somewhat stiff after exercising, especially when you first start, but this stiffness will gradually lessen as your body becomes accustomed to the movements. Although the exercises are gentle, you may find that if you have a bad back or a tricky knee, some exercises may be difficult or painful. Don't worry – leave them out. As you begin to enjoy moving your body, you will find that there are lots of other activities that you can enjoy – walking, swimming, dancing, all great fun, and good for you as well! If you really catch the exercise bug, there are many exercise books around from which you can enlarge your repertoire. There are, however, certain types of movement that you should avoid.

● *Avoid anything that calls for leaping, jumping, landing heavily on your feet.* Our extra weight landing heavily on weak joints can lead to serious injury.

● *Avoid toe touching or bending forward from the waist.* This can be risky for anyone if not done carefully. Many back problems are caused by people swooping down to touch their toes – it puts strain on the supporting ligaments of the spine and on the discs. For those of us who are large the dangers are even more pronounced. We have extra weight to lift as we bring our body back to the upright position and the risk of back injury is even greater.

● *Avoid lying flat on your back with straight legs.* Whenever you lie on your back on the floor, your knees should be bent to eliminate pull on your lower back. Do not be tempted to do these exercises or any other exercises (including various versions of sit-ups) with straight legs, especially if you have a bad back. Raising the knees relaxes the back and is a good trick to remember if you suffer from backaches. Lying on a firm bed with one or more pillows under your knees can lead to speedy relief.

Breathing is an essential part of any exercise programme. Proper breathing relaxes the whole body, carries oxygen to the muscles and prepares them for working. Each time you breathe deeply you are exercising and strengthening the stomach muscles, which in turn will give support to your back and help avoid spinal injury. Before you begin your exercises practise proper breathing.

Sit straight in a chair with one hand on your chest and the other on your stomach. Breathe in as deeply as possible through the nose. Your stomach should be the first to expand. You should try and consciously push it out against your hand. This expansion of the abdomen indicates that your diaphragm is lowered, allowing your lungs to take in their full complement of oxygen.

If your chest is the first to expand, then your breathing is too shallow and you should practise a few more times until you feel this bellowing of the stomach each time you inhale. When you exhale contract the stomach muscles and squeeze them against your back until every bit of 'stale' air is expelled. Once you have mastered this breathing technique it will come naturally and become a pleasurable part of your routine. You should always begin any exercise session with five or six good deep breaths.

In the exercises that follow it is important that you stand in the proper position.

STAND UP STRAIGHT

Stand up very straight and tall, with your feet slightly apart, so that you are comfortable and your thighs are not pushing together. Your feet should be parallel, your knees aligned directly over your feet – do not let your knees sag inwards. Your weight should be equally distributed between your heels and the balls of your feet. Don't tip forwards or backwards. Imagine that you have a thread pulling you up by the top of your head and your body is very long, very tall. This is the correct position for the exercises which follow.

● Always remember to breathe deeply and rhythmically as you do the following exercises.

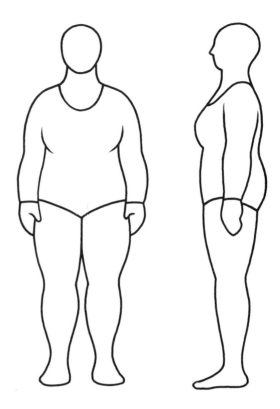

The three following exercises are especially good for releasing tension in the back of the neck and between the shoulders. Do them any time you feel tense and tight or feel a headache coming on, and remember to always breathe deeply and rhythmically as you do them.

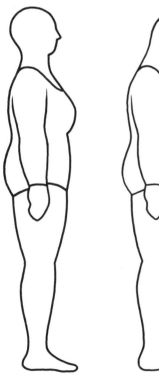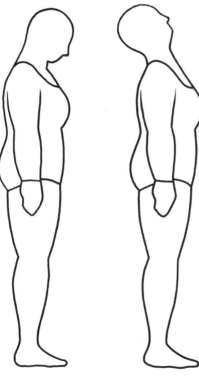

NECK LOOSENER

(Left) Stand up straight, with your shoulders relaxed and your arms and hands hanging loosely by your sides. Lower your head slowly forward as far as you can with your chin aiming to reach your chest. Hold for a second as you feel the stretch down the back of your neck. Slowly raise the head to the starting position. Now lower your head as far back as you can. Feel the stretch down the front of your jaw and neck. Do not let the head drop suddenly but always be in control of this slow gentle movement. Repeat five times each way.

(Exercise continues overleaf)

● I prefer this neck stretcher to the more common headrolls which make me dizzy and which are very hard to do without scrunching up your shoulders.

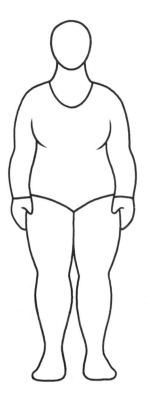 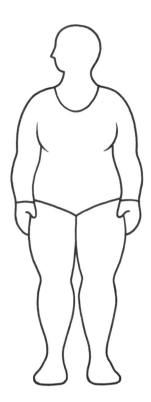 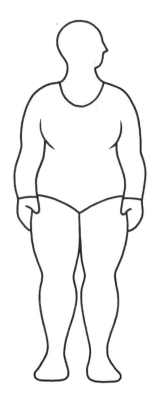

(Above) From 'eyes front' starting position turn the head slowly to the right as far as you can, hold for a second, then turn slowly to the left as far as you can. Repeat five times.

(Below) Next, looking straight ahead, lower head to the side and try to touch right ear to right shoulder. Be sure to keep your shoulders loose and relaxed as you do this, do not allow them to hunch up. Now slowly lift head and repeat, this time to the left. Repeat five times.

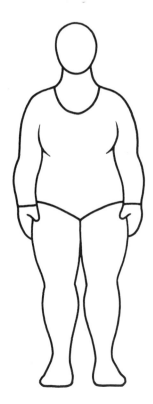 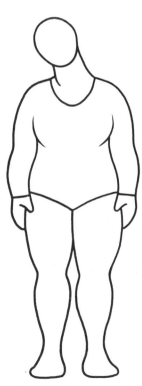 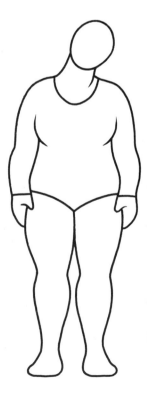

SHOULDER ROTATIONS

Stand up straight. Bring the right shoulder forward, then up to the right ear, then as far back as you can, pushing the shoulder towards the spine, then bring it slowly down to the starting position. While working the right shoulder try and keep the left shoulder and the head absolutely still. Just think of isolating the 'working' shoulder from the rest of your body. It helps to watch yourself in a mirror as you do this. Repeat four times. Repeat with left shoulder.

Reverse. This time begin by bringing the right shoulder back, then up to the ear, then forward, and then gently down. Repeat four times. Repeat with left shoulder.

Both shoulders. Bring both shoulders together, first forward, then up to the ears, then back – bringing the shoulder-blades as close together as you can, then down and relax. Shake out the arms and shoulders and legs.

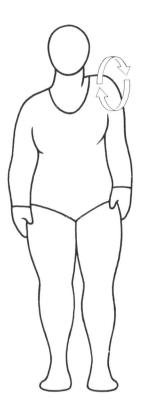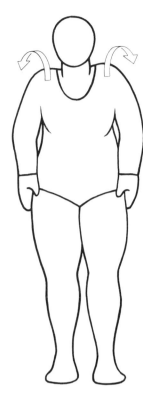

● It's always a good idea to have a *gentle* shake-out between exercises to relax all the working muscles and get them ready for the next exercise.

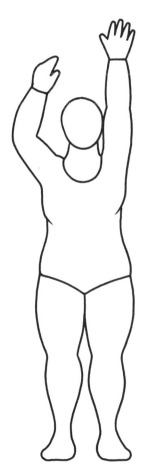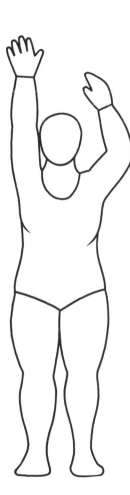

ARM AND SIDE STRETCHES

Stand up straight. Raise both arms high above the head. Stretch up with the right arm, straightening the elbow and extending the fingers towards the sky. Feel the stretch all along the right arm and down the right side to your waist. As you reach up with the right arm, make sure the left shoulder and arm are relaxed. Now stretch up with the left arm as you relax the right. Repeat eight times with each arm. Relax and shake out.

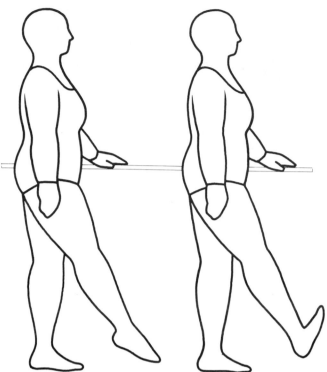

FLEX-POINT

Stand up straight. Supporting yourself on the back of a chair or kitchen counter raise the right leg about 6 in/15 cm off the floor. Point the foot forward and feel the stretch along the top of your foot and ankle; then flex the foot, pulling your toes up towards the body, feel the stretch down the back of your leg. Repeat six times. Change legs and repeat with left foot. Be sure that the supporting leg is kept absolutely straight, with the muscles 'pulled up' so that it feels like an iron rod. Relax and shake out legs.

ANKLE ROLLS

Same starting position as Flex-point. Raise the right leg. Flex the foot and slowly rotate the ankle, to the right, down towards the floor, in to the left then up. Repeat four times. Change feet and repeat four times with left foot. Go back to right foot and this time rotate in the opposite direction. Repeat four times with each foot. Relax and shake out the feet and legs.

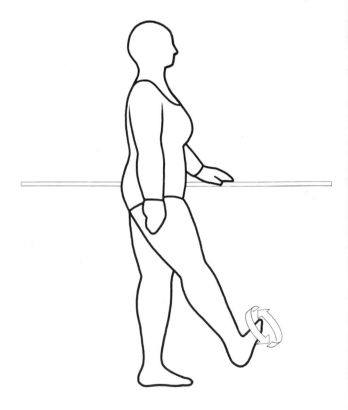

We're now going to move down on to the floor. It's important to remember to move slowly and smoothly when you are getting down to or up from the floor. Don't fling yourself down or leap up suddenly, but once again move deliberately, as if you were pushing through quicksand, and you will be unlikely to injure yourself. To lie down on the floor on your back, always start in a sitting position. Gently lower yourself until you are lying first on your *side*. Then roll over on to your back. Reverse this procedure for sitting up. Roll from your back over on to your side, then use your arms to push yourself up to a sitting position. Sitting straight up without first turning on to your side can lead to back injury.

● *Always use a mat or lie on a thick carpet when you are working on the floor.* You can also fold several blankets together to make a cushioned surface. In spite of our natural padding, it is easy to bruise yourself at pressure points if you exercise on a bare floor. It's also very uncomfortable!

STOMACH STRENGTHENER (basic breathing)

Lie on the mat or carpet, knees bent, feet about 8 in/20 cm apart so that your legs feel comfortably balanced, toes slightly turned in, hands on stomach. Breathe in deeply through your nose, expand the stomach as you breathe in, feel the air filling your stomach and then breathe out very slowly. As you breathe out, contract the stomach muscles and press the spine down against the floor. Repeat five times.

Not only is this excellent for relaxing the whole body and increasing the flow of oxygen to the muscles but it is an excellent stomach strengthener.

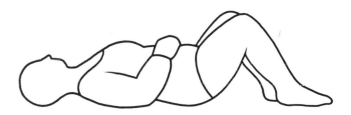

● In some of the exercises that follow I will give specific breathing instructions. It may seem complicated at first, but if you remember always to exhale on the exertion portion of the movement you will soon get the hang of it.

PELVIC TILT

Maintain the same starting position as in the previous exercise. Slowly inhale and fill the stomach with air. As you exhale, contract the stomach muscles, tighten the buttocks and the thighs, and, keeping the waist pressed against the mat, tilt the pelvis forward in a very gentle movement. Your lower spine should only come off the floor about 1 in/2·5 cm. Inhale as you relax and gently roll down on to the floor again. Repeat eight times.

This is great for lower back pain; it releases all the tension that tends to collect there, especially if you have back problems as many of us do. It was first taught to me as a teenager when I had injured my back lifting a heavy paint can while lying on my stomach! – smart, hey? In addition to being great for the back it also strengthens the thighs and the buttocks.

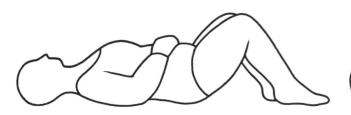

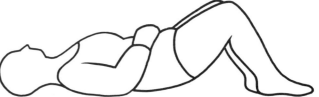

SMALL NECK-STRETCHER

Lying in the same beginning position as in the previous exercise lace your fingers behind your head. Inhale, feel the stomach expand. Exhale, contract the stomach, and bring the head, neck and upper spine up and forward, pointing the elbows towards your knees and looking through the knees. Keep the stomach muscles contracted as you hold this stretch for a second. Inhale, relax and slowly roll down again. This is not a sit-up, but a very small movement, just lifting the head, neck and upper spine. Repeat eight times.

This exercise releases the tension in the neck and shoulders, and strengthens the upper and middle back and the stomach.

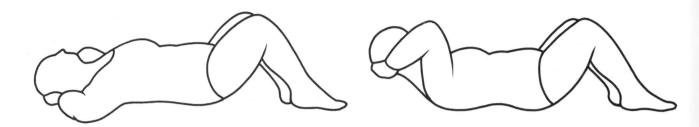

I had been very inactive for a long time when I decided to start exercising. I started by going for long, brisk walks – too long for my body as it turned out. My knees started to bother me – they just weren't used to the strain of carrying my body around for such long periods of time. My doctor suggested I do some leg-strengthening exercises to build up the leg muscles and take pressure off my knees, and to ease up a bit on the walking until my legs were stronger. The flex-points and ankle rolls described earlier are excellent for building up flexibility of the legs and ankles, as are the leg exercises which follow. The simple leg raises are excellent for building up the quadriceps muscles that support the knees. If my knees do start to bother me, I do these raises twice a day. Do as many raises as you can until your thighs feel tired. Remember to do them slowly and rhythmically. As with all of these exercises, if you rush them, you will negate the effect.

LEG RAISES

Sit with legs outstretched in front of you, several inches apart to allow room for your thighs. Rest your weight on your hands, which you place on the floor just behind you. Bend your left leg. Inhale. As you exhale flex the right foot, push out through the heel and slowly raise the right leg about 8–12 in/20–30 cm. Inhale as you slowly bring the foot down again and relax. Repeat eight times or until your muscles feel tired. Then repeat with the left leg.

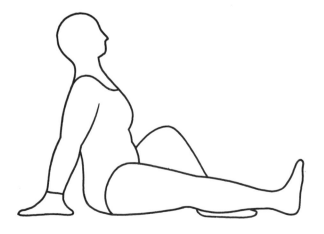
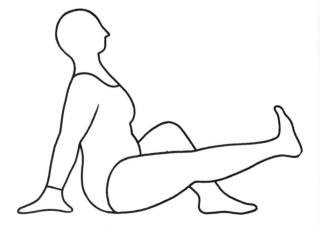

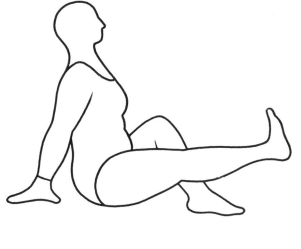

SEATED FLEX-POINTS AND ANKLE ROLLS

You may prefer to do the flex-points and ankle rolls in this seated position instead of standing up as I described them earlier. In that case begin with the leg raised as in previous exercise, and with your foot raised do the flex-points first with your right foot, then with the left, then go on to the ankle rolls as described for the standing versions. Make sure you give your legs a gentle shake-out between each exercise to relax them. Breathe deeply and rhythmically throughout the flex-points and ankle rolls.

You may find that your neck and shoulders tense up a bit while doing this. Relax them with a few head turns and shoulder rotations before going on to the next exercise.

● Always remember to give yourself a gentle shake-out after you've exercised a particular part of the body.

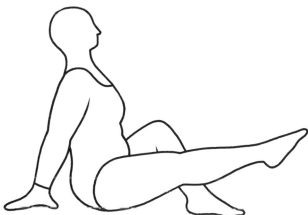

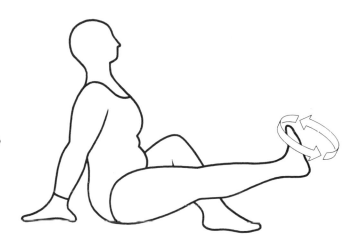

SIDE LEG LIFT

Lie on your right side with your head propped up in your right hand, and your left hand on the floor in front of your chest supporting your body. Extend your legs in front of you, ideally at a 90° angle to your body, or at an angle that is comfortable. Flex the feet and straighten the legs. Inhale and feel the stomach expand. Exhale and very slowly raise the left leg to just above hip height. Inhale as you slowly lower the leg. Repeat five times, then turn over and repeat with other leg. Do as many of these as you can until the muscles tire; build up to about fifteen repetitions with each leg.

This one strengthens the outer thighs and buttocks as it works the hip joint.

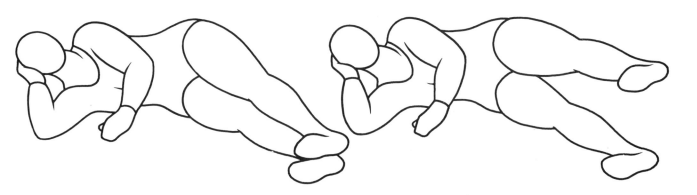

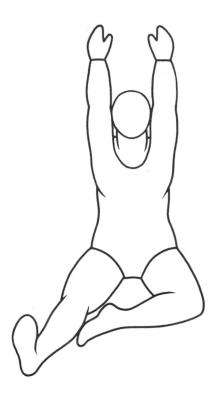

SINGLE LEG STRETCH

Sit on the floor, legs stretched out in front of you and feet about 2 ft/60 cm apart. Bend the left knee and place the sole of the left foot against the inside of the right leg. Keep the right foot flexed, the hips aligned and the back very straight. Inhale and raise the arms above the head towards the ceiling. Exhale, lower the head against the chest and stretch out along the extended leg, past the flexed foot. Inhale and reach up. Repeat five times to the right side. Then change sides and repeat five times to the left.

This one stretches the lower back, the inner thighs and the backs of the legs (the hamstring muscles).

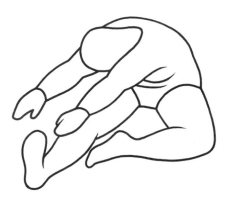

TWO-LEGGED STRETCH

Sit up with your legs apart in a 'V' and the knees straight, the feet flexed. Spread your legs apart as far as you can without losing your balance. With the back straight inhale and bring the arms up above the head with the palms facing each other. Inhale, lower the chin to the chest. Exhale, contract the stomach and stretch out over the right leg, reaching towards the right foot with both hands. Inhale as you come up. Turn towards the left leg. Exhale and stretch out over the left leg. Repeat three times to each side.

This is great for overall flexibility and to stretch and tone the inner thighs.

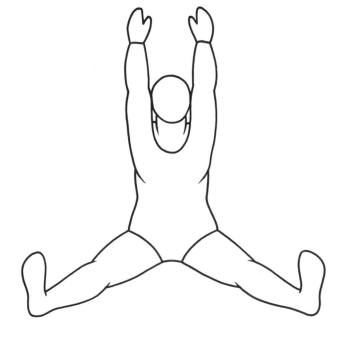

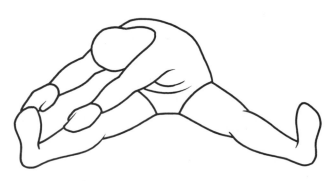

WAIST STRETCHER

Sit up with the legs in the same position as in the previous exercise. Inhale as you raise both arms until they are outstretched at shoulder level. Exhale as you lift one arm up over your head and stretch over towards opposite foot.

Keep your spine 'long' and don't allow it to collapse forward. Inhale as you return to centre position. Exhale and repeat to other side. Repeat three times.

This stretches and tones the waist area and inner thighs.

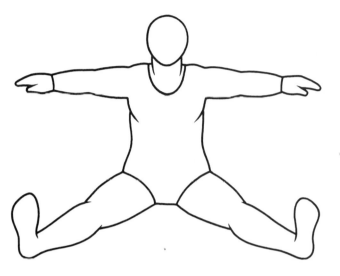 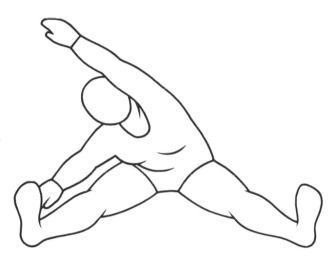

SUPER-STRETCH

This exercise is in two parts. First, sit up straight, legs straight out, feet flexed and slightly apart. Inhale as you reach up towards the ceiling with both arms and back straight. Exhale and reach out over your legs and grab your ankles (or any part of your legs that you can reach!). Relax. Inhale, feel the stomach expand, and still hold on to your legs. Exhale, contract the stomach, bend the elbows and pull your head down closer to your knees. Inhale and straighten the elbows, still holding on to the legs. Exhale and pull yourself down again. Repeat five times.

This releases tension and stretches the back and the backs of the legs.

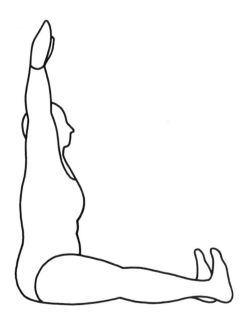 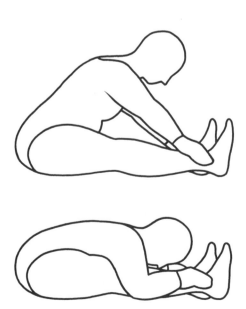

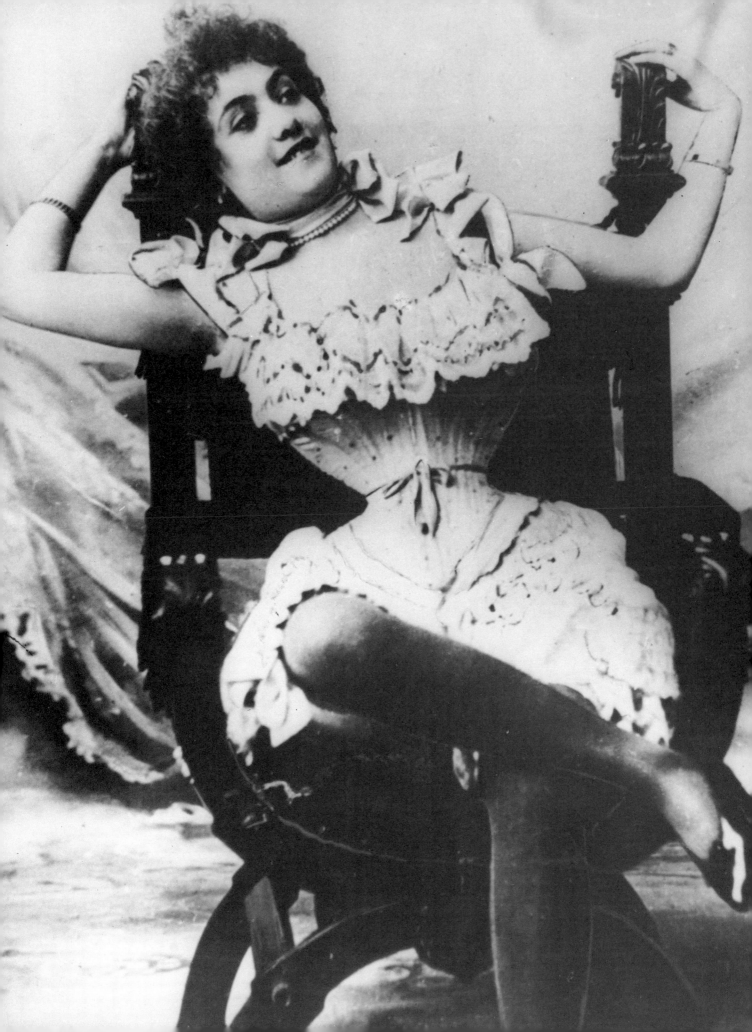

13

THE HISTORICAL PERSPECTIVE

Throughout this book I've been talking about two things – compulsive eating and body size, and how the first has been the sad consequence of trying to alter the second. I'm suggesting that the time has come to end the torture that women put themselves through in their quest for the fashionable shape, an end to this twentieth-century madness that leaves so many of us with disabling eating disorders and cripplingly low self-esteem.

It might seem that the present-day predilection for doing battle with our bodies is something new. It isn't. Fashion has, seemingly forever, decreed that we alter our basic contours. The shape we were born with has rarely been seen to be good enough and throughout the centuries people have tortured themselves to achieve what was thought to be fashionable at the time. In retrospect, and from a different cultural perspective, many of these attempts seem bizarre and barbaric: think of the painful binding of women's feet in China, the head-flattening practised by the ancient Egyptians and the American Indians, the neck-stretching and massively distorted lips and earlobes prized by some African tribes. These are only a few examples of the many painful alterations that people throughout the ages have made to their bodies. Very often the distortion achieved by these practices singled out the bearer as a member of a more privileged stratum of society, in much the same way as today being slim and beautiful is a prerequisite for entry into the jet-set. When considering the fashions of our own time, it is important to remember that passing fashions are simply that – passing.

Nevertheless, looking back over the history of fashion is fascinating, for it is the history of people's attempts to make their 'imperfect' natural shapes conform to a current ideal. Until this century, the more drastic means of altering this form were mainly mechanical. A vast variety of devices were worn: corsets to make you smaller, padding to make you bigger, straps, laces and constructions of all sorts were employed.

We certainly don't think of the fashions of antiquity as requiring rigid undergarments – their loose flowing lines seem the ultimate in unrestricted, comfortable style. Yet even in ancient Crete women and men wore tight girdles around

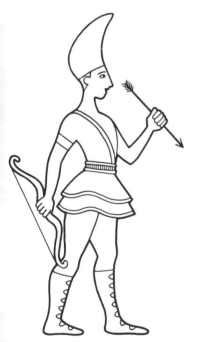

Above: The wasp waist: Cretan warrior of 1500 BC

Opposite: The definitive hourglass figure considered fashionable during Victorian times could be achieved by surgical removal of the bottom ribs (1900)

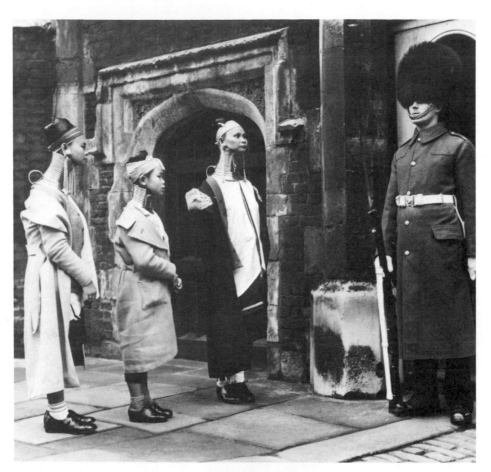

Left: Neck-stretching. Another culture's idea of beauty

Below left: Chinese foot-binding. Tiny feet were an indication of a woman's inability to work and therefore of her husband's wealth

Below right: Head-flattening among Indian tribes – an elongated head was useless for carrying heavy burdens and so singled out the bearer as a member of the leisured class

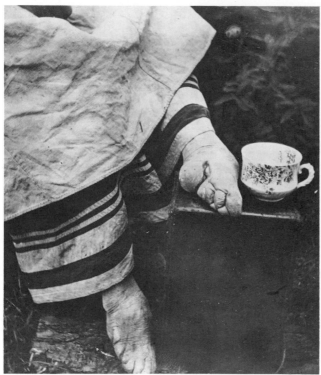

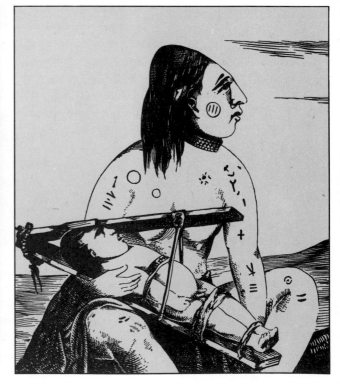

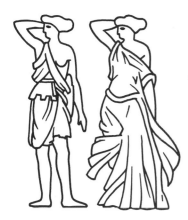

The flowing fashions of antiquity

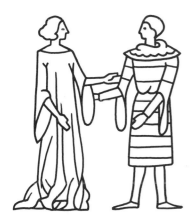

Loose-flowing dress before tight lacing became all the rage

their waists and, surprisingly, in Greece, not during the finest epochs of Greek history but rather during the time of Greek decadence, women wore corsets. They were designed not to make the waist appear smaller, a small waist never having appealed to the Greeks, but to make the hips appear larger.

Until the thirteenth century, clothes remained mainly loose and flowing, togas, mantles, tunics, until one development influenced much of future fashion. This was the widespread adoption of the button. Until that time clothes had been draped over the body or slipped on over the head, but now the use of the button made it possible to cut the garment to fit the shape of the body underneath. It was at this time that the waist attained its position as 'queen of the erogenous zones', and in the fourteenth century both women and men were defined by contemporary sources as being 'tightly laced'.

With the Renaissance came new ideas in most spheres of creative endeavour, and fashion was no exception. Fashions changed radically during this period and for the first time the ideal fashionable shape departed entirely from the natural shape and curves of the body. Women were muffled up in voluminous layers of heavy fabrics with enormous sleeves and monumental crinolines over layer upon layer of petticoats.

Not all artificial aids were designed to *restrict* size. Padding of strategic areas has often been in style. During the Renaissance vast hip cushions and false breasts, sometimes made of tin and wax, were worn to emphasize the ideal X shape of the time. The only people who looked thin were servants and others too poor to afford all the extensive layers of clothes – they couldn't have worked decked out in that manner anyway. Of course, the fashionable lady didn't have to worry about work. She hardly even moved and, as her clothing became more and more restricted, so the image of woman as decorative object developed.

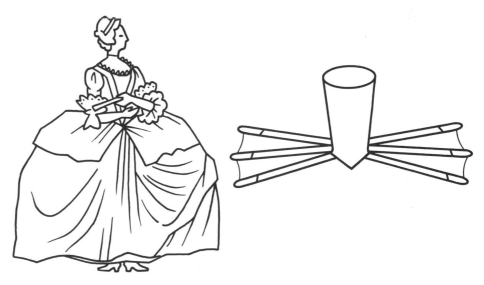

English dress of 1759 with matching undergarment!

In the eighteenth century, when vast hooped skirts that turned their wearer into a walking lampshade were popular, corsets were terrifying items, more like suits of armour than underwear. There was a very brief respite for the waist during the Empire period, but even under those high-waisted, neoclassical styles a type of corset was worn, this time designed to push the breasts up and out.

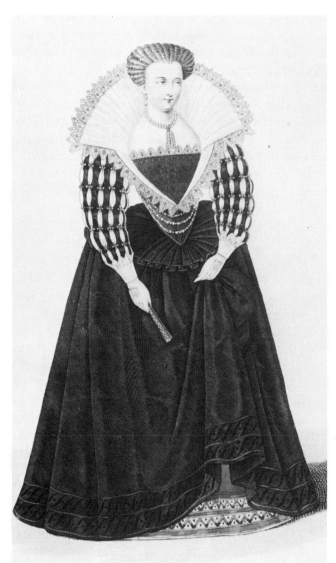

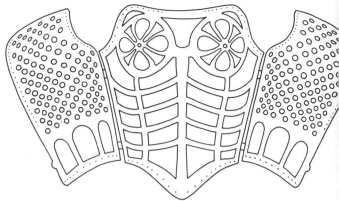

Steel corset of the early sixteenth century from Venice

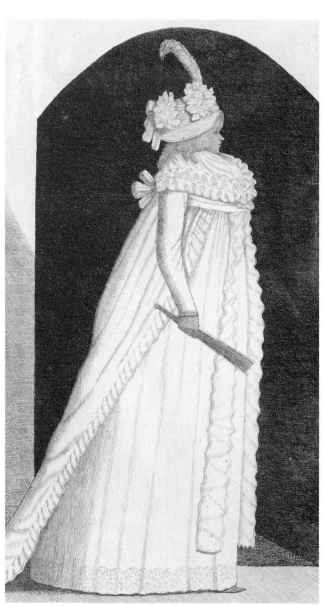

Above: During the Renaissance the ideal fashionable shape
departed entirely from the natural shape and curves of the body

Right: During the Empire period corsets were worn to push the
breasts up and out

This relatively unrestricted period was, however, short-lived, and by 1830 tight corseting of the waist was back with a vengeance. It was in this year that a young girl calling herself 'Mignonette' wrote to a popular ladies' magazine, saying that since the age of thirteen she had been wearing and *sleeping* in a very tight corset. Another girl at a fashionable London school wrote to say that she wore corsets laced at the back so that she wouldn't be tempted to loosen them. Both these girls were highly pleased with the results, and thoroughly recommended the method. At this time, the right kind of corset was a topic for endless discussion, in much the same way that today we discuss the right kind of diet.

The harmful effects of corseting. This drawing, which dates from 1793, shows the difference between a normal chest and one deformed by tight lacing

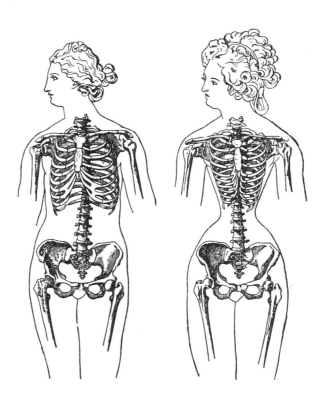

Despite the enthusiasm of Mignonette and her contemporaries, corsets were terribly dangerous. Their dangers had been known for some time; deformities and curvature of the spine, respiratory problems and fits of fainting, serious digestive disorders and childbirth complications could all be caused. Yet still, in their pursuit of the fashionable ideal, women continued to strap themselves in. And for some, the corset was not enough. The definitive hourglass figure could be achieved by surgical removal of the bottom ribs, an operation which allowed the corset of the fortunate recipient of this latest medical advance to be laced even tighter. This sounds horrifying, doesn't it? Almost like foot-binding or head-flattening? Yet today's fat removal procedures, intestinal bypass operations, and jaw-wiring seem no less barbaric.

It seems fairly certain that, apart from all the other ills caused to the female form by the era of the corset, anorexia nervosa was a killer long before it was medically identified. The delicate Victorian heroine 'dying of a broken heart' and 'wasting away' sound to our post-Freudian ears remarkably like adolescent trauma and anorexia nervosa. The attitudes of the time towards women and food are ones we can see mirrored today.

It was considered indelicate for ladies to eat much in public. Lord Byron, a style-setter for the sentiments of his time, could not bear to see a woman eating and tight corsets made it physically impossible, if not actually dangerous, to do more than toy with a few mouthfuls. An American handbook on etiquette published in 1855 stated that 'Tea and toast is all ladies may eat nowadays. We do not expect a lady to eat beefsteak.' Victorian ladies used to eat several hours before they went out to dinner, giving them time to digest. They then spent up to half an hour clinging to the bedpost and gritting their teeth while someone laced them in. In 1902 a guidebook to social behaviour in England stated: 'Some men are very fastidious about the appetites displayed by ladies and would have them reject the entrées and dine upon a thin slice of chicken or a spoonful of jelly.' How women were supposed to develop the large and voluptuous contours that came into vogue at the end of the nineteenth century is somewhat of a mystery.

Towards the end of the 1800s, reaction against the constrictions of corseting began. There was the Rational Dress Society, who promoted sensible, loose, 'artistic' dress for women – and who were mercilessly lampooned by the press. The Pre-Raphaelites had begun to promote an image of womanhood, loose, graceful, natural and definitely uncorseted, that had not been seen for centuries.

But, despite the efforts of the reformers, the ideal woman of the last thirty or forty years of the nineteenth century was still for the most part firmly corseted.

'A correct view of the new machine for winding up the ladies', 1820

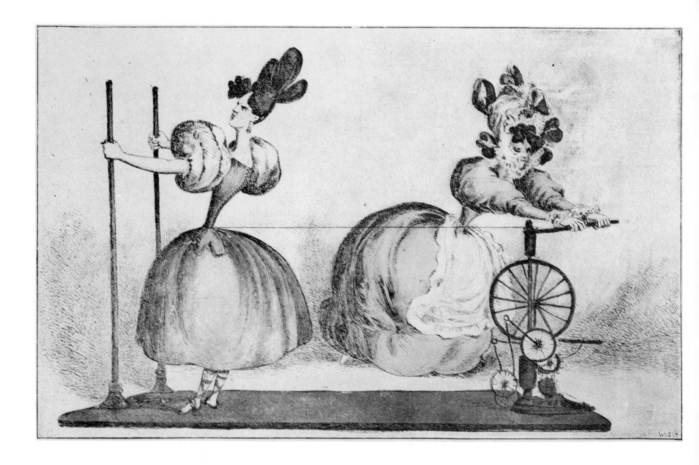

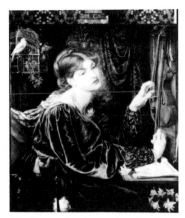

The loose, flowing unrestricted dress of the Pre-Raphaelites

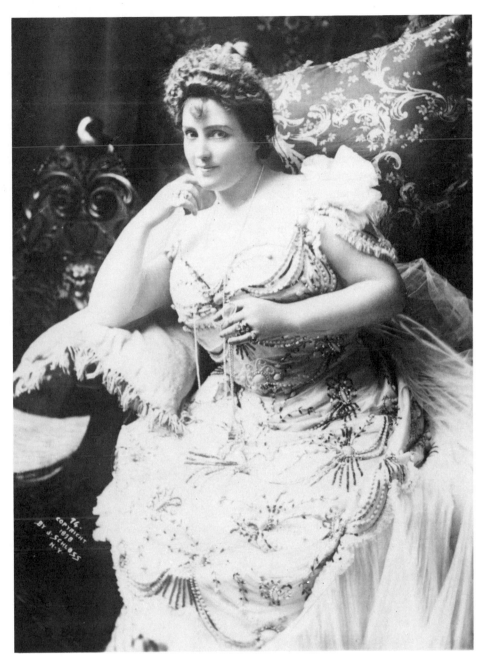

Lillian Russell, 1862–1922 – the archetypal, voluptuous woman – a great beauty of her time

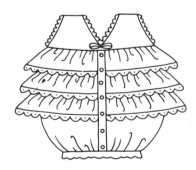

The false bosom: the Amplificateur, 1908

She was also large and voluptuous and padding of the hips and bosom came back into style. A big bust was needed to fill out the ample fronts of the bloused dresses in vogue during the early years of the twentieth century and the Amplificateur, the forerunner of the padded bra, was a godsend to the flat-chested.

An English visitor to America in 1880 was surprised by the number of 'fine, buxom, matronly women', another by young American women's fear of being too thin. 'They are constantly having themselves weighed,' he wrote, and 'every ounce of increase is greeted with delight, and talked about with the most dreadful plainness of speech. When I asked a beautiful Connecticut girl how she liked the change, "Oh, immensely!" she said, "I have gained eighteen pounds in flesh since last April"' (Louis W. Banner, *American Beauty*, Knopf, New York, 1983).

Corsets were still widely worn up to and including the 1920s when straight boyish figures came into fashion, skirts went up for the first time ever and legs attracted all the attention. Breasts were out, and tight bandaging of the chest to give the impression that you were flat as a pancake was in. In spite of the appeal of the natural look, tight corsets were still worn to achieve a long boyish silhouette over the hips and thighs. In fact, girdles and roll-ons lived on in a big way up to the 1960s, when tights arrived on the scene and skirts got so short that it was almost impossible to wear any underwear at all. Yet even in the early seventies, when increasing freedom for women and the blue-jean revolution had become firmly entrenched, a survey carried out in Spain claimed that 60 per cent of Spanish girls still wore girdles – under their jeans!

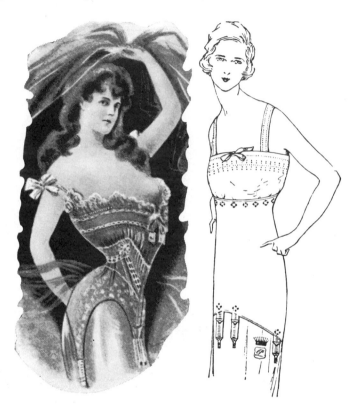

Corset advertisements 1913 (left) and 1924 (right). Women's bodies have always been expected to change shape according to current fashions

Dieting

With the coming of the twenties and the new natural look, the time for radically altering the figure by means of artificial aids was largely over. There were no more layers and layers of clothes to hide what was underneath, a long thin line was essential, but more flesh was on display. It was the era of the DIET.

People must have always known that the intake of food affects our health and body size in various ways. In the eleventh century it first became fashionable for noblemen to have a *regimen sanitatis* (rules of eating, etc., for good health) drawn up for them by learned men or physicians. One regimen drawn up for 'Dame Isabelle, queene of England' in the fourteenth century, contained the following advice about things that were 'bad for ye stomak': 'Alle swete things, for why, thei swellen, notes [nuts], old chese…all fryed things…To eten [eat] or [before] thou have hunger…To drynke, having no thirst.' And they even understood about stress, because the list of bad things includes 'hevines' (violence), 'drede' (dread), 'besines' (business)…

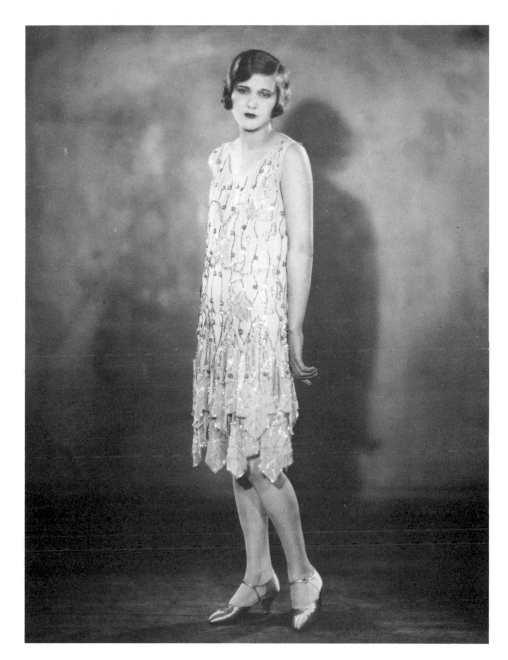

1920s fashions emphasized a flat, boyish shape

But the reducing diet as we know it seems to be a fairly recent phenomenon – only about 120 years old. Until then the equivalent of the modern 'binge and diet' could have been 'gorge and spa'. Spas were, of course, the grandmothers of present-day health farms, with hot-bath treatments, immersions in mud for the skin, and all sorts of other beauty and curative treatments. They also developed into major social centres, the height of fashion for anyone who could afford them. Spas were usually centred on natural springs of water which were supposed to have health-giving properties. At the spas you could avail yourself of the latest methods of hydrotherapy, which were reckoned to cure everything you could imagine and consisted of the rather bizarre application of cold water to all parts of the body. The patient was subject to violent showers, jets of water, buckets emptied over the head repeatedly and contraptions to bathe specific areas of the body. Women even stood over jets of water for hours in an attempt to cure barrenness.

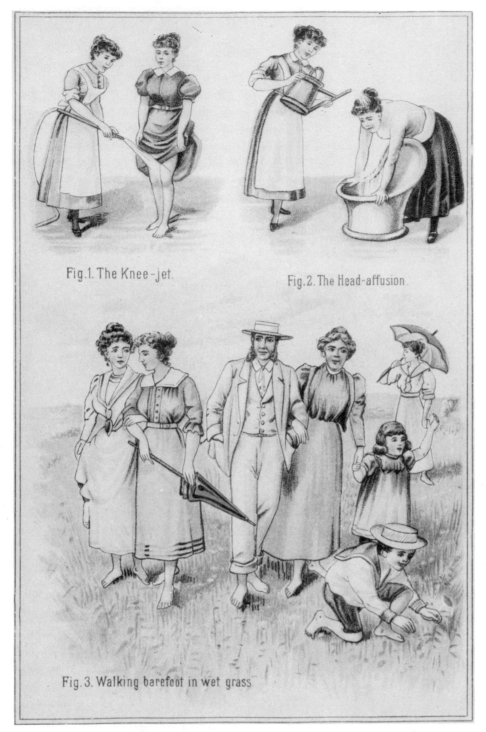

Fig.1. The Knee-jet.

Fig.2. The Head-affusion.

Fig.3. Walking barefoot in wet grass

A major function of 'taking the waters' was to purge oneself periodically of the excesses of food and drink indulged in during the rest of the year. Violent fasting regimes were rigorously adhered to under the watchful eye of the spa doctor, who told patients exactly what to eat and how much water to drink. The Bath Oliver biscuit, still sold today, was originally a slimming biscuit of a sort, patented by Dr Oliver of Bath. It was in fact derived from a ship's biscuit. Every day at the spa, you ate your biscuits and drank a few glasses of nasty tasting water and waited for it to do you good. More recently, Michel Guérard first developed his *cuisine minceur* at the spa of Eugénie-les-Bains: clients could go and lose up to 10 lb/4·5 kg in three weeks while eating superlative food at only 400–500 calories a meal.

The reducing diet proper started in a big way with an Englishman, William Banting, who in 1863 published his influential 'Letter on Corpulence Addressed To The Public'. Having suffered all his life from 'extreme obesity', he was finally advised by an eminent surgeon, William Harvey, to go on a diet that restricted the intake of starch and sugar – a treatment Harvey had worked out for use with diabetics. Banting's work went through twelve editions in America between 1863 and 1902; so well known was he that 'dieting' for many years was known as 'banting'. His popular diet consisted of:

Breakfast: 5–6 oz/140–170 g of meat – either beef, mutton, kidneys, bacon or boiled fish (no pork or veal). Cup of tea or coffee, no milk or sugar. One biscuit or 1 oz/30 g dry toast.

Dinner: 5–6 oz/140–170 g any fish except salmon, herring or eel, any meat except pork or veal. Any vegetable except potatoes, parsnips, beet, turnip or carrot (and absolutely no green peas). 1 oz/30 g dry toast. Fruit, not sweetened. 2–3 glasses of good claret, sherry or madeira (champagne, port and beer are forbidden).

Tea (6 p.m.): 3–4 oz/85–115 g meat or fish, as above. 1–2 glasses claret or sherry and water.

Nightcap: Grog (whisky, gin or brandy, without sugar) or claret or sherry.

It is not clear that Banting's theories, as taught to him by Harvey, were revolutionary – it may be that knowledge of low-starch and low-sugar diet effects already existed. Yet it's fairly certain that Banting made them popular with the general public for the first time. The letters from 'satisfied customers' published in the later editions of his book bear this out.

Quote from one letter: 'My own medical man, in 1854, recommended me to try and live on meat alone, but after trying it for a week I could not endure the sight of it. The redeeming point, to my mind, in your dietetic table, is the ounce of toast that you are allowed.'

Another quote from a 'lady of quality': 'I certainly have been rather troubled with constipation, but I find that returning to my old diet one day in the week removed this.'

Banting was, of course, subjected to the usual envious remarks from other members of the medical profession. One correspondent reported that his doctor had told him that Banting's ideas were 'as old as the hills', but the correspondent wondered why, if that were true, his doctor had never suggested them to him himself.

Through Banting's work the omission of bread, potatoes and sugar as a means to weight loss became widespread. It was a theory that formed the linchpin of most famous diets, and was to remain in favour until very recently.

Scientific findings about weight gain and loss and dietary theories abounded and, by the turn of the century, it seems, the whole circus was on the road. Dieting, exercising, steam baths and massage were seen as the 'secret of youth' by leaders of New York society by 1900; in 1912 *Vogue* satirized the diet mania by advising its readers to 'pirouette while you peel potatoes' in order to lose weight.

Lillian Russell, whose voluptuous beauty had been the ideal some years earlier, started dieting at the end of the century, and kept her flagging career alive by stories of her epic struggles to lose weight, trying every new diet and reporting on them gleefully – sometimes tongue in cheek – including one system that involved the dieter rolling over 250 times every morning before breakfast.

It seems that the diet craze hit Britain a bit later than the USA, despite Banting's work. One English writer claims that diets were a novelty in the 1920s. But it caught on quickly – reducing pastes, facial rejuvenators, special exercisers, patent rubber rolling pins to whittle down curves (made in two sizes, one exclusively for work on double chins and thick ankles) reducing salts, gland extracts – the whole works.

The coming of the Second World War and the food restrictions suffered by Europe had a calming effect on the enthusiasm to diet – on a ration of 2 oz/55 g of butter per person per week, Britain was on a low-fat diet for six or seven years without having any choice in the matter.

Then in the 1960s Twiggy burst on the scene, dieting was in with a vengeance, and most of the post-pubertal females of the Western world went running for the nearest lettuce leaf. Super-thin was in, and it has remained that way ever since, with its attendant miseries and self-deprivation.

Achieving the fashionable shape, whatever it is, has always involved some kind of misery and suffering. Why women have done it is the subject of much debate. Why the 14 in/36 cm waist, for example? To show that you were not pregnant – therefore virginal, therefore available and desirable? Why the vast crinolines of the eighteenth century – to show that you didn't work (you couldn't possibly, since you couldn't even get through a door except sideways) and therefore were rich, leisured and desirable? And why, now, the 8 st/112 lb/51 kg exercise goddess, stripped almost naked to show – what? Maybe future generations will be able to see her in her proper perspective, and maybe they will also see that, with the ferocious pressures she faces to exercise and diet, her 'lot' is not all that different from her sisters in previous centuries. Maybe they will see that she is really no more free, no more unrestricted, no less a victim of the fashionable ideal than were they.

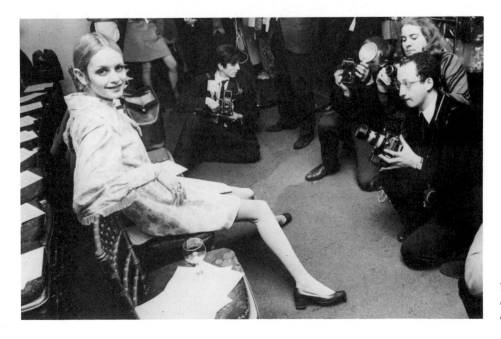

Twiggy, her child-like, emaciated looks set the standard of beauty for years to come

Perhaps to future generations the silhouette of the slimmer (right) will look just as bizarre as the Victorian bustle (left)

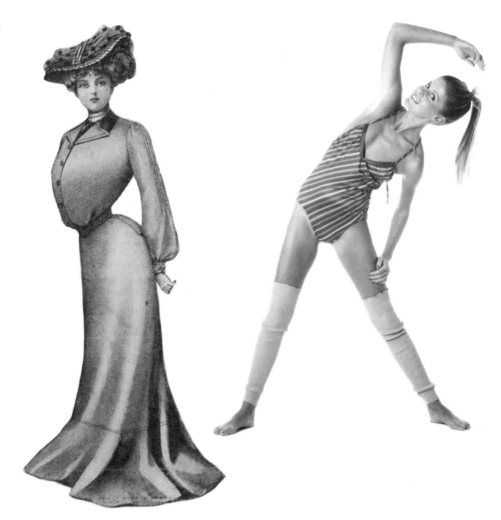

Women have started to say no to all the traditional stereotypes into which we have been squeezed. We now assume that it is our right to choose the kind of life we lead. We choose our careers, our mates, the age at which we bear our children, or whether we become mothers at all. We're saying no every day to outdated concepts of womanhood. Is it not also time to say no to an age-old convention that dictates that we spend a great deal of time and energy trying to conform to the fashionable body shape of the moment?

Is it not time to accept ourselves no matter what our shape or size, and to reject any school of thought that insists that to be acceptable we have to conform to its particular idea of beauty? It's time to look beyond our size, beyond our shape, to the women we are – to the women we can become.

> ❛ There aren't any limits if you're fat, there's no reason why you can't go swimming or dancing or stay out all night and look glamorous. There's nothing that says you've got to look like a mouse or hide in the corner and be a wallflower or do the washing up for everybody after the party. If you're an extrovert, be an extrovert. If you want to have pink streaks in your hair, have pink streaks in your hair. You can be just like everybody else. ❜
>
> *Janis Townes*

14

POSITIVE ACTION

Once we accept that we have a right to a full and happy life, free from discrimination, we can do much to effect positive change in the world around us. We can make our influence felt within the many spheres in which, until now, big women have been shabbily treated.

It is up to us to re-educate the people around us on their attitude to big women. If we don't do it, nobody else will.

The personal

> ❛ There's always going to be some times when you feel awful, everyone does, and it's ridiculous to blame it on your weight. If you weren't overweight you would have a big nose or a spotty back or ingrowing toenails.
>
> I suggest being very firm with people who tell you that you look awful. Just tell them that they're wrong! I really resent it if I'm feeling good in something and someone says to me, 'You ought to be wearing vertical stripes or a nice two-piece.' They don't think I'm entitled to flop around in my baggy dungarees, because I look twice the size in them. Well, that's neither here nor there. Size isn't what makes you look good, bad or indifferent, it's just the restrictions of the kind of clothes that are available – that and people's prejudices. ❜
>
> *Denise Smith*

Dealing with friends and family can be difficult. They often believe that the only way we can be happy is to be thin. Even though they believe their concern to be in our best interests, the well-meaning remarks and suggestions they make about our size or our eating habits can be painful and distressing. Don't grin and bear it! It's vital to discuss the issues with those we care about and to make them aware of the realities concerning size and dieting. Talk to them openly about the problems that we face in dealing with the rest of society and explain to them that their support and understanding is invaluable.

Remember that if you have a fat child, life at school for him or her can be hell, so it's essential that at home you provide a positive and supportive atmosphere.

❛ Across the road there's a family who are all big, so my father thinks, 'That's OK, it runs in the family', but because I'm the only big one in our house, he thinks there's something wrong with me. ❜
Liz Birru

❛ I have rows with some of the other teachers because they think they should say something to the fat child who is eating crisps, and I say, 'Let him eat crisps because if you tell him not to, he'll eat them in secret and eat three bags instead of one.' If they see food as something you are trying to take away from them they just get obsessed about it and eat more.

Sometimes the children say to me, 'Why don't you go on a diet?' And I answer, 'Why should I , what's wrong with me?' And they say, 'Well, you're big.' 'And you're small,' I say. Then they say, 'But you've got such a pretty face,' and I say, 'I'm lucky then aren't I?' ❜
Elizabeth Osborne

❛ When talking to the parents of a young child who is fat I would say, first of all, if they're really worried about it, they need to look at their own eating and cooking habits. Some kids are fat because they're meant to be, but it's no good going on about the kid being fat if you feed them on rubbish. So you establish the right kind of eating habits, but after that you lay off them. Don't make their lives hell. Some kids are born to be big; some of us are. If they're compulsive nibblers and over-eaters, and there's a reason, the child is unhappy, then deal with that. Don't deal with the fatness as a problem in itself. You may regard it in some settings as a symptom of disorder. Sometimes it can be the symptom of an unhappy child. Sometimes it just is the symptom of a child being the grandchild of a particular person. The last thing you do is make dramas about it. Why make the kid miserable? That way you're setting the pattern for lifelong dieting and making him fatter. ❜
Claire Rayner

The public

Fat discrimination has become rampant in the last few years. It is to the advantage of the slimming industry and the publishers of books and articles about dieting that this be so. It is important to protest against any example that comes to your attention. Fat discrimination has, in some cases, even become institutionalized.

Recently in Britain one of the largest restaurant groups announced a scheme for modernizing all its branches. As part of this facelift, all of their waiters and waitresses were to be fired. When the re-hiring procedure commenced, no waitress above a size 14 and no waiter with a waist measurement bigger than 36 in/ 91 cm would be re-employed.

The public excuse given for this outrage was financial; it was uneconomic for the company to order their stylish new uniforms in the larger sizes. A less publicized justification was that the sight of the bigger waiters and waitresses made customers aware of the negative aspects of over-indulgence and discouraged them from eating.

If all of us whose measurements coincided with those of the unfortunate waiters and waitresses who stood to lose their jobs had written to the managing director of this chain stating our intention of boycotting all the restaurants in his group, and if we had encouraged our friends and families to do the same, they would have had to reconsider this policy.

In another recent incident, which was, unfortunately, barely publicized, a part-time tea-lady at a major international company applied for full-time employment. After the company doctor had given her the required physical examination, not only was her application turned down, but she lost her part-time position as well. The reason given for this was that she was overweight and that, like all overweight people, she would tend to have an unacceptable level of absenteeism.

All too often stories like this appear as afterthoughts hidden in a small column at the back of our newspapers. If people are to appreciate fully the level of sanctioned prejudice that we face, then it is important that these injustices are exposed, challenged and publicized. Write to newspapers and to current affairs programmes, news programmes, and chat shows, both on television and radio, insisting that they deal with these incidents.

It is essential that we bring the issue out into the open. Fat people have been hiding behind a veil of embarrassment for too long. Just hearing the problems discussed in public can help people gain strength and self-confidence, so that, eventually, they too can join in the fight.

❛ Those of us who feel better about ourselves have a responsibility to show those who don't that life can be better. Some successful big women, women in the public eye, refuse to talk about their size. They refuse to discuss it because they say they don't want to make an issue of it, *they've* coped. I can see their point but I don't agree with it. After all it is a very real issue and a lot of people *can't* cope. I don't like this analogy because it's rather a cliché, but it would be like a black person saying, 'I refuse to discuss racial prejudice because personally I haven't suffered from it.' If a woman is in the public eye with the power to influence public opinion that that implies, then I think it's very helpful to a lot of unhappy people if she at least discusses the issues. It helps to bring the whole thing out in the open. ❜ *Elizabeth Osborne*

❛ Society has to see and hear big women, and get used to the fact that we are not just a tiny minority that can be locked away. ❜ *Janis Townes*

❛ I had a long-running part in a TV series. It was refreshing because although the part had been written as a dumb blonde secretary, the producer had seen me and thought, 'I like this girl, I like whatever quality she's got and I will use that instead.' But by the second series, they started putting lines in about my size, and made my character the butt of jokes about dieting. So I told the producer that I thought it was diminishing the character and the material – working towards the lowest common denominator. It happens quite unintentionally. Even bright, informed people just don't realize that they are, in fact, conforming to a preconceived notion of a fat person. So I pointed out that we were pushing it in the direction of a cliché-cum-stereotype. The producer agreed and rewrote the script. So, instead of being the girl who couldn't climb the stairs, or was caught eating Mars Bars, I ended up riding bikes and being very active – and much more interesting. ❜ *Annette Badland*

The media

You can influence what you see on television and what you read in magazines and newspapers. Write and complain about endless dieting features. TV programmes and commercials can be the worst culprits when it comes to ridiculing fat people. We are all too often seen as the butt of cheap, easy humour. If you see a programme that is offensive, write to the producer, or the head of the network. If it is a commercial, write to the managing director of the company that makes the product.

As you will no doubt have noticed I am a great believer in writing letters. If every woman who reads this book were to write just one letter a month I believe we could effect a radical change. There is only one golden rule of letter-writing. Always go straight to the top. Don't waste time writing to underlings in the customer-relations or public-relations department. Write to the managing director of the company. You can always call up and find out his name. He may pass the letter back down the line, and your reply may not come from him, but you will know that he or someone in his office has at least read your letter and is aware of your complaint.

The fashion industry

❛ Clothes are the one thing that really irritate me. You see something you like, and you look at it and you think 'No, I am not going to get into that.' And you think, 'Why don't they make them bigger, why don't they just make them bigger?' ❜ *Helen Terry*

❛ Everyone who is in any kind of manufacturing is there in order to survive and keep other people in work. For a company to go from a size 8, or a size 4, the way some companies do in America, up to a size 20, is an awful lot to deal with. Every pattern has to be graded so that it fits each size. So you may have the ideal basic shape for a 12 or even a 14, but when it comes to going further up, to an 18 or a 20, then the set of the garment won't be the same. It will need to be adapted. Let's face it, there are a lot of large women and girls who are afraid of having fashiony things. It may well be that one becomes more conservative, more shy, being large. Well, the women won't necessarily buy these new garments and the manufacturer will be left having expended his time and money on a collection which is good, but doesn't sell. ❜ *Joanne Brogden*

❛ When I'm buying for my shop and I ask the manufacturers why they don't do larger sizes, they say it's too expensive, the extra cloth, cutting the patterns, etc., and when you get above a size 20 the proportions can be completely out of kilter. It's mainly the British manufacturers who say this. Some foreign manufacturers go from a size 6 to a 26. Everything is graded accordingly and there is no extra cost involved. Another thing they say is 'There isn't the demand.' Well, there isn't the demand because every big woman is terrified of asking. If we had a rally and went round all the stores *en masse* they'd do something about it. In the final analysis, it has to come from us. ❜ *Angela Troak*

If outsize manufacturers are wary about improving their lines because they are afraid that we won't buy better clothes, then, as Angela says, it is up to us to convince them that they are wrong. Let's face it, it's easier and cheaper for them to turn out shapeless tents than it is to design and manufacture interesting, fashionable clothes. And if we go on buying inferior merchandise, why should the outsize manufacturers provide us with anything better?

The size discrimination that goes on within the fashion industry is perhaps the easiest for us to combat. It is an area where we do have power, financial power. There is a tangible product involved that we can accept or reject. It is essential that we start to vote with our wallets, we must only buy what is decent, and leave those things that are little more than abominations where they belong, on the rails in the outsize department. But before you leave, check the label, find out who the manufacturer is and write directly to him. Tell him you didn't buy his clothes, tell him why and tell him what kind of clothes you would buy. Send this same letter to the manager of the outsize department or shop and to the managing director of the outsize chain.

But don't stop at outsize. Write to any shop or department store where you would like to shop, but who doesn't carry your size. Ask them why. Tell them they're losing out on a substantial amount of business by not catering for larger sizes. After all, their business, like any other, is only about money and profit, and we can improve the quality of the clothes on offer to us by convincing the fashion industry that their retrogressive attitudes are costing them money.

> ❛ It would be marvellous if the better department stores had a stylish, elegant department that didn't have a coy name like 'big girls', and that stocked things from the good manufacturers. It might have to cost a little bit more, because it's obvious that for me a skirt or a jacket, or whatever it is, is going to take a bit more fabric, but I'm prepared to pay for it, because that's just the way it is. ❜
>
> *Joanne Brogden*

Write to designers and manufacturers of 'standard' size clothes and tell them that you'd be a good customer if only they made things in your size.

> ❛ There'd be a chance of the clothing situation improving if people did special lines. Say one bullied Jasper Conran into doing a 'large ladies' collection. Now that would be very interesting, and if it was seen to make money, that might reduce the prejudice against larger sizes. ❜ *Meredith Etherington-Smith*
>
> ❛ One really should write to all the fashion pages and say 'Why the hell do you think you're doing us a favour by doing one page a year on bigger sizes?' And how often do they do a big clothes feature for someone who's seventeen? Fashion writers could use a bit of imagination instead of excluding us from fashion, after all we're always being told almost 50 per cent of women are over a size 14. Every newspaper runs a fashion article each and every week, and I don't see why they couldn't have one garment each week for somebody big. ❜
>
> *Sue Formston*

It is also essential to write not only to the fashion editors but to women's page editors and to overall editors of newspapers and magazines. They are the ones in control of what we read every day. Tell them that you are a large woman *and* one of their readers and that you demand to see big clothes on big models and you demand to see them regularly, not once every six months. Remind them just how many big women there are and just how many of us they are ignoring by following their present strategy of excluding us from their pages. If enough of us put pressure on the right people we can get results.

> ❛ **Big women have to lead the way. By going out and showing people how great you can look, that's how to change things.** ❜
> *Kate Franklin*

*　　　*　　　*

I n this chapter I've outlined just a few of the specific ways in which we can take positive action to better our lot.

People are always asking me if I really think the situation is improving for big women, or if the ever-increasing thrust of the diet and exercise industry are daily making things more unbearable. I, for one, am filled with optimism for our future. The women I've met through my work of the past five years, and the thousands of other women who've written to me of their past pain and their present determination, speak to me of a new anger and a new refusal to accept that we should take second place to those whose proportions are less generous than our own.

This says to me that things are getting better, that the days of hiding ourselves away are ending. Everywhere out there, women like you, like me, are struggling towards a new level of self-acceptance and of self-respect. I believe wholeheartedly that it is within our power to bring about changes, not just in the way we feel about ourselves, but in the rules that have kept us outside the mainstream of society for so long. And I believe that if we stand and fight together we can and will win. I believe that no matter what our weight, no matter what our size, we can be anything that we want to be.

It's hard for me to finish this book, to write the last page. With every word I've felt that I was reaching out and talking to so many of you who would understand. To be able to speak with other women through the years was what enabled me to put an end to the painful isolation that I felt for so long as a compulsive eater. I hope that this book has helped you to see that *you* are not alone.

I hope it has given you the strength and the courage to face the world and to fight back against anyone or anything who tries to deny you your basic right to live the happy, healthy, successful life to which each and every one of us is entitled – no matter what our size.

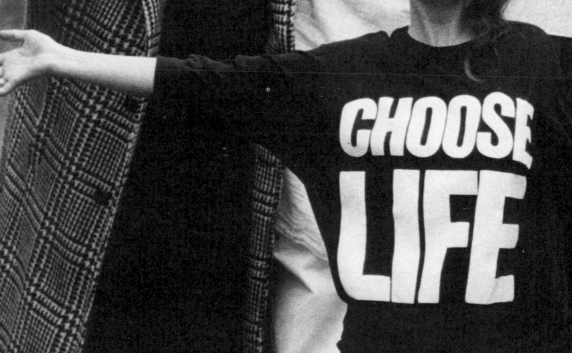

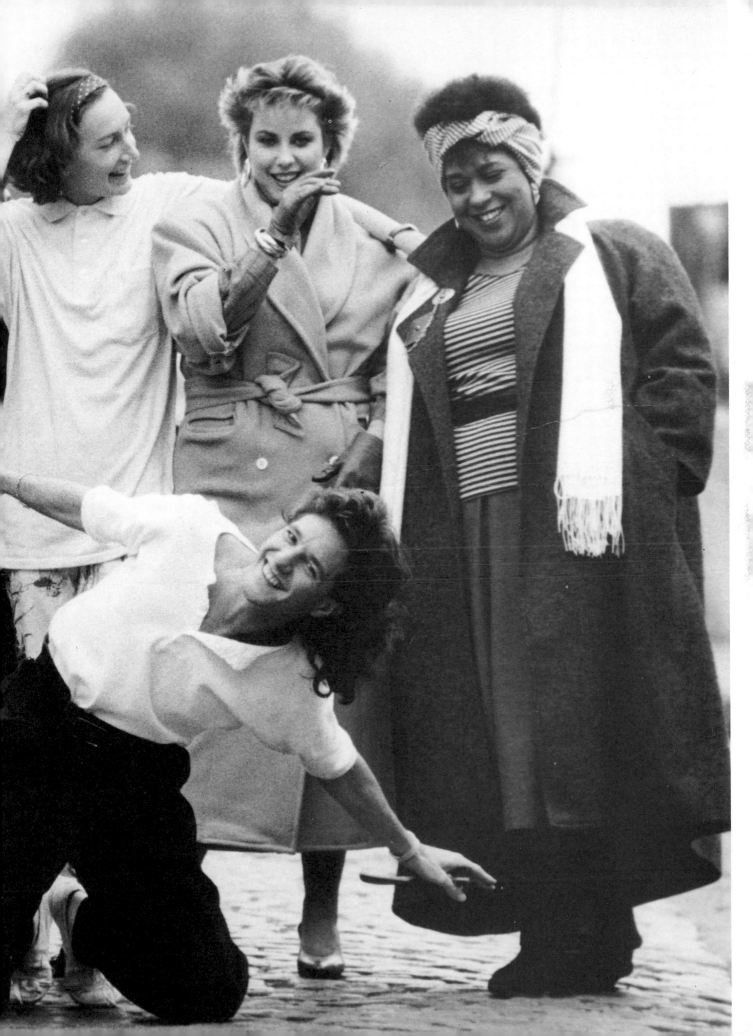

CREDITS

Styling: Julia Fletcher

Hair: Paula Mann and Gregory Cazaly at Joshua
and Daniel Galvin; Paul Yacomine at Neville Danielle;
Gianni at Strands; Carmel at Clifford Stafford; Dar

Make-up artists: Paula Owen, Kim Jacobs, Mark Easton,
Mark Hayles, Lynne Easton

Make-up: With many thanks for their help to Max Factor;
Elizabeth Arden; and to Rimmel for shades from their
'Dark Colour Collection' – a range specially formulated
for darker skins

*   *   *

CHAPTER 7

Facing p. 88
White tops, yellow sweep, black skirt by Bodymap

Between pp. 88–9
White layers all by Wendy Dagworthy
Trenchcoat by Burberry
Rose suède skirt by Nigel Preston for Maxfield Parrish,
pink linen blouse by Sheridan Barnett, cashmere sweater
from Selfridges
Black suit by Monica Chong, hat by Philip Somerville, fur
by Edelson Furs at Selfridges

Facing p. 89
Ball-gown by Ken Smith

Facing p. 96
Red jumpsuit by Barbara Jones of Features
Navy jacket by Calvin Klein, striped T-shirt from Macy's,
hat from Gieves and Hawkes

Facing p. 97
Brocade jacket by Sassa, caftans by Soraya Imports
Charcoal jacket and flannel skirt by Sheridan Barnett,
shirt and tie by Hawes and Curtis

CHAPTERS 9 AND 10

Clothes: Wendy Dagworthy, Michiko Koshino, Dorothée Bis,
Betty Jackson, Joseph Tricot, Kenzo, Sheridan Barnett,
Bill Gibb, Jennifer Kiernan, Sulka, Shi Cashmere,
Gloria Vanderbilt, Sharon Minetta, Miss Selfridge, Flip,
Lawrence Corner, Marks and Spencer, Jean Renard, Alkit,
Dickens and Jones, Macy's, Issey Miyake; 'outsize' clothes
from the Base, London, and Ashanti, New York.

Antique clothes: Lunn Antiques, Gallery of Antique Clothing
and Textile, American Classics

Shoes: Ravel, Maud Frizon, Charles Jourdan,
Pineapple Dance Shop, Accessoire, Xanier Danaud, Bertie,
London Espadrille Centre, Mulberry, Soraya Imports,
Diego Della Valle

Jewellery: Butler and Wilson, Margaret's Jewel Box, Rocks,
Merola, Adrien Mann, Corocraft, Imanginca, Harvey Nichols,
Christian Dior, Dreams of the Orient, Vendôme, Ken Walker

Belts: Malcolm Parsons, Metal Duck Company

Scarves: Cornelia James, N. Peal, Hermès

Hats: The Hat Shop

Head-wrapping: fabric by Steve Wright

Gloves: Cornelia James

Handbag and watch: Hermès

Set dressing and furniture: Liberty's, Harrod's,
Harvey Nichols, Homelights

Bikes: Raleigh

CHAPTER 10 (PATTERN DESIGNS)

One-size top and trousers by Barbara Hollingum
Dot-dash sweater by Jennifer Kiernan

ILLUSTRATION ACKNOWLEDGEMENTS

While every effort has been made to trace the copyright holders of the photographs reproduced in this book, some of those which did not bear identification remain uncredited. The publishers will be pleased to make the correct acknowledgement in any future edition.